Intraocular Tumors

Intraocular Tumors

Gholam A. Peyman, M.D.

Dept. of Ophthalmology
The University of Illinois
Eye and Ear Infirmary/Chicago, Illinois

David J. Apple, M.D.

University of Iowa Hospitals
Dept. of Ophthalmology
Iowa City, Iowa

Donald R. Sanders, M.D.

Dept. of Ophthalmology
The University of Illinois
Eye and Ear Infirmary
Chicago, Illinois

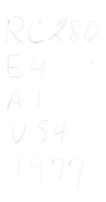

APPLETON/CENTURY/CROFTS   New York

77 78 79 80 81 / 10 9 8 7 6 5 4 3 2 1

Prentice-Hall International, Inc., London
Prentice-Hall of Australia, Pty. Ltd., Sydney
Prentice-Hall of India Private Limited, New Delhi
Prentice-Hall of Japan, Inc., Tokyo
Prentice-Hall of Southeast Asia (Pte.) Ltd., Singapore
Whitehall Books Ltd., Wellington, New Zealand

Library of Congress Cataloging in Publication Data
University of Illinois Symposium on Intraocular
    Tumors, Chicago, 1975.
    Intraocular Tumors.
    Includes index.
    1. Eye—Tumors—Congresses. 2. Melanoma—
Congresses. I. Peyman, Gholam A. II. Apple,
David J., 1941–   III. Sanders, Donald R.
IV. University of Illinois at the Medical Center.
V. Title.
RC280.E9U54   1975   616.9′94′84   77-24269
ISBN 0-8385-4302-2

Text design: The Old Typosopher
Cover design: Kristin Herzog

PRINTED IN THE UNITED STATES OF AMERICA

Contributors

Daniel M. Albert, M.D.
Professor
Dept. of Ophthalmology
Harvard Medical School
Massachusetts Eye and Ear Infirmary
Boston, Massachusetts

David J. Apple, M.D.
Associate
Dept. of Ophthalmology
University of Iowa Hospitals and Clinics
Iowa City, Iowa

Devron H. Char, M.D.
Assistant Professor
Dept. of Ophthalmology
School of Medicine
University of California, San Francisco
San Francisco, California

Wallace H. Clark, M.D.
Professor and Chairman
Dept. of Pathology
Temple University Health Sciences Center
Philadelphia, Pennsylvania;
Professor
Fels Research Institute
Philadelphia, Pennsylvania

John B. Constantine, M.D.
Dept. of Ophthalmology
University of Iowa Hospitals and Clinics
Iowa City, Iowa

Frederick H. Davidorf, M.D.
Associate Professor
Dept. of Ophthalmology
Director of Retina Service
Ohio State University
Columbus, Ohio

James G. Diamond, M.D.
Assistant Professor
Dept. of Ophthalmology
University of Iowa Hospitals and Clinics
Iowa City, Iowa

Robert M. Ellsworth, M.D.
Edward S. Harkness Institute
Columbia Presbyterian Medical Center
New York, New York

Jay L. Federman, M.D.
Associate Surgeon
Retina Service
Wills Eye Hospital
Philadelphia, Pennsylvania;
Associate Professor
Dept. of Ophthalmology
Jefferson Medical College of
Thomas Jefferson University
Philadelphia, Pennsylvania

Gerald A. Fishman, M.D.
Associate Professor
Dept. of Ophthalmology
University of Illinois
Eye and Ear Infirmary
Chicago, Illinois

Marcel Frenkel, M.D.
Associate Professor
Dept. of Ophthalmology
University of Illinois
Eye and Ear Infirmary
Chicago, Illinois

David K. Gieser, M.D.
Assistant
Dept. of Ophthalmology
University of Illinois
Eye and Ear Infirmary
Chicago, Illinois

Morton F. Goldberg, M.D.
Professor and Head
Dept. of Ophthalmology
University of Illinois
Eye and Ear Infirmary
Chicago, Illinois

Nancy A. Hamming, M.D.
Assistant
Dept. of Ophthalmology
University of Illinois
Eye and Ear Infirmary
Chicago, Illinois

Janet R. Lang, M.S.
Dept. of Ophthalmology
Ohio State University
Columbus, Ohio

Donald R. May, M.D.
Instructor
Dept. of Ophthalmology
University of Illinois
Eye and Ear Infirmary
Chicago, Illinois

Ian W. McLean, M.D.
Dept. of Ophthalmic Pathology
Armed Forces Institute of Pathology
Washington, D.C.

Karl C. Ossoinig, M.D.
Professor
Head of Ultrasound Service
Dept. of Ophthalmology
University of Iowa Hospitals and Clinics
Iowa City, Iowa

Gholam A. Peyman, M.D.
Professor
Dept. of Ophthalmology
University of Illinois
Eye and Ear Infirmary
Chicago, Illinois

Jeffrey Rutgard, M.D.
Dept. of Ophthalmology
University of Illinois
Eye and Ear Infirmary
Chicago, Illinois

Donald R. Sanders, M.D.
Chief of Ophthalmology
Dept. of Surgery
Westside Veterans Administration Hospital;
Assistant Professor of Ophthalmology
The University of Illinois
Eye and Ear Infirmary
Chicago, Illinois

Delia N. Sang, M.D.
Research Fellow
Dept. of Ophthalmology
Harvard Medical School
Massachusetts Eye and Ear Infirmary
Boston, Massachusetts

Jerry A. Shields, M.D.
Senior Assistant Surgeon
Oncology Unit
Retina Service
Wills Eye Hospital
Philadelphia, Pennsylvania;
Associate Professor of Ophthalmology
Jefferson Medical College of
Thomas Jefferson University
Philadelphia, Pennsylvania;
Consultant on Ocular Oncology
Lankenau Hospital,
Children's Hospital, and
U.S. Naval Hospital
Philadelphia, Pennsylvania

Anatol Stankevych, M.D.
Dept. of Ophthalmology
Cook County Hospital
Chicago, Illinois

Mano Swartz, M.D.
Instructor
Dept. of Ophthalmology
University of Illinois
Eye and Ear Infirmary
Chicago, Illinois

Martin H. Vogel, M.D.
Oberarzt der Universitats-Augenklinik
Gesamthochschule Essen
West Germany

Robert C. Watzke, M.D.
Professor
Head of Retina Service
Dept. of Ophthalmology
University of Iowa Hospitals and Clinics
Iowa City, Iowa

Thomas A. Weingeist, M.D., Ph.D.
Assistant Professor
Dept. of Ophthalmology
University of Iowa Hospitals and Clinics
Iowa City, Iowa

Lorenz E. Zimmerman, M.D.
Chairman
Dept. of Ophthalmic Pathology
Armed Forces Institute of Pathology
Washington, D.C.

Participants—Tumor Symposium

Daniel M. Albert, M.D.
Professor
Dept. of Ophthalmology
Harvard Medical School
Massachusetts Eye and Ear Infirmary
Boston, Massachusetts

David J. Apple, M.D.
Associate Professor
Dept. of Ophthalmology
University of Iowa Hospitals and Clinics
Iowa City, Iowa

Devron H. Char, M.D.
Assistant Professor
Dept. of Ophthalmology
School of Medicine
University of California, San Francisco
San Francisco, California

Frederick H. Davidorf, M.D.
Associate Professor
Dept. of Ophthalmology
Director of Retina Service
Ohio State University
Columbus, Ohio

James G. Diamond, M.D.
Assistant Professor
Dept. of Ophthalmology
University of Iowa Hospitals and Clinics
Iowa City, Iowa

Robert M. Ellsworth, M.D.
Edward S. Harkness Institute
Columbia Presbyterian Medical Center
New York, New York

Jay L. Federman, M.D.
Associate Surgeon
Retina Service
Wills Eye Hospital
Philadelphia, Pennsylvania;
Associate Professor
Dept. of Ophthalmology
Jefferson Medical College of
Thomas Jefferson University
Philadelphia, Pennsylvania

Gerald A. Fishman, M.D.
Associate Professor
Dept. of Ophthalmology
University of Illinois
Eye and Ear Infirmary
Chicago, Illinois

Marcel Frenkel, M.D.
Associate Professor
Dept. of Ophthalmology
University of Illinois
Eye and Ear Infirmary
Chicago, Illinois

Morton F. Goldberg, M.D.
Professor and Head
Dept. of Ophthalmology
University of Illinois
Eye and Ear Infirmary
Chicago, Illinois

Karl C. Ossoinig, M.D.
Professor
Head of Ultrasound Service
Dept. of Ophthalmology
University of Iowa Hospitals and Clinics
Iowa City, Iowa

Gholam A. Peyman, M.D.
Professor
Dept. of Ophthalmology
University of Illinois
Eye and Ear Infirmary
Chicago, Illinois

Jerry A. Shields, M.D.
Senior Assistant Surgeon
Oncology Unit
Retina Service
Wills Eye Hospital;
Associate Professor of Ophthalmology
Jefferson Medical College of
Thomas Jefferson University;
Consultant on Ocular Oncology
Lankenau Hospital,
Children's Hospital, and
U.S. Naval Hospital
Philadelphia, Pennsylvania

Mano Swartz, M.D.
Instructor
Dept. of Ophthalmology
University of Illinois
Eye and Ear Infirmary
Chicago, Illinois

Martin H. Vogel, M.D.
Oberarzt der Universitats-Augenklinik
Gesamthochschule Essen
West Germany

Robert C. Watzke, M.D.
Professor
Head of Retina Service
Dept. of Ophthalmology
University of Iowa Hospitals and Clinics
Iowa City, Iowa

Lorenz E. Zimmerman, M.D.
Chairman
Dept. of Ophthalmic Pathology
Armed Forces Institute of Pathology
Washington, D.C.

Contents

Preface

This book documents the proceedings of a recent symposium on intraocular tumors that was held at the University of Illinois Eye and Ear Infirmary, Chicago. Emphasis was on a clinically relevant approach to differential diagnosis and management of intraocular tumors. In addition, the most recent concepts on pathogenesis and the role of the immune system in prognosis and therapy were discussed.

The first section of this book deals with the diagnostic techniques used in differentiating tumors of the uveal tract and therapeutic modalities presently in use for the treatment of uveal malignant melanoma.

The second section includes the most recent information on the immunodiagnostic and immunotherapeutic aspects of intraocular tumor management.

The third section is a discussion of the differential diagnosis of leukocoria with special emphasis on clinical presentation, management, and continuing research of retinoblastoma.

The clinical and pathologic aspects of other less common intraocular tumors such as von Hippel-Lindau angiomatosis and ciliary body tumors are also discussed.

The primary intent for publishing this symposium is to share the expertise of the participants, to aid the ophthalmologist in tumor detection, differentiation, and management, and to give the reader insight into the behavior and prognosis of these intraocular tumors.

We wish to thank primarily all of the participants of the symposium for their valuable contributions to this book. We thank Dr. Morton F. Goldberg for his support and encouragement. Special recognition is due to Jane Lantz and Maxine Gere for their editorial assistance. We would also like to thank the Lions Club of Illinois for their financial support of our tumor research.

Intraocular Tumors

Jerry A. Shields

1 The Differential Diagnosis of Malignant Melanoma of the Choroid

One of the most difficult diagnostic problems in ophthalmology is the clinical differentiation of choroidal melanoma from certain lesions that may clinically simulate melanoma. Even in eyes with clear media, where the lesion may be easily visualized ophthalmoscopically, the diagnosis may be quite difficult.[1,2] The use of ancillary diagnostic procedures, such as fluorescein angiography, ultrasonography, and the radioactive phosphorus uptake (^{32}P) test, has helped to alleviate some of these diagnostic difficulties.[3,4] This discussion will consider some of the lesions that are known to simulate posterior uveal melanomas and outline the ophthalmoscopic criteria that may differentiate them from true melanomas. The use of ancillary tests, such as ultrasonography,[5] fluorescein angiography,[6] and the ^{32}P test[7-9] will be alluded to in this section, but will be discussed in detail in other chapters. The sequence used here is the order of frequency of eyes enucleated for so-called pseudomelanomas as derived from the two large series reported by the Armed Forces Institute of Pathology.[1,2]

RHEGMATOGENOUS RETINAL DETACHMENT

The rhegmatogenous retinal detachment (RRD) was the most common lesion leading to enucleation as a suspected melanoma in the two large series reported from the Armed Forces Institute of Pathology.[1,2] Our more recent clinical experience, however, suggests that it is now rather uncommon for an RRD to be diagnosed as a melanoma. The opposite situation, in which a patient with a malignant melanoma is referred for retinal detachment surgery, occurs rather frequently. In these cases, the lesion is usually recognized as a melanoma and the retinal surgery is cancelled.

Certain ophthalmoscopic features help to differentiate a detachment secondary to a melanoma from an RRD: the presence of a retinal break, the surface appearance, and the presence of shifting fluid.

A retinal break is present in all cases of RRD, but it is very rare in a detachment secondary to a melanoma. Although a number of cases have been reported,[10,11] I have carefully examined several hundred choroidal melanomas, and to date, have

This study was supported in part by the Retina Research and Development Foundation, Philadelphia.

1

not observed a peripheral retinal break in such cases. Since peripheral retinal holes are occasionally observed as incidental findings in otherwise normal eyes, it would not be surprising to observe occasionally an unrelated retinal break in an eye with a melanoma.

In an RRD, the surface of the retina usually has a rippled appearance. The normal choroid can be seen through the detachment and the subretinal fluid does not shift. In the case of choroidal melanoma, the surface of the detachment is smooth, and the normal choroidal pattern cannot be seen in the area of the tumor. In detachments secondary to tumors, the subretinal fluid shifts with the movement of the patient's head, a phenomenon not observed in an RRD. In cases with hazy ocular media, transillumination and ultrasonography should readily differentiate a melanoma from an RRD. If doubt still exists, a ^{32}P test is negative in an RRD, but positive in a choroidal melanoma.

SENILE EXUDATIVE MACULOPATHY

Senile exudative maculopathy ("disciform macular degeneration") is frequently confused clinically with a malignant melanoma.[12] Helpful differentiating features include the location of the lesion, the presence of hemorrhages and exudates, and the status of the opposite eye.

This lesion is usually located in the center of the macular area, a somewhat unusual site for a melanoma. The extensive hemorrhages and exudates associated with this lesion are unusual for a comparable-size melanoma. The condition is often bilateral, although frequently asymmetric, and the opposite eye shows macular drusen or pigmentary disturbances. Fluorescein angiography reveals hypofluorescence in the areas of hemorrhage and perhaps transmission through retinal pigment epithelial defects, but not the pattern observed with melanomas.

INTRAOCULAR INFLAMMATION

Several inflammatory processes may occasionally be confused with a choroidal melanoma. Examples include certain types of choroiditis, sarcoid granulomas, granulomatous sclerouveitis, and presumed ocular histoplasmosis. We have observed several patients with choroiditis of undetermined cause associated with a retinal detachment that simulated a choroidal tumor. These lesions, however, are nonpigmented and are often associated with inflammatory cells in the vitreous or anterior chamber, whereas melanomas are usually pigmented and rarely have inflammatory cells. Sarcoidosis may occasionally produce a focal choroidal mass simulating a tumor.[13] In contrast to melanoma, however, it is more common in blacks.

Granulomatous sclerouveitis may produce such massive thickening of the retina and choroid, with overlying retinal detachment, that it resembles a choroidal tumor. In some cases, it may be virtually impossible to differentiate such a lesion from a melanoma.[2, 14] These patients, however, often have diffuse or focal episcleritis, a rare finding with melanoma. The maculopathy associated with presumed ocular histoplasmosis has been mistaken for a malignant melanoma in the posterior pole on rare occasions.[1] The associated peripapillary and focal peripheral lesions should provide a clue to the true diagnosis.

DEGENERATIVE RETINOSCHISIS

Degenerative or "senile" retinoschisis, especially the bullous type, has occasionally been mistaken for a malignant melanoma.[1, 2, 15] The clinical appearance, location, bilaterality, and presence of holes are helpful in the diagnosis. It appears clinically as a smooth, thin-walled bullous lesion, associated with extensive peripheral cystoid degeneration. White dots represent interrupted Müller's cells on the inner surface of the retinoschisis cavity. The fluid within the cavity is usually clear and typical outer layer holes may occur. Retinoschisis is most commonly located in the inferotemporal quadrant peripherally, and is usually bilateral and symmetric. Melanomas, on the other hand, are unilateral, solid, and do not have the typical white dots and associated holes. In cases where the clinical diagnosis is still uncertain, transillumination and ultrasonography readily differentiate retinoschisis from melanoma. Although the ^{32}P test is not usually necessary in such cases, the results are negative in retinoschisis.

LESIONS OF THE RETINAL PIGMENT EPITHELIUM

Certain lesions of the retinal pigment epithelium may be clinically confused with choroidal melanoma. These lesions include congenital hypertrophy, reactive hyperplasia, adenomas, and hamartomas of the retinal pigment epithelium.

Congenital hypertrophy of the retinal pigment epithelium is a flat, well-delineated, pigmented lesion due to excess pigment within the affected cells.[16, 17] Those in the posterior segment are small, often only 1 to 2 disk diameters in size, while those in the periphery may be larger. With time, focal areas of hypopigmentation within the lesion occur, superficially resembling drusen or lipofuscin pigment seen over some choroidal melanomas. A surrounding hypopigmented halo is frequently present.[16, 17]

These lesions are easily differentiated from choroidal nevi and small choroidal melanomas because they are completely flat and well delineated, and they have the typical halo and depigmentation. In contrast to melanomas, they occur rather commonly in blacks. When they occur in the far periphery, they are usually larger and give the false impression of being elevated. The well-delineated scalloped margin, however, easily distinguishes the lesion from melanoma. Occasionally, this condition occurs as multiple flat pigmented lesions, known as congenital grouped pigmentation of the retina.[18] These lesions should not be confused with melanoma.

Reactive hyperplasia of the retinal pigment epithelium may occur secondary to ocular trauma, inflammation, or other insults, and may simulate a choroidal melanoma.[19, 20] Although it may take a variety of forms, it is usually jet black and may develop rapidly after the appropriate stimulus. Melanomas, on the other hand, are usually less deeply pigmented and progress more slowly in eyes with no history of trauma or inflammation.[21]

Benign tumors of the retinal pigment epithelium are quite rare, but a number of cases have been reported.[22] In most instances, it has been impossible to differentiate clinically adenomas of the retinal pigment epithelium from choroidal melanomas. In contrast to melanomas, however, they are usually jet black, have no associated retinal detachment, are slowly progressive or unchanging, and are more common in blacks. The role of fluorescein angiography, ultrasonography, ^{32}P uptake, and other ancillary tests is still unproved in such cases. Malignant tumors of the retinal pigment epithelium are extremely rare and are difficult or impossible to differentiate from malignant melanoma of the choroid.

Combined hamartoma of the retinal pigment epithelium may present as a pigmented fundus lesion located at the posterior pole or in the periphery.[14] It differs from melanomas in that it is nonprogressive and often exhibits tractional phenomena with dragging of the retina toward the lesion. This effect is probably due to shrinkage of the mass secondary to gliosis. Histologically these lesions exhibit a benign proliferation of retinal pigment epithelium, glial cells, and blood vessels.[14]

CHOROIDAL DETACHMENT

The choroidal detachment appears clinically as a smooth, elevated lesion extending from the ciliary body region for a variable distance posteriorly. Superficially, it may closely resemble a ciliary body melanoma.[2] In most cases, however, the lesion is annular, involving all quadrants of the fundus—an extremely rare occurrence for melanomas. There is usually a history of recent surgical or nonsurgical trauma with hypotony. The demonstration of a wound leak through the surgical incision is helpful in the differential diagnosis. In some cases, however, a recently operated eye may contain an unsuspected melanoma that resembles a choroidal detachment, leading to confusion in diagnosis.[23]

Choroidal detachments permit transmission of light, whereas melanomas usually cause a dense shadow. If the diagnosis is still uncertain, ultrasonography and the ^{32}P test may easily make the distinction.

Choroidal detachments are occasionally seen in eyes with no history of trauma, as a part of the uveal effusion syndrome.[24, 25] These eyes present with an elevated smooth lesion in the ciliary body and peripheral choroid, associated with a large bullous retinal detachment and dramatically shifting subretinal fluid. They often demonstrate peculiar brown pigment clumping at the level of the retinal pigment epithelium.

Although the choroidal effusion syndrome may simulate melanoma, the extent of the retinal detachment is usually much greater than one would expect for a melanoma of comparable size. In addition, the typical scattered pigment at the level of the retinal pigment epithelium is atypical for melanoma.

As in the case of postoperative choroidal detachments, transillumination is helpful in differentiating the lesion from melanoma, as are ultrasonography and the ^{32}P test.

Hemorrhagic choroidal detachments may be particularly difficult to distinguish from melanoma. There is usually a history of recent surgery or trauma. Transillumination is of limited value in such cases because a dense hematoma often casts a shadow similar to a melanoma. Ultrasonography and the ^{32}P test are helpful in these cases.[23]

CHOROIDAL HEMANGIOMA

Choroidal hemangiomas may be very difficult to differentiate from amelanotic choroidal melanomas.[2, 26, 27] These tumors are typically nonpigmented, but they may have scattered clumps of pigment on the surface. They are red-orange or yellow-orange and are usually located in the posterior pole, either nasal or temporal to the optic disk. Accumulation of subretinal fluid may cause a serous detachment of the fovea. Fluorescein angiography and ultrasonography may be helpful in differentiating choroidal hemangioma from amelanotic choroidal melanoma.[27] If the diagnosis is still in doubt, the ^{32}P test is usually negative in choroidal hemangiomas.

The Sturge-Weber syndrome is frequently associated with a choroidal hemangioma. In these cases, the choroidal hemangioma is more diffuse and the affected eye often has glaucoma. These findings, in association with the facial angioma, are evidence in favor of choroidal hemangioma rather than melanoma.[27]

METASTATIC TUMORS TO THE CHOROID

A tumor metastatic to the choroid is probably the lesion most difficult to differentiate clinically from melanoma.[3, 4] It usually occurs as a nonpigmented choroidal mass, most often in the posterior pole.

Ferry and Font[28] have listed the most common primary sites of tumors metastatic to the eye. In the case of breast carcinoma, the patient usually gives a history of mastectomy, suggesting the proper diagnosis. In the case of tumors arising in the lung or gastrointestinal tract, however, the ocular symptoms may be the first manifestation of systemic disease. In these cases, ophthalmoscopic differentiation may be difficult.

There are certain ophthalmoscopic features that suggest the possibility of metastatic tumor rather than primary choroidal melanoma. The metastatic tumor is more likely to have a flat or diffuse configuration. The mass itself is amelanotic with typical brown pigment clumping on the surface. It is often located just temporal to the fovea and causes visual symptoms by encroaching on the fovea. Metastatic tumors frequently cause a serous retinal detachment, which is usually more extensive than expected for a melanoma of comparable size.[29] Although these features are helpful in differentiating metastatic tumor from melanoma, they are not absolute, and exceptions do occur. For example, a diffuse amelanotic melanoma, although a rare occurrence, may be virtually impossible to differentiate from metastatic tumor.

When the diagnosis of tumor metastatic to the choroid is entertained, a complete systemic evaluation to locate the primary lesion is mandatory. Recent studies suggest that plasma carcinoembryonic antigen levels may be useful in distinguishing metastatic tumors from melanoma in some instances.[30, 31]

CHOROIDAL NEVUS

The choroidal nevus may be difficult or impossible to differentiate from a small melanoma.[1, 2] The presence of elevation, overlying lipofuscin pigment, drusen, subretinal fluid, and a visual field defect are suggestive of early melanoma, although such changes may be seen with benign nevi as well.[32] In borderline cases, some authorities choose to do fluorescein angiography, ultrasonography, and a ^{32}P test to help establish the diagnosis,[3, 4, 33, 34] and others prefer to observe the lesion periodically for evidence of growth.[34, 35]

MELANOCYTOMA

The melanocytoma (magnocellular nevus) is a benign pigmented lesion, typically located over the optic nervehead.[36] Its dark black appearance and superficial location, often within the nerve fiber layer, differentiates it from melanoma. In contrast to melanoma, it occurs with equal frequency in blacks and whites.

Although typically located on the optic nervehead, the melanocytoma may be located anywhere in the uveal tract.[32,37] When located in the choroid, it may be impossible to differentiate from any other nevus or small melanoma.[32]

HEMORRHAGIC DETACHMENT OF RETINAL PIGMENT EPITHELIUM

Hemorrhagic detachment of the retinal pigment epithelium appears as a smooth dark fundus mass that may simulate a melanoma.[12] The typical smooth dark appearance differs from the usual melanoma, which has a mottled appearance due to overlying retinal pigment epithelium alterations. Since this lesion often occurs as a part of senile macular degeneration, macular changes in the opposite eye are often helpful in suggesting the diagnosis. If the diagnosis remains uncertain, fluorescein angiography shows hypofluorescence of the lesion.

VITREOUS HEMORRHAGE

Vitreous hemorrhage, from any cause, sometimes assumes a globular configuration and resembles a melanoma. Indirect ophthalmoscopy usually indicates the true location of the lesion and suggests the diagnosis. It is also helpful to have the patient move the eye in different directions with the lesion under indirect ophthalmoscopic observation. A vitreous hemorrhage moves back and forth and then assumes its original position, whereas a melanoma remains fixed and does not show such movement.

OTHER LESIONS SIMULATING MELANOMA

Central serous chorioretinopathy, subluxated lens, and retained intraocular foreign bodies may occasionally simulate melanoma. In most cases, however, careful clinical evaluation leads to the correct diagnosis.

REFERENCES

1. Ferry AP: Lesions mistaken for malignant melanoma of the posterior uvea. Arch Ophthalmol 72:463, 1964
2. Shields JA, Zimmerman LE: Lesions simulating malignant melanoma of the posterior uvea. Arch Ophthalmol 89:466, 1973
3. Shields JA, McDonald PR: Improvements in the diagnosis of posterior uveal melanomas. Arch Ophthalmol 91:259, 1974
4. Shields JA, McDonald PR, Sarin LK: Problems and improvements in the diagnosis of posterior uveal melanomas. In Croll M, Brady LW, Carmichael PL, Wallner RJ (eds): Nuclear Ophthalmology. New York, Wiley, 1976, pp 37–49

5. Coleman DJ, Abramson DH, Jack RL, Franzen LA: Ultrasonic diagnosis of tumors of the choroid. Arch Ophthalmol 91:344, 1974
6. Norton EWD, Smith JL, Curtin VT, Justice J Jr: Fluorescein fundus photography: an aid in the differential diagnosis of posterior ocular lesions. Trans Am Acad Ophthalmol Otolaryngol 68:755, 1964
7. Hagler WS, Jarrett WH II, Humphrey WT: The radioactive phosphorus uptake test in the diagnosis of uveal melanoma. Arch Ophthalmol 83:548, 1970
8. Shields JA, Sarin LK, Federman JL, Mensheha Manhart O, Carmichael PL: Surgical approach to one ^{32}P test for posterior uveal melanomas. Ophthalmic Surg 5:13, 1974
9. Shields JA, Hagler WS, Federman JL, Jarrett WH II, Carmichael PL: The significance of the ^{32}P uptake test in the diagnosis of posterior uveal melanomas. Trans Am Acad Ophthalmol Otolaryngol 79:297, 1975
10. Bedford MA, Chegnell AH: U-shaped retinal tear associated with presumed malignant melanoma of the choroid. Br J Ophthalmol 54:200, 1970
11. Robertson DM, Curtin VT: Rhegmatogenous retinal detachment and choroidal melanoma. Am J Ophthalmol 72:351, 1971
12. Zimmerman LE: Macular lesions mistaken for malignant melanoma of the choroid. Trans Am Acad Ophthalmol Otolaryngol 69:623, 1965
13. Letocha C, Shields JA, Goldberg RE: Retinal changes in sarcoidosis. Can J Ophthalmol 10:184, 1975
14. Gass JDM: The Differential Diagnosis of Intraocular Tumors. St. Louis, Mosby, 1974
15. Zimmerman LE, Spencer WH: The pathologic anatomy of retinoschisis. Arch Ophthalmol 63:34, 1960
16. Buettner H: Congenital hypertrophy of the retinal pigment epithelium. Am J Ophthalmol 79:177, 1975
17. Purcell JJ, Shields JA: Hypertrophy with hyperpigmentation of the retinal pigment epithelium. Arch Ophthalmol 93:1122, 1975
18. Shields JA, Ts'o MOM: The histopathology of congenital grouped pigmentation of the retina. Arch Ophthalmol 93:1153, 1975
19. Kurz GH, Zimmerman LE: Vagaries of the retinal pigment epithelium. Int Ophthalmol Clin 2:441, 1962
20. Frayer WC: Reactivity of the retinal pigment epithelium: an experimental and histopathologic study. Trans Am Ophthalmol Soc 64:587, 1966
21. Shields JA, Green WR, McDonald PR: Uveal pseudomelanoma due to post-traumatic pigmentary migration. Arch Ophthalmol 89:519, 1973
22. Garner A: Tumors of the retinal pigment epithelium. Br J Ophthalmol 54:715, 1970
23. Shields JA, Leonard BC, Sarin LK: Multilobed uveal melanoma simulating a postoperative choroidal detachment. Br J Ophthalmol, 60:386, 1976
24. McDonald PR, de la Paz V, Sarin LK: Nonrhegmatogenous retinal separation with choroidal detachment (uveal effusion). Trans Am Ophthalmol Soc 62:226, 1964
25. Brockhurst RJ, Schepens CL: Uveal effusion. Arch Ophthalmol 70:101, 1963
26. Jarrett WH II, Hagler WS, LaRose JH, Shields JA: Clinical experience with presumed hemangioma of choroid: radioactive phosphorus uptake studies as an aid in differential diagnosis. Trans Am Acad Ophthalmol Otolaryngol, in press
27. Canny CLB, Shields JA: Choroidal hemangiomas. Surv Ophthalmol, in preparation
28. Ferry AP, Font RL: Carcinoma metastatic to the eye and orbit. Arch Ophthalmol 92:276, 1974
29. Shields JA: Metastatic tumors to and from the eye. In Croll M, Brady LW, Carmichael PL, Wallner RJ (eds): Nuclear Ophthalmology. New York, Wiley, 1976, pp 151–60
30. Michelson JB, Felberg NT, Shields JA, Foster L: Carcinoembryonic antigen positive metastatic adenocarcinoma of the choroid. Arch Ophthalmol 93:794, 1975

31. Michelson JB, Felberg NT, Shields JA: Carcinoembryonic antigen in the evaluation of intraocular malignancies. Arch Ophthalmol, 94:414, 1976
32. Shields JA, Font RL: Melanocytoma of the choroid clinically simulating a malignant melanoma. Arch Ophthalmol 87:396, 1972
33. Shields JA, Annesley WH, Totino JA: Nonfluorescent malignant melanoma of the choroid diagnosed with the ^{32}P test. Am J Ophthalmol 79:634, 1975
34. Shields JA: The management of small malignant melanomas of the choroid. In Brockhurst RJ (ed): Controversy in Ophthalmology. Philadelphia, Saunders, in press
35. Curtin VT, Cavender JC: The natural course of selected malignant melanomas of the choroid and ciliary body. Mod Probl Ophthalmol 12:523, 1974
36. Zimmerman LE, Garron LK: Melanocytoma of the optic disc. Int Ophthalmol Clin 2:431, 1962
37. Howard GM, Forrest AW: Incidence and location of melanocytomas. Arch Ophthalmol 77:61, 1967

Gerald A. Fishman

2 The Value of Fluorescein Angiography in the Differential Diagnosis of Choroidal Melanomas

Several reports[1-10] have described characteristic features noted on fluorescein angiography in patients with choroidal melanomas. This report evaluates the sensitivity and specificity of these angiographic findings by comparing the angiographic changes in retinal and choroidal lesions that ophthalmoscopically resemble choroidal melanomas.

NORMAL FLUORESCEIN ANGIOGRAM

The sequence of events in a normal angiogram begins with the injection into the antecubital vein of 5 ml of a 10 percent solution of sodium fluorescein dye or, occasionally, 10 ml of a 5 percent solution. Light from a fundus camera passing first through a blue filter (Wratten 47 or Baird Atomic B5) enters the eye and "excites" fluorescence from the dye passing through retinal and choroidal vessels. Excitation is maximal in the ranges of 485 to 500 nm. The maximum fluorescence returning from the fundus is within 520 to 530 nm. A yellow "barrier" filter (Wratten 15 or 12), which transmits maximally at the above wavelengths, is interposed between the emerging light and the camera film, thus allowing maximal film exposure at the most optimal wavelengths. The majority of fluorescent light is emitted from free fluorescein in the plasma which is not bound to serum protein. Notably, 50 to 85 percent of fluorescein is bound to serum protein, in which state its efficiency in emitting fluorescein when excited by the appropriate wavelength of light is only approximately 26 percent, compared to approximately 80 percent efficiency of unbound fluorescein. An additional loss in fluorescence results from its absorption by hemoglobin. Figures 2.1 through 2.4 illustrate the sequence of fluorescein dye accumulation within the choroid. The rest of this chapter is a description of the manner in which choroidal lesions disrupt this normal pattern. In this regard, the following questions seem most pertinent:

1. How do various lesions modify normal choroidal fluorescence?
2. Are these modifications specific for individual lesions?
3. Are these modifications detectable in the majority of cases (sensitivity)?

This study was supported in part by training grant EY 24-16 from the National Eye Institute, NIH, and by the National Retinitis Pigmentosa Foundation.

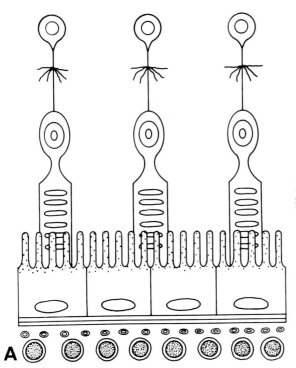

FIG. 2.1A. Initial stages of fluorescein angiography with dye in the larger choroidal vessels. **B.** Early phase angiogram with dye in larger choroidal vessels.

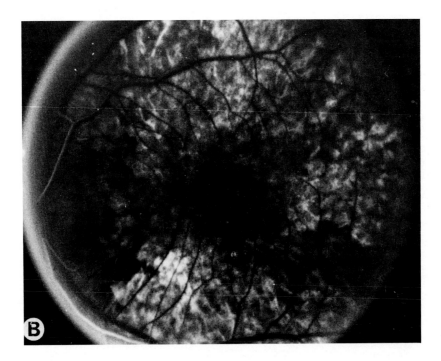

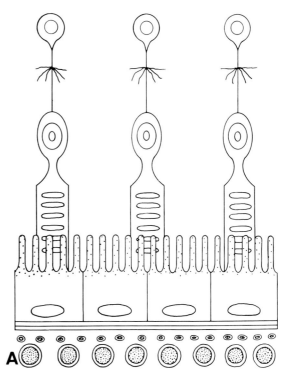

FIG. 2.2. Dye within both large choroidal vessels and the choriocapillaris. **A.** Drawing. **B.** Angiogram.

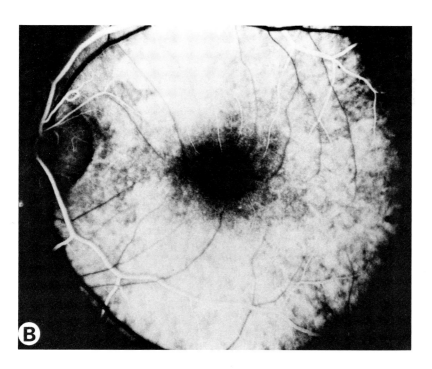

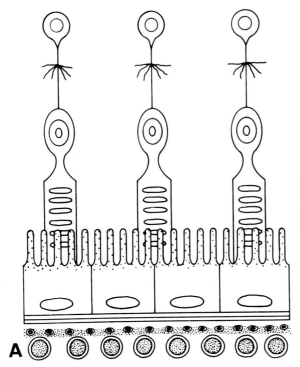

FIG. 2.3. Dye has leaked out from choriocapillaris vessels and is accumulating within interstitial tissue. **A.** Drawing. **B.** Angiogram.

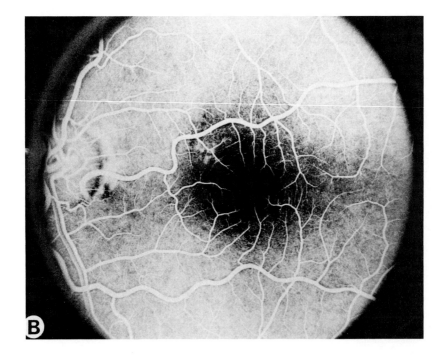

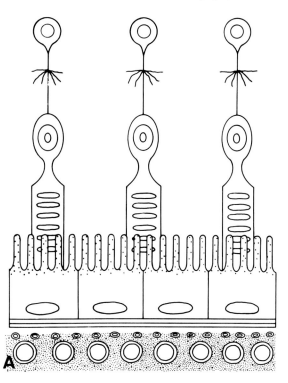

FIG. 2.4. Larger choroidal vessels are seen in silhouette by contrast with fluorescein accumulation within the connective tissue of the choroid. **A.** Drawing. **B.** Angiogram.

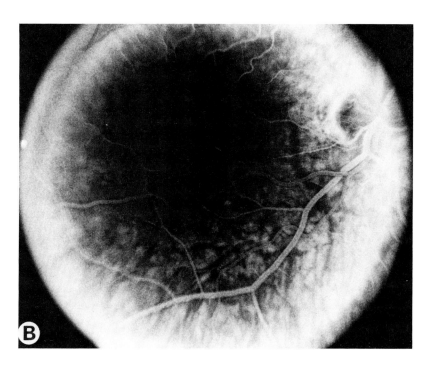

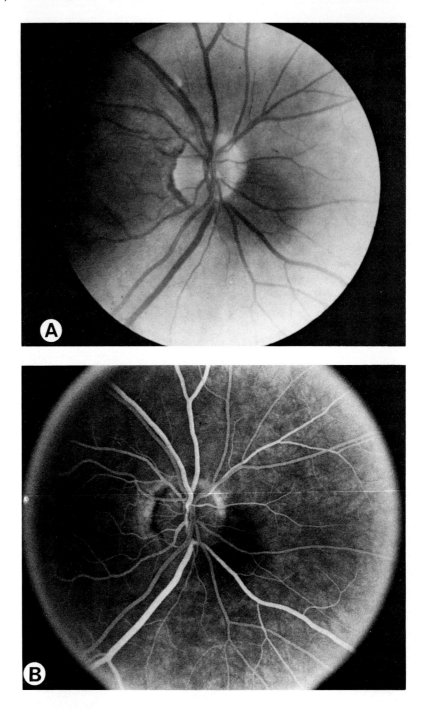

FIG. 2.5A. Typical slate gray, flat, choroidal nevus. **B.** Corresponding zone of hypofluorescence on fluorescein angiogram.

CHOROIDAL NEVI

Most choroidal nevi, which result from a focal collection of benign choroidal melanocytes, cause a localized area of relative hypofluorescence. This effect results from absorption of both the excitation stimulus and emitted fluorescence by the uveal melanocytes within the lesion. If the lesion resides exclusively within the deeper layers of the choroid, only fluorescence from larger choroidal vessels is absorbed and the localized hypofluorescence may be minimal. If the nevus is more superficial and also involves choriocapillaris vessels, the hypofluorescence may be more evident. In one series, choriocapillaris involvement was noted in one-third of 102 nevi studied histologically.[11] Figure 2.5 shows a typical pattern of hypofluorescence associated with a choroidal nevus. Some choroidal nevi disrupt the overlying retinal pigment epithelium (Fig. 2.6). Resultant changes include hypopigmentation and drusen formation. In one series,[12] 10 percent of cases showed hyperfluorescence from window defects associated with atrophy of the overlying retinal pigment epithelium. Hale and co-workers[13] reported the occurrence of drusen in approximately 80 percent of choroidal nevi examined histologically. Naumann et al[12] cite a 50 percent incidence noted angiographically.

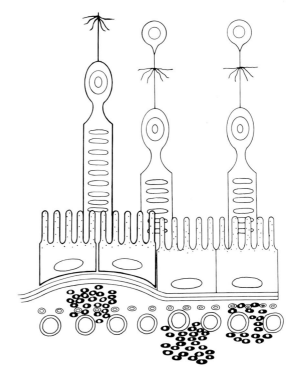

FIG. 2.6. Geographic relationships between nevus cells and the retinal pigment epithelium and choriocapillaris.

CHOROIDAL MELANOMA

Double Circulation

Choroidal melanomas with large tumor vessels near their surface manifest a double circulation, which consists of the simultaneous visibility of both retinal and tumor vessels at the tumor site. Also important in distinguishing this finding, first emphasized by Charamis and associates,[14] is the absence of heavy pigmentation in the tumor. Fluorescein dye progressively leaks from the tumor vessels and causes a late staining of the tumor tissue. Since Edwards and associates[5] saw these vessels only when tumors were elevated 6 mm or more, their presence presumably indicates a more advanced stage. Other changes associated with melanomas include the accumulation of fluid in the subretinal space and outer plexiform layers (Fig. 2.7). These findings are recognized angiographically in later photographs as the dye accumulates into overlying subretinal fluid and outer plexiform spaces (Figs. 2.8, 2.9). Figure 2.10 shows a large choroidal melanoma with double circulation noted on fluorescein angiography.

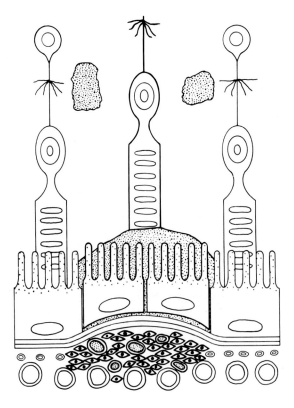

FIG. 2.7. Choroidal melanoma: tumor vessels, disruption of the retinal pigment epithelium, and dye accumulation within the subretinal space and outer plexiform layers.

Tumor Staining

In most choroidal melanomas a double circulation is not evident. The majority of cases show late staining of the tumor, presumably resulting from the leakage of normal choroidal vessels and tumor vessels located deep within the lesion. Optimal fluorescence is facilitated by concurrent overlying hypopigmentation and atrophy of the retinal pigment epithelium. Dye probably accumulates both in necrotic or extracellular spaces and intracellularly.[4] In late-phase angiograms, some eyes show punctate hyperfluorescent dots, which are most apparent at the periphery of the lesion (Fig. 2.11). The exact anatomic change within the choroid or retinal pigment epithelium causing this appearance is uncertain. Loewer-Sieger and Oosterhuis[15] and Oosterhuis and Waveren[3] have associated these changes with capillary dilatations in the choroid. Yanko[16] attributed the punctate hyperfluorescence to blood channels having a course perpendicular to the tumor surface, while Hayreh[2] suggests a positive correlation with localized areas of subretinal or sub-pigment epithelial exudation.

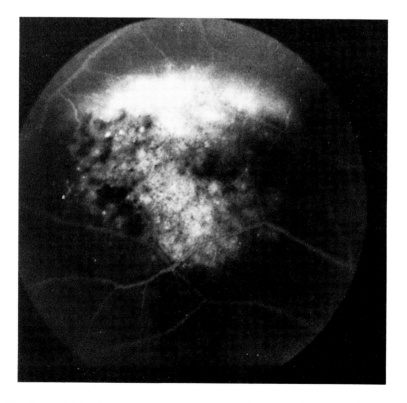

FIG. 2.8. Upper third of late-stage angiogram shows dye accumulation within the subretinal space.

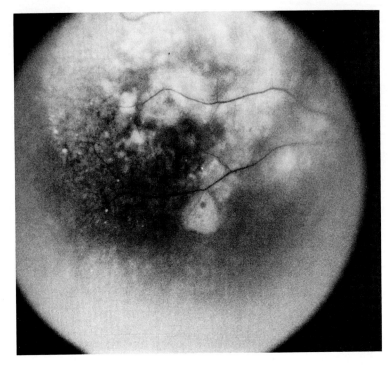

FIG. 2.9. Late-stage angiogram shows dye accumulation within the outer plexiform layer.

Lipofuscin

Clumps of macrophages, which contain pigment released from destroyed retinal pigment epithelium or retinal pigment cells containing similar pigment, can accumulate on the surface of the tumor and within the outer retina. Some investigators have described the presence of this orange pigment (lipofuscin) overlying choroidal melanomas.[17-19] By denying the blue excitation light access to the tumor, its presence causes a hypofluorescence on angiography that corresponds in location to the orange pigment. Similarly, any substantial pigment accumulation, hemorrhage, or optically opaque exudate within or overlying the tumor reduces its degree of fluorescence.

No Abnormal Fluorescence

Recently Shields and co-workers[20] described a case of malignant melanoma within the macula in which there was no abnormal fluorescence. Histologic sections showed that there was no destruction of the overlying retinal pigment epithelium, which contributes significantly to the hyperfluorescence seen in choroidal melanomas. Nadel and co-workers[21] reported a nonfluorescent melanoma in which the lack of fluorescence was attributed to hemorrhage overlying the tumor. Some tumors may invade through the retina and into the vitreous. In these cases there may be a relative absence of tumor fluorescence and staining as dye leaks into the vitreous.[5]

Factors contributing to the fluorescence of choroidal melanomas include the degree of disruption of the overlying retinal pigment epithelium and the presence of tumor vessels that leak dye and, along with leakage from normal choriocapillaris vessels, contribute to late staining of the tumor tissue. Edwards et al[5] found no positive correlation between cell type and particular fluorescein angiographic patterns. The presence of visible tumor vessels is related to the size and location of the vessels. The degree of pigmentation within the lesion also contributes to the degree of fluorescence by absorbing fluorescein. Although disruption of the retinal pigment epithelium is seen in choroidal nevi, clinically identifiable tumor vessels and late staining of these lesions are atypical; when present, they arouse suspicion of a more malignant lesion. The presence of abnormally permeable vessels and late staining of the lesion, although characteristic, is not pathognomonic for a choroidal melanoma. The presence of hyperfluorescent dots at the periphery of the lesion suggests the increased possibility of a choroidal lesion being a melanoma, but is not pathognomonic. Lipofuscin pigment on the surface of the lesion may also be seen in metastatic lesions and hemangiomas of the choroid. Small choroidal melanomas that do not disrupt the overlying retinal pigment epithelium or have tumor vessels may not present angiographic findings characteristic of choroidal melanomas.

MELANOCYTOMA

Most reported melanocytomas are jet black lesions within the optic nerve. They represent a benign type of nevus, although on rare occasions melanocytomas have been reported to undergo malignant change.[22] On fluorescein angiography in cases of melanocytoma of the optic nervehead,[23, 24] the lesion typically demonstrates blockage of fluorescence similar to most nevi of the choroid. Shields and Font[25] described a choroidal melanocytoma that showed hyperfluorescence associated with disruption of the retinal pigment epithelium as well as staining of the lesion and subretinal fluid accumulation inferior to the lesion. All three features were also noted as characteristically seen in choroidal melanomas (Fig. 2.12).

METASTATIC CHOROIDAL LESIONS

Lesions metastatic to the choroid occur most frequently from primary sites within the breast, lung, or gastrointestinal tract. The lesions are often yellow-orange with an overlying pigment mottling. They can be flat or moderately elevated. Often, an extensive serous detachment of the retina is seen. Fluorescein angiographic changes vary considerably depending on both the overlying retinal pigment epithelial changes and the presence of tumor vessels (Fig. 2.13). Some metastatic lesions may, therefore, show minimal or no hyperfluorescence,[26, 27] while others manifest extensive hyperfluorescence and late tumor staining, not unlike that seen in primary choroidal melanoma (cf. Fig. 2.11). The presence of large choroidal vessels within a tumor or late localization of fluorescein within areas of retinal cystoid edema both weigh against the diagnosis of choroidal metastases.[28]

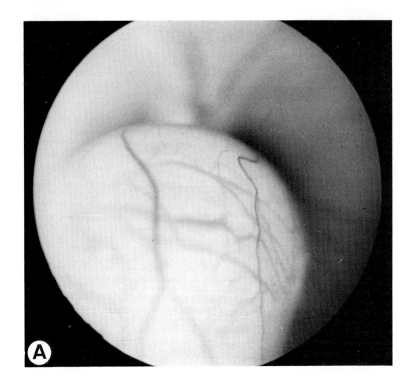

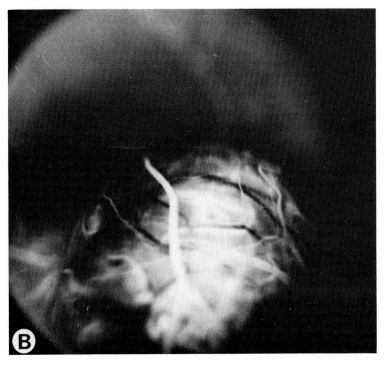

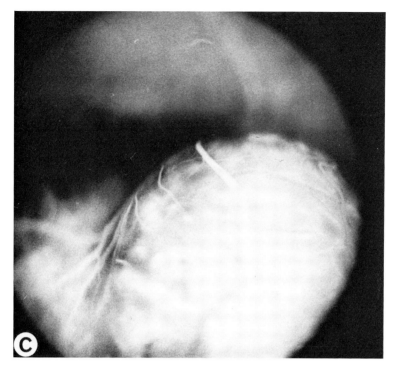

FIG. 2.10A. Mushroom-shaped choroidal melanoma with large tumor vessels. **B.** Double circulation with tumor and retinal vessels visible simultaneously. Note leakage of dye from within the tumor. **C.** Staining of tumor tissue in late-stage angiogram.

CHOROIDAL HEMANGIOMAS

Choroidal hemangioma, a vascular hamartoma, occurs as either a localized choroidal tumor in a patient with no other evidence of vascular malformation, or as a diffuse cavernous hemangioma of the choroid, associated with the Sturge-Weber syndrome (Fig. 2.14). Isolated choroidal hemangiomas show a salmon-colored localized fundus lesion. On fluorescein angiography dilated vascular channels can be seen during early stages (Fig. 2.15A). There is a progressive leakage of dye with resultant staining of interstitial choroidal tissue (Fig. 2.15B). Overlying disruption of the retinal pigment epithelium facilitates visibility of the choroidal fluorescence in a pattern similar to that of malignant melanomas. Serous detachment of the retina and cystoid changes in the outer plexiform layer, both also seen in choroidal melanomas, are frequently associated. Fluorescein angiography cannot conclusively differentiate between this lesion and an amelanotic melanoma. The small hyperfluorescent spots in some melanomas are not a feature seen in choroidal hemangiomas.

In the Sturge-Weber syndrome the choroid on the same side as the facial lesions is diffusely thickened and exhibits a more red-orange color than the opposite normal eye. In the majority of cases the overlying retinal pigment epithelium and retina

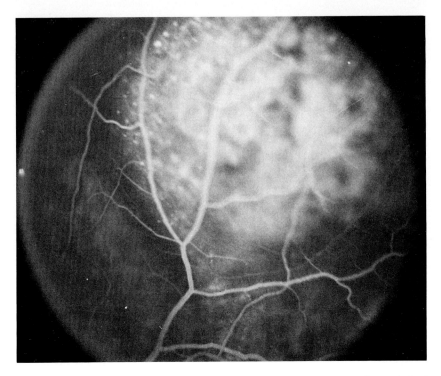

FIG. 2.11. Multiple punctate hyperfluorescent spots most evident at the periphery of the lesion.

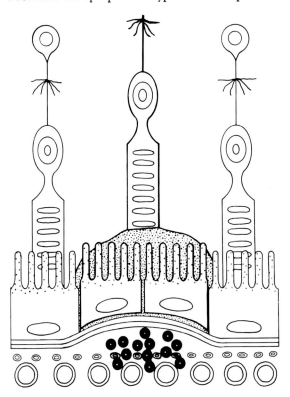

FIG. 2.12. Disruption of the retinal pigment epithelium and dye accumulation within the subretinal space associated with a choroidal melanocytoma.

are normal. In typical cases an exaggerated choroidal flush is seen during the early stages of dye perfusion.

DISCIFORM DEGENERATION OF THE MACULA

Disciform degeneration of the macula implies the detachment of the retinal pigment epithelium and/or sensory retina with neovascular tissue present generally within both the subretinal and subpigment epithelial spaces. Frequently hemorrhage and variable degrees of gliosis are also present (Fig. 2.16). Figure 2.17 shows a sequence of angiograms from a patient with presumed ocular histoplasmosis showing subretinal neovascularization. The delicate frondlike appearance of these vessels is angiographically different from the large tumorlike vessels seen in choroidal melanomas. Their presence is reassurance of nonmalignancy in a specific lesion.

CHOROIDAL HEMORRHAGES

Hemorrhages below the retinal pigment epithelium consistently show hypofluorescence on angiography (Fig. 2.18). As suggested, the fluorescence is absorbed by the extravascular hemoglobin. This pattern of hypofluorescence is, as noted,

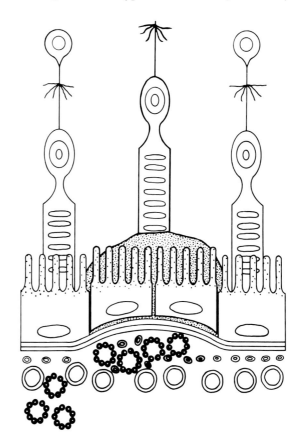

FIG. 2.13. Changes within the retinal pigment epithelium and dye accumulation within the subretinal space associated with a lesion metastatic to the choroid.

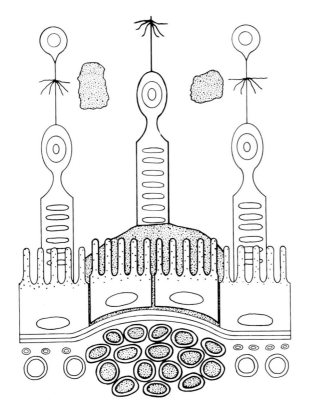

FIG. 2.14. Choroidal hemangioma with associated disruption of the retinal pigment epithelium and fluid accumulation within the subretinal space and outer plexiform layer.

unusual in choroidal melanomas. If the diagnosis is uncertain, a suspicious lesion can be followed. Most choroidal hemorrhages resorb within ten days to two weeks after the onset.[29] Figure 2.19 shows a choroidal hemorrhage with characteristic angiographic pattern.

CHOROIDAL DETACHMENT

Choroidal detachments, which usually present as a round, elevated, brown mass extending from the peripheral fundus, are most frequently associated with postoperative hypotony. They do not show hyperfluorescence, abnormal permeable vessels, or late staining. Therefore, angiographic studies are helpful in differentiating these lesions from ciliary body or choroidal melanomas. However, in most instances clinical features, including the patient's history, are adequate to make this distinction. These lesions, which often have a scalloped or multilobed configuration, transilluminate, in contrast to pigmented melanomas, which do not.

RETINAL MACROANEURYSMS

Retinal macroaneurysms[30, 31] resulting in secondary intraretinal and subretinal hemorrhages with subsequent resolution may resemble a choroidal melanoma (Fig. 2.20A). Hemorrhages usually resorb over a six- to eight-week period. Some cases

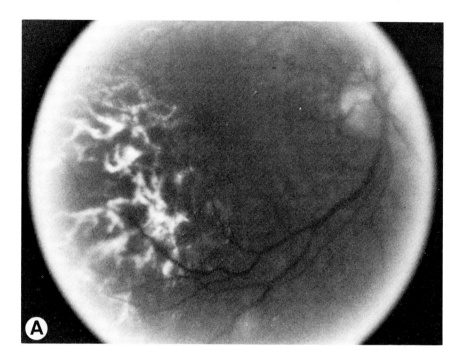

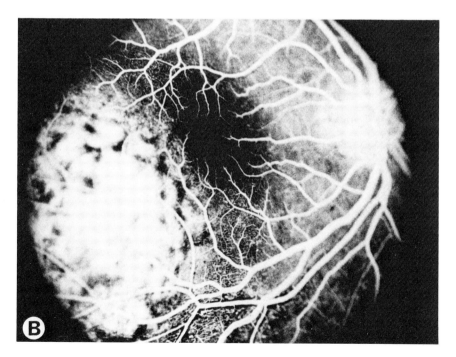

FIG. 2.15A. Early-stage angiogram shows large vessels comprising the lesion. **B.** Leakage of fluorescein from hemangioma with staining of the lesion.

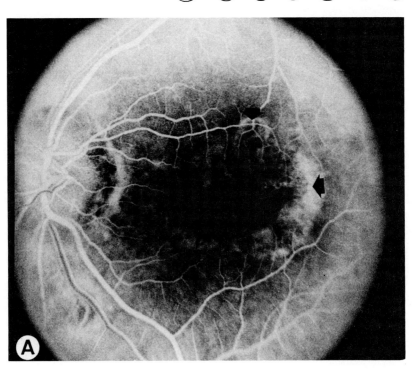

FIG. 2.16. Disciform lesion with subpigment epithelial and subretinal neovascularization and dye accumulation.

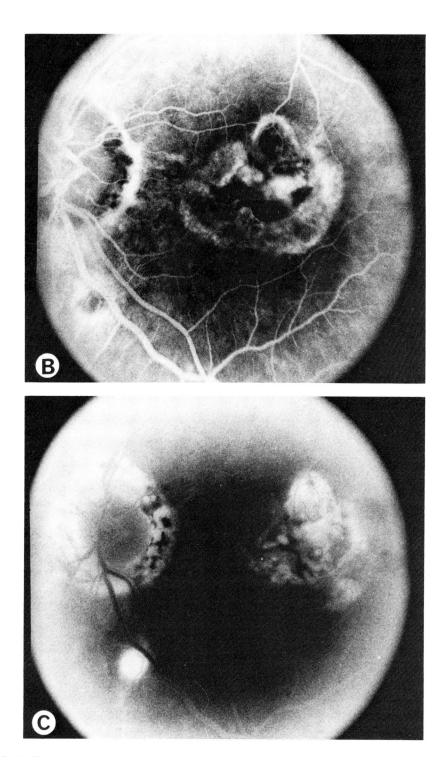

FIG. 2.17A. Early-stage angiogram with subretinal and/or subpigment epithelial neovascularization (arrows). **B.** As angiography continues, dye leaks from the neovascular tissue. **C.** Late-stage angiogram with staining of glial and fibrous tissue associated with the disciform lesion.

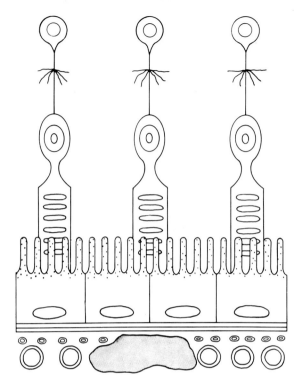

FIG. 2.18. Choroidal hemorrhage.

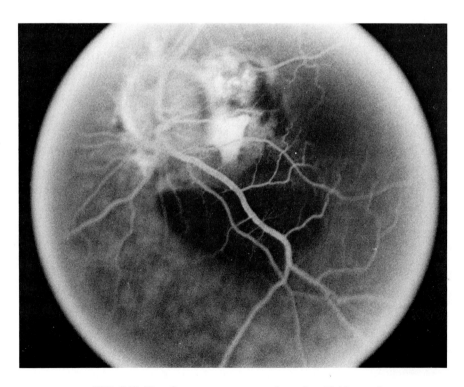

FIG. 2.19. Hypofluorescence corresponds to choroidal hemorrhage.

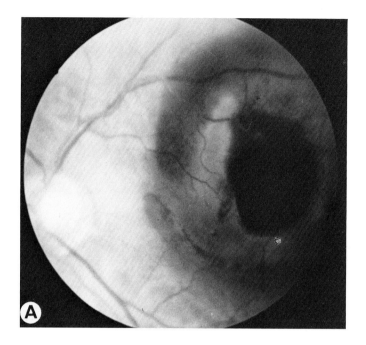

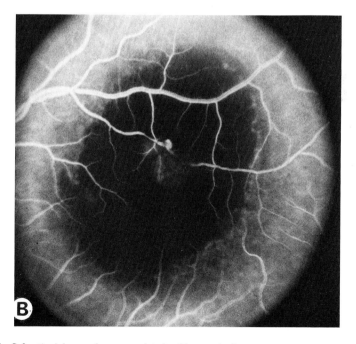

FIG. 2.20A. Subretinal hemorrhage associated with a retinal macroaneurysm. First indication of disorder was visual loss. **B.** Small vascular dilatation on retinal arteriole (macroaneurysm). Large zone of hypofluorescence corresponds to subretinal hemorrhage.

may show macular edema and intraretinal exudates in the absence of hemorrhage. Fluorescein angiography (Fig. 2.20B) shows a localized saccular dilatation, which presumably was the source of the initial hemorrhage. While the visual prognosis in patients with hemorrhage is good, it is considerably less optimistic in those patients with macular edema. There is a natural tendency for most macroaneurysms to resolve spontaneously with resultant fibrosis.[30] The presence of spontaneous pulsation may indicate impending vessel rupture and serious bleeding.[32] Etiologic factors in these macroaneurysms include aging, hypertension, and arteriosclerosis, which were present in many of the reported cases.

HYPERTROPHY AND HYPERPIGMENTATION OF THE RETINAL PIGMENT EPITHELIUM

Cases of hypertrophy and hyperpigmentation of the retinal pigment epithelium were recently reported by Buettner.[33] Lesions are typically flat, gray-brown or black, often with rounded margins and a hypopigmented halo border (Fig. 2.21). Fluorescein angiography shows hypofluorescence from the lesion because of dye absorption by the pigment. Leakage within or late staining of the lesion is not seen. In some cases a normal choriocapillaris is seen through hyperpigmented lacunae

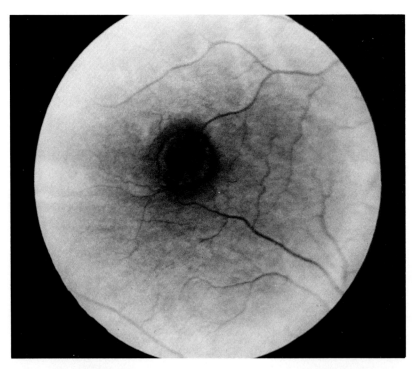

FIG. 2.21. Discrete black lesion with halo border is typical of hypertrophy and hyperpigmentation of the retinal pigment epithelium.

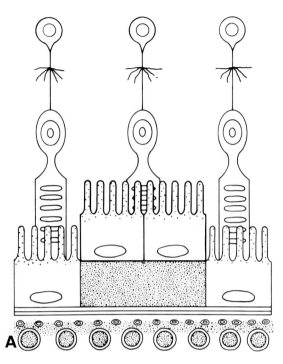

FIG. 2.22A. Detachment of the retinal pigment epithelium. **B.** Localized hyperfluorescence corresponds to detachment of the retinal pigment epithelium.

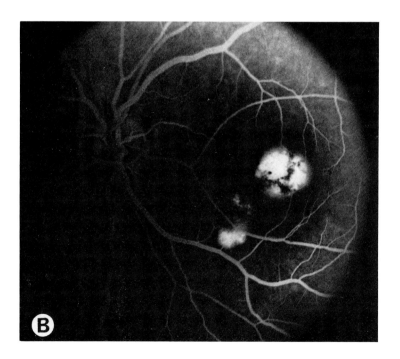

within the lesion or through areas corresponding to the hypopigmented halo. Histologic changes include hypertrophic retinal pigment epithelial cells having large, round pigment granules. Overlying photoreceptor cell inner and outer segments show marked degeneration.[33]

RETINOSCHISIS AND RETINAL DETACHMENT

Angiographic findings in retinoschisis and retinal detachment patients do not show hyperfluorescence or late staining, as noted in choroidal melanomas or some of the other choroidal diseases described.[10] In some earlier cases the area of detachment or schisis is relatively hypofluorescent due to partial obscuration of the background choroidal fluorescence. In long-standing detachments, secondary defects within the retinal pigment epithelium may cause a hyperfluorescence.

SEROUS DETACHMENT OF THE RETINAL PIGMENT EPITHELIUM

Characteristic angiographic findings are seen in detachment of the retinal pigment epithelium. A circumscribed hyperfluorescence corresponds to the detached retinal pigment epithelium. The fluorescence increases in intensity but not in area as the study progresses. Residual fluorescence often remains for over an hour as the dye accumulates in the subpigment epithelial space (Fig. 2.22).

CONCLUSION

In summarizing the preceding examples the following conclusions warrant further emphasis.

1. The ability of blue excitation light to reach the fluorescein within a lesion is at least as important as its histopathologic characteristics in determining the lesion's degree and pattern of fluorescence.
2. The histopathologic characteristics of the lesion do influence its pattern of fluorescence, determining the various factors within the lesion that either impede or facilitate this excitation.
3. Because some similar secondary (disruption of the retinal pigment epithelium) and primary (presence of tumor vessels) histologic changes that facilitate excitation are seen in different choroidal lesions, fluorescein angiography does not in all cases provide a conclusive diagnosis.
4. Fluorescein angiography studies can, however, offer additional information regarding general anatomic and physiologic alterations caused by a lesion in question.

ACKNOWLEDGMENT

Norbert Jednock provided photographic assistance, and Kathy Sisson graciously contributed the drawings.

REFERENCES

1. Rosen ES, Garner A: Benign melanoma of the choroid. Br J Ophthalmol 53:621, 1969
2. Hayreh SH: Choroidal melanoma: fluorescence, angiographic and histopathological study. Br J Ophthalmol 54:145, 1970
3. Oosterhuis JA, Waveren CHWV: Fluorescein photography in malignant melanoma. Ophthalmologica 156:101, 1968
4. Sollom AW: Fluorescence in malignant melanoma of the choroid. Ophthalmologica 156:117, 1968
5. Edwards WC, Layden WE, MacDonald R Jr: Fluorescein angiography of the choroid. Am J Ophthalmol 68:797, 1969
6. Flindall RJ, Gass JDM: A histopathologic fluorescein angiographic correlative study of malignant melanomas of the choroid. Can J Ophthalmol 6:258, 1971
7. Hayreh SS: Choroidal tumors: role of fluorescein fundus angiography in their diagnosis. Curr Concepts Ophthalmol 4:168, 1974
8. Gitter KA, Meyer D, Sarin LK, Keeney AH, Justice J: Fluorescein angiography of metastatic choroid tumors. Arch Ophthalmol 89:97, 1973
9. Pettit TH, Barton A, Foos RY, Christensen RE: Fluorescein angiography of choroidal melanomas. Arch Ophthalmol 83:27, 1970
10. Snyder WB, Allen L: Fluorescence angiography of ocular tumors. Trans Am Acad Ophthalmol Otolaryngol 71:820, 1967
11. Naumann G, Yanoff M, Zimmerman LE: Histogenesis of malignant melanomas of the uvea. Arch Ophthalmol 76:784, 1966
12. Naumann G, Hellner K, Naumann LR: Pigmented nevi of the choroid: clinical study of secondary changes in the overlying tissues. Trans Am Acad Ophthalmol Otolaryngol 75:110, 1971
13. Hale PN, Allen RA, Straatsma BR: Benign melanomas (nevi) of the choroid and ciliary body. Arch Ophthalmol 74:532, 1965
14. Charamis J, Kalsourakis N, Mandras G: The study of the cerebroretinal circulation by intravenous fluorescein injection. Am J Ophthalmol 61:1078, 1966
15. Loewer-Sieger DH, Oosterhuis JA: Melanoma or hemangioma of the choroid. Ophthalmologica 163:32, 1971
16. Yanko L: An angiographic and histologic study of the vasculature of choroidal malignant melanoma. Acta Ophthalmol 51:12, 1973
17. Wallow IHL, Ts'o MOM: Proliferation of the retinal pigment epithelium over malignant choroidal tumors: a light and electron microscopic study. Am Ophthalmol 73:914, 1972
18. Smith LT, Irvine AR: Diagnostic significance of orange pigment accumulation over choroidal tumors. Am J Ophthalmol 76:212, 1973
19. Font RL, Zimmerman LE, Armaly M: The nature of the orange pigment over a choroidal melanoma. Arch Ophthalmol 91:359, 1974
20. Shields JA, Annesley WH, Totino JA: Nonfluorescent malignant melanoma of the choroid diagnosed with the radioactive phosphorus uptake test. Am J Ophthalmol 79:634, 1975
21. Nadel A, O'Connor P, Lincoff H: Nonfluorescent melanoma. Am J Ophthalmol 70:748, 1970
22. Thomas CI, Purnell EW: Ocular melanocytoma. Am J Ophthalmol 67:79, 1969
23. Balestrazzi E: Melanocytoma of the optic disc. Ophthalmologica 166:289, 1973
24. Wiznia RA, Price J: Recovery of vision in association with a melanocytoma of the optic disk. Am J Ophthalmol 78:236, 1974
25. Shields JA, Font RL: Melanocytoma of the choroid clinically simulating a malignant melanoma. Arch Ophthalmol 87:396, 1972
26. Norton EWD, Smith JL, Curtin VT, Justice J: Fluorescein fundus photography: an aid in the differential diagnosis of posterior ocular lesions. Trans Am Acad Ophthalmol Otolaryngol 68:755, 1964

27. Harner RE, Smith JL, Reynolds DH: Fluorescein fundus study of metastatic breast carcinoma. Arch Ophthalmol 78:300, 1967
28. David DL, Robertson DM: Fluorescein angiography of metastatic choroidal tumors. Arch Ophthalmol 89:97, 1973
29. Tredici TJ, Fenton RH: Hematoma beneath the retinal pigment epithelium. Arch Ophthalmol 72:796, 1964
30. Robertson DM: Macroaneurysms of the retinal arteries. Trans Am Acad Ophthalmol Otolaryngol 77:55, 1973
31. Cleary PE, Hohner EM, Hamilton AM, Bird AC: Retinal macroaneurysms. Br J Ophthalmol 59:355, 1975
32. Shultz WT, Swan KC: Retinal aneurysms. Am J Ophthalmol 77:304, 1974
33. Buettner H: Congenital hypertrophy of the retinal pigment epithelium. Am J Ophthalmol 79:177, 1975

James G. Diamond
Karl C. Ossoinig

3 Contact A-Scan and B-Scan Ultrasonography in the Diagnosis of Intraocular Lesions

Ultrasound in ophthalmic diagnosis utilizes a beam emitted from a pencil-like probe in a fashion similar to a pen light. Such an ultrasound beam can be made visible by a special photographic technique (Fig. 3.1). The energy of the ultrasound beam is reflected and scattered by the acoustic interfaces encountered along its path. This occurrence is more or less comparable to the properties of light interacting at optical interfaces. The energy returning to the probe as an echo is amplified, processed, and displayed on an oscilloscope screen as an echogram (ultrasonogram). Echograms differ from each other principally in number, distribution, and intensity of echos. Tissues that differ in degree of acoustic reflection, size, and distribution of interfaces can be categorized on the basis of the echo patterns that each reflects. This effect is analogous to the different color characteristics produced by objects when struck by the same light beam.

INSTRUMENTATION

In ophthalmic diagnosis, the contact A- and B-scan methods are mainly used. The A-scan linearly displays the acoustic structures of the tissues encountered along the path of the beam. Figure 3.2 illustrates the typical A-scan echograms from a normal eye. The contact or "dead" zone corresponds to a distance of up to 5 μsec (7.5 mm) in front of the probe. One can therefore use only the right three-quarters of the pattern for accurate interpretation. Immersion B-scan units are far superior in detailing the anterior globe as this contact zone is eliminated. When an ultrasound beam directed into a tissue is shifted, the resulting echogram changes according to the characteristics of the newly encountered structures. The number, position, height, width, and movement of the underlying echo spikes indicate the number, location, density, size, and consistency of the individual anatomic structures.[1-3]

The B-scan echograms in Fig. 3.3 depict a cross section through the tissue examined. With a reduction in decibels, a corresponding loss of tissue detail occurs. In A-scan, single decibel unit changes are possible; 10-dB increment variations are the minimum in B-scanning. This feature allows wider latitude for quantitation

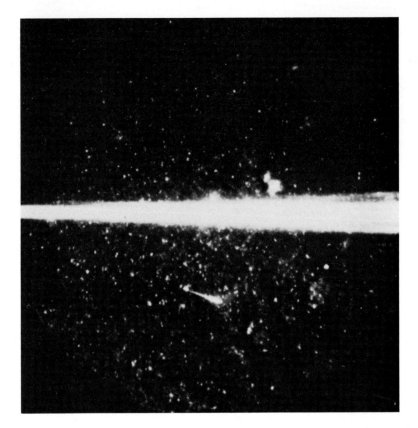

FIG. 3.1. Schlierfield technique revealing the pencil-like path of an A-scan ultrasound beam. (Courtesy of E. W. Purnell and A. Sokollu, Cleveland Clinic.)

with the A-scan unit as will be discussed later. The wedge-shaped empty space (Fig. 3.3) is the result of the shadowing effect of the optic nerve. This display illustrates the topography (shape and lateral extension) of the anatomic structures better than the A-scan method. However, it does not indicate other important information about reflectivity, mobility, and tissue consistency to the same degree as the A-scan display. Table 3.1 lists the advantages and disadvantages of the two

Table 3.1

Comparison of Contact A- and B-Scan Echographic Techniques

Technique	Advantage
A-scan	Higher efficiency in the orbit and posterior pole, useful in detection, differentiation, and measurements Faster performance Better applicability
B-scan	Easier demonstration of shape, topography, and size Higher efficiency in the anterior globe, useful in detection and differentiation

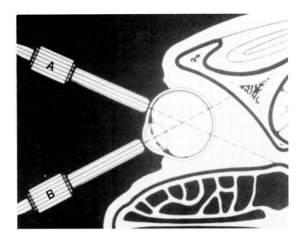

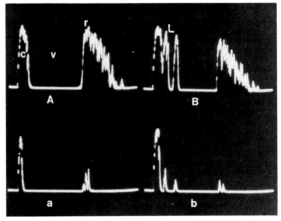

FIG. 3.2. Top: A-scan probe with beam direction bypassing lens (A) and aimed through it (B). **Bottom:** Contact A-scan echograms of normal globe at tissue sensitivity (tracings A and B) and at measuring sensitivity (tracings a and b) settings. The horizontal axis of the echogram represents the path of the beam while the vertical axis depicts structures hit by the beam. Tracings A and a were made bypassing the lens and show the contact or "dead" zone (c), empty vitreous cavity (v), and normal retinal–choroidal–scleral layers (r). Tracings B and b were made through the lens and have additional lens spikes (L). The contact or dead zone commences with the initial spike at the left border of the echogram and covers one-quarter to one-third of the display at tissue sensitivity.

systems. The combined use of A- and B-scan displays, applying the major attributes of each instrument, provides maximum clinical information.[4, 5]

The method practiced at the University of Iowa combines the use of the Kretz unit 7200 MA (the only standardized A-scan unit available) and the Bronson-Turner contact B-scan.[6, 7]

INDICATIONS

The indications for echography can be classified as absolute and relative. The absolute indications include (1) opaque ocular media, (2) clear ocular media in the presence of tumors of the posterior segment presenting problems in a differential diagnosis (eg, subretinal hemorrhage versus melanoma), and (3) the need for exact measurements of axial length. The relative indications include (1) senile cataracts, prohibiting fundus evaluation prior to surgery, and (2) miosis and anterior chamber abnormalities prohibiting fundus evaluation on a follow-up basis (eg, in glaucoma patients).

CLINICAL EXAMINATION

The combined A- and B-scan technique consists of a basic screening examination followed, when applicable, by special examination techniques for tissue diagnosis.

Basic Examination

The purpose of the basic examination[7] is to detect lesions. The equipment used for the basic examination consists primarily of the A-scan unit, set at "tissue sensitivity." This adjustment differs and is a defined setting of each standardized Kretz 7200 MA unit. It emits a wide, intense sound beam, insuring detection of low reflective lesions (Fig. 3.2, echo displays A and B). One starts the examination by placing the probe at the 6 o'clock limbus, moving slowly inferiorly toward the fornix. This maneuver is repeated in each of eight meridians, equally spaced for 360° around the globe. The patient is asked to look in the direction in which one wishes to examine. The beam must be aimed through the center of the globe, bypassing the lens (Fig. 3.2, echo display A). Otherwise, lens spike patterns will appear adjacent to the contact zone, making interpretation more confusing (Fig. 3.2, echo display B). One must also continuously angle the probe so that the sound beam reaches the most perpendicular point opposite that of the probe. It is this area that is being examined, which must be kept in mind throughout the procedure.

After the basic examination with the scanner set at tissue sensitivity, the setting is decreased by 24 dB, to what is termed measuring sensitivity (T-24 dB). The sound beam is narrower, and the resolution capacity is increased, thereby insuring detection of flat fundus lesions that may have been missed at the tissue sensitivity setting (Fig. 3.2, echo displays a and b). Figure 3.2 shows three separate spikes at the right of echogram a, which are the retina, choroid, and sclera. However, when the beam is directed through the lens, there occurs in addition to the normal lens spike pattern a decrease in number and height of the retinal–choroidal–scleral echos (Fig. 3.2, echo display b). The lens has absorbed some of the energy from the ultrasound beam, thereby decreasing its resolution potential. Again, this information is a reminder that one must bypass the lens when evaluating the posterior segment of the eye.

The results at the completion of this part of the examination are interpreted as either normal, abnormal, or equivocal. In the case of a normal evaluation, as in Fig. 3.2, the patient can be discharged with a reported normal echogram. However, if there is a questionable or positive finding, one continues the evaluation with special ultrasonographic examination techniques. These techniques elucidate a presumptive final tissue diagnosis by means of a process of exclusion.

Special Examinations

The special examination techniques[7,8] include (1) topographic echography for the location, shape, and border of lesions (primarily by B-scan); (2) quantitative echography for the determination of the reflectivity pattern, structure, and sound

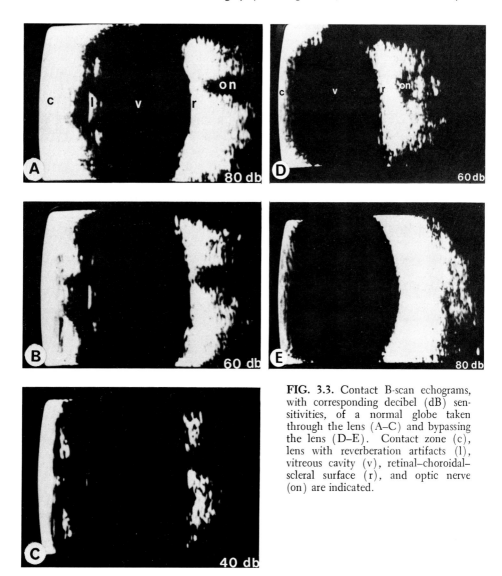

FIG. 3.3. Contact B-scan echograms, with corresponding decibel (dB) sensitivities, of a normal globe taken through the lens (A–C) and bypassing the lens (D–E). Contact zone (c), lens with reverberation artifacts (l), vitreous cavity (v), retinal–choroidal–scleral surface (r), and optic nerve (on) are indicated.

attenuation of lesions (primarily by A-scan); and (3) kinetic echography for the evaluation of the consistency and vascularity of lesions (by A-scan).

In topographic echography, the B-scan is the preferred instrument as it allows for easier demonstration of the shape and size of lesions (Fig. 3.3). Nevertheless, A-scan may be required to complete the information. The objective of topographic echography in the case of intraocular tumors is to differentiate well-circumscribed mass lesions—ie, malignant melanoma, exophytic retinoblastoma, choroidal hemangioma, metastatic carcinoma, and hemorrhagic disciform degenerations—from diffuse mass lesions—ie, vitreous hemorrhage, membranes, retinal detachment, and point-like echo sources of foreign bodies. Once a well-outlined mass lesion in suspected or proved, one performs quantitative echography.

Quantitative echography uses the tissue sensitivity setting as in the basic examination (Fig. 3.2, echo display A). At this setting tumor mass echograms present with a steeply rising, 100 percent high (overloaded) surface spike, which is followed by single "tumor mass spikes" from the inner tumor structure (Fig. 3.4). The weaker echo spikes from the inner tumor substance contrast with the surface spikes, which are always stronger. The intensity of tumor mass spikes depends on the acoustic architecture of the lesion. Tumors with "coarse grain" (ie, hemangiomas) have a high inner reflectivity; those with a "fine grain" (ie, melanomas) have a low inner reflectivity. While all four lesions in Figure 3.5 have similar surface spikes, only the mass lesions have inner spikes.[9–12]

In addition to the quantitative behavior of a mass lesion, its consistency (solid versus nonsolid) and blood supply (more versus less vascular) are of significant value in our exclusion method of differential diagnosis of tumors. Mobility and vascularity are evaluated by kinetic echography. In kinetic echography the behavior of the lesion is best evaluated during the examination by observing the display screen from which it can be videotaped. Kinetic echography I reveals spontaneous movement, as seen in blood flow. Kinetic echography II deals with aftermovement and its relationship to the consistency of the lesion. In kinetic echography I the probe and the eye to be examined are kept immobile. Any motion of single tumor spikes indicates blood flow in the tumor mass. During kinetic echography II eye movements are used to produce aftermovement. During an eye movement all echo spikes are in motion. When the motion stops, the signals from the ocular wall and from any scleral, choroidal, or retinal lesion attached to the wall stop immediately (solid lesion). Mobile lesions, in contrast, continue to move after the eye motion has stopped. This effect is a consequence of the inertia imparted to a mobile structure (nonsolid lesions). The A-scan echogram from an eye with a vitreous hemorrhage and solid tumor, ie, malignant melanoma, is shown in

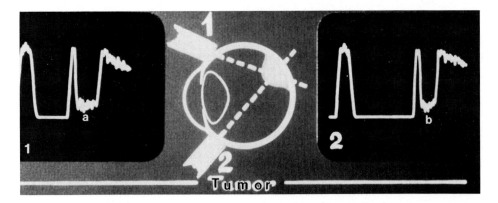

FIG. 3.4. Contact A-scan echograms of suspect tumor mass. High surface spikes are followed by wider (tracing 1a) and narrower (tracing 2b) inner spikes dependent on sound beam direction.

Figure 3.6 (top). Immediately after eye movement has been induced, the echo spikes associated with the vitreous hemorrhage are blurred due to their aftermovement. Simultaneously, the tumor mass spikes from the "melanoma" are focused, indicating no aftermovement (Fig. 3.6 middle). Thus, dual presence of a circumscribed and diffuse mass lesion is verified.

Topographic echography locates the lesion. Quantitative echography determines the reflectivity pattern of the lesion, which can be documented by photography and compared to known patterns. Kinetic echography evaluates the behavior of the lesion during the examination by observing the display screen from which it can be videotaped. A still photograph, such as Figure 3.6 (middle), is not adequate to differentiate spontaneous movement from aftermovement. The movement must be evaluated at the time of the kinetic examination.

By means of the combined findings of the special techniques described above, close to 30 different intraocular lesions can be differentiated. Any lesion can be detected, provided it is at least 50 μm in size in the vitreous cavity or 1 μsec (0.75 mm) elevated from the sclera in fundus lesions. To further differentiate fundus tumors, they must have an elevation from the sclera of at least 2 μsec (1.5 mm).

MALIGNANT MELANOMA

The single most frequent and dangerous tumor in the eye of an adult is malignant melanoma of the choroid and ciliary body.[13-15] Most malignant melanomas can be diagnosed conclusively or tentatively on the basis of their ophthalmoscopic appearance. In these cases ultrasound provides supportive evidence for the diagnosis by evaluating deeper structures unreachable by other means. We have examined with echography approximately 200 histologically proved malignant melanomas prior to enucleation. Of these cases, 86 percent were diagnosed or highly suspected by clinical examination. Under these circumstances ultrasound served as an adjunct in the final diagnosis. In 13 percent (26 cases) of the histologically proved melanomas, echography played a major role in the diagnosis. Opaque ocular media, ie, cataract or vitreous hemorrhage, hampered or prevented evaluation by optical means. In almost 3 percent of the cases evaluated, the presence of a malignant melanoma was not suspected and was only detected by echography. The preliminary diagnoses in these cases included cataract, irritable eye, vitreous hemorrhage, and acute angle closure glaucoma. These findings indicate that all eyes with opaque media should have an ultrasound examination prior to any surgery.

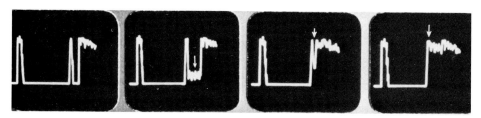

FIG. 3.5. Typical contact A-scan echogram patterns of intraocular lesions with differentiating inner spike patterns (arrows). Echograms show (from left to right): serous retinal detachment; malignant melanoma; Kuhnt-Junius lesion; hemangioma.

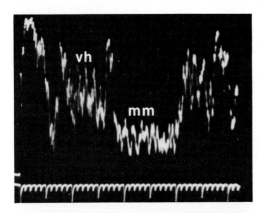

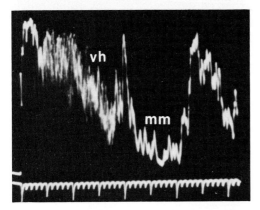

FIG. 3.6 **Top.** Contact A-scan: malignant melanoma (mm) associated with vitreous hemorrhage, (vh). **Middle.** Contact A-scan: aftermovements of vitreous hemorrhage (vh) with focused tumor spikes (mm). **Bottom.** Contact B-scan: vitreous cavity filled with blood (vh) and suspect tumor mass (mm).

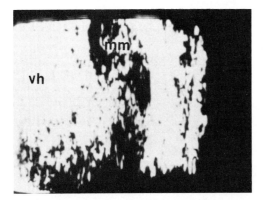

The differential acoustic criteria of malignant melanoma are listed in Table 3.2. The hallmark of malignant melanoma is the low to medium reflectivity of its inner tumor spikes at tissue sensitivity (5 to 60 percent in small and up to 80 percent in large tumors) combined with solid consistency (no aftermovement of the surface tissue spikes during kinetic echography) and regular structure (Figs. 3.6, 3.7). The B-scan (Fig. 3.8 top) shows the massive dome-shaped elevation of the

Table 3.2

Echographic Characteristics of Malignant Melanoma of the Choroid and Ciliary Body with Preferred Unit for Their Determination (A- or B-Scan)

Unit	Characteristics
A	Reflectivity: low to medium (10%–60%)
A	Mobility: solid (no aftermovements)
A	Vascularity: fast spontaneous vertical movements
BA	Sound attentuation: shadow; weaker scleral echo; choroidal excavation
AB	Location: subretinal
BA	Shape: relatively prominent
A(B)	Growth during follow-up: significant
A	Remote serous detachment of retina

pedunculated tumor with an associated marked shadowing effect evidenced by the acoustic void. The echogram in Figure 3.8 (middle) shows the high surface signals with low reflectivity of the inner tumor spikes characteristic of a melanoma. The A-scan echogram in Figure 3.8 (bottom) is taken at measuring sensitivity (T-24 dB); as a result, the low reflective inner tumor spikes have disappeared. More than 80 percent of malignant melanomas present, in addition, with definite signs of vascularity evidenced by spontaneous movement in the echogram. While none of these criteria alone establishes the diagnosis of malignant melanoma, in combination they are pathognomonic for such a lesion.

A number of other A- and B-scan criteria as listed in Table 3.2 are helpful but not necessary or specific for melanoma. If the tumor structure is irregular or the lesion is not large enough, the echographic diagnosis may be equivocal. Under these circumstances, ultrasound can detect growth during a follow-up period. Such measurement is best done with the A-scan unit. The low reflectivity of the malignant melanoma lesion is explained by its histologic appearance, devoid of large reflecting surfaces.

A subretinal hemorrhage, however, like a malignant melanoma, possesses interfaces that are small, so that the reflectivity is likewise low (Fig. 3.9). In spite of the large number of cells present in these two lesions, it is their associated small

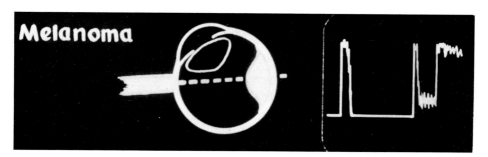

FIG. 3.7. Contact A-scan echogram of melanoma with high surface spike and low-medium reflectivity.

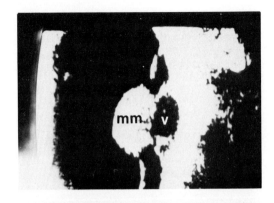

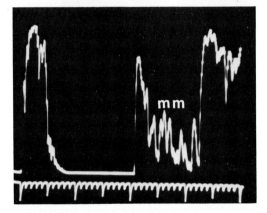

FIG. 3.8 **Top.** Contact B-scan echogram of mushroom-shaped (pedunculated) melanoma (mm) showing acoustic void (v). **Middle.** Contact A-scan at tissue sensitivity with typical pattern of inner tumor spikes (mm). **Bottom.** Contact A-scan at lowered sensitivity (approximately T-24 dB) with loss of weak inner tumor spikes.

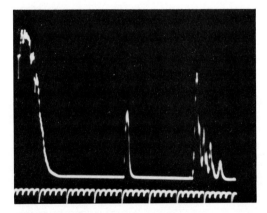

interfaces that are responsible for their low reflectivity patterns. However, during kinetic echography, a subretinal hemorrhage presents marked aftermovement not found in malignant melanoma (Fig. 3.9). Other fundus lesions that may be confused with malignant melanoma clinically, eg, choroidal hemangioma and hemorrhagic disciform lesions, are characterized by high reflectivity. A-scan echograms from choroidal hemangiomas and disciform macular degeneration document the high reflectivity found (Fig. 3.5). Choroidal hemangiomas possess the typically

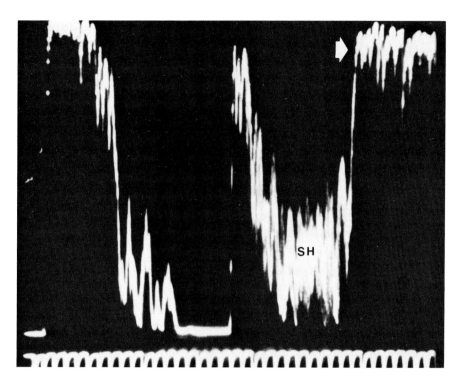

FIG. 3.9. Contact A-scan of subretinal hemorrhage with nonfocused inner tumor mass spikes (SH) and focused scleral signal (arrow) indicating aftermovement.

high spikes (100 percent) at tissue sensitivity on A-scan and elevated irregular contour on B-scan (Fig. 3.10). In the case of Kuhnt-Junius lesions, two high echo spikes are typically obtained, one from the retina and the other from the pigment epithelium (Fig. 3.11). When follow-up examinations show a decrease in the size of the mass, the diagnosis of melanoma is unlikely.

With the combined A- and B-scan techniques (with emphasis on a standardized A-scan method), malignant melanomas of the choroid and ciliary body have been diagnosed correctly in 97 percent of the 200 cases examined. The two false-negative diagnoses were caused by atypically heterogeneous lesions that produced high reflectivity and were diagnosed as metastatic tumors rather than malignant melanomas. In addition, four false-positive diagnoses of malignant melanoma have occurred. These eyes were practically blind due to extensive disciform macular degeneration and vitreous hemorrhage (two cases), organized hemorrhage in retinoschisis (one case), and panophthalmitis with destruction of the sclera (one case).

RETINOBLASTOMA[15, 16]

Bilateral retinoblastoma can be most often diagnosed by ophthalmoscopy and biomicroscopy. Unilateral retinoblastoma may cause considerable diagnostic difficulty. Table 3.3 presents the acoustic differential criteria for the echographic

Table 3.3

Echographic Characteristics of Retinoblastoma with Preferred Unit for Their Determination (A- or B-scan)

Unit	Characteristics
A	Reflectivity: high (80–100%)
AB	Sound attenuation: very strong; shadow; weak scleral signal
A	Vascularity: fast spontaneous movements (vertical, at low sensitivity)
A	Mobility: solid (at least partly; no aftermovements)
BA	Location: retina
A(B)	Growth during follow-up: significant
A	Axial length measurement

diagnosis of a retinoblastoma. The few hallmarks of retinoblastoma are an extremely high reflectivity (80 to 100 percent spike height at tissue sensitivity) and strong sound attenuation (Fig. 3.12). Kinetic echography usually plays a minor role, since aftermovements are difficult to elicit in these young patients, who require general anesthesia for evaluation. The other criteria listed in Table 3.3 help in the echographic diagnosis but are not in themselves specific. The histologic explanation for

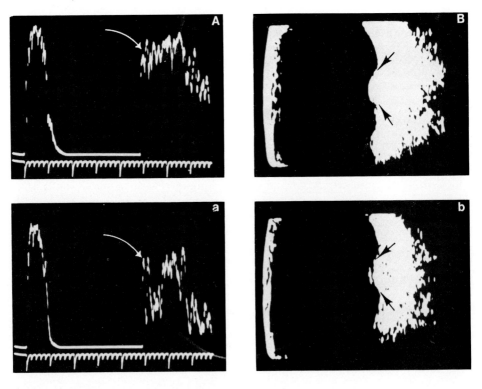

FIG. 3.10. Contact A- and B-scan of choroidal hemangioma indicating tissue sensitivity (tracings A and B) and measuring sensitivity (tracings a and b). Tumor mass is indicated by arrows.

the high reflectivity of this type of tumor is the rosette arrangement of the tumor cells, the frequently large vessels, and the necrosis that produce large interfaces between areas having great acoustic differences. Most important are the calcium deposits that behave like foreign bodies, reflecting and scattering the sound waves more strongly than any biologic tissue. Ultrasound will detect such calcifications in 80 percent of retinoblastomas even when the calcifications are not visible by conventional x-ray. If a retinoblastoma is of sufficient size and contains calcium deposits, it will produce a pattern typical of retinoblastoma on acoustic grounds. Lesions without calcium, however, are not likely to produce high enough reflectivity to be reliably diagnosed by ultrasound. The only false-negative response in our series of 18 cases was obtained from a homogenous retinoblastoma that was erroneously diagnosed as Coats' disease. In only the last 11 cases of suspected retinoblastoma were the criteria listed in Table 3.3 applied. There have been no erroneous diagnoses in any of these patients. The A- and B-scans in Figure 3.12 are of a retinoblastoma in the only eye of a child whose other eye was enucleated with a large retinoblastoma. Echograms may play a useful role in follow-up of such lesions both during and after treatment. Echography becomes even more important when

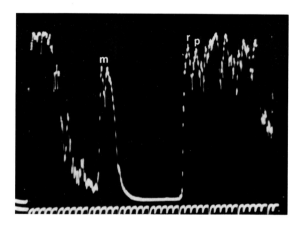

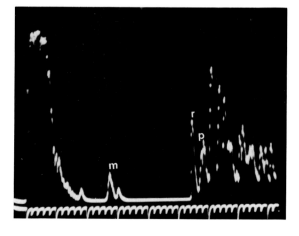

FIG. 3.11. Contact A- and B-scan echograms of Kuhnt-Junius lesion and anteriorly located membrane (m). Two high echo spikes typically occur in Kuhnt-Junius, one from the retina (r) and one from the pigment epithelium (p).

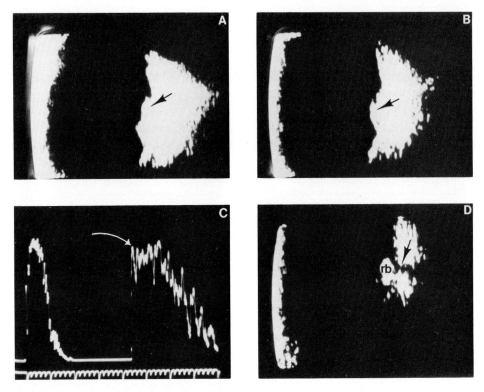

FIG. 3.12. Contact A- and B-scan of retinoblastoma. **A.** Contact B-scan: high sensitivity (80 dB) with posterior lesion (arrow). **B.** Contact B-scan: medium sensitivity (60 dB) with decrease in posterior signals and retention of tumor mass echos (arrow). **C.** Contact A-scan: tissue sensitivity with high (100 percent) lesion spike (arrow). **D.** Contact B-scan: low sensitivity (40 dB) with persistence of tumor signals (rb), shadowing effect (arrow), and general loss of posterior signals.

opaque ocular media secondary to cataract and/or vitreous hemorrhage develop following radiation treatment.

In the differential diagnosis of the more common causes of leukocoria, ie, persistent hyperplastic primary vitreous (PHPV), retrolental fibroplasia, and Coats' disease, an echographic differentiation can be made. In PHPV and retrolental fibroplasia, a membranous structure is encountered instead of the solid lesion of retinoblastoma. In Coats' disease, a subretinal mass lesion is found as an exophytic retinoblastoma, but it is of much lower reflectivity. The late stages of these and other causes of leukocoria tend to contain calcium deposits and bone spicule formation that may make it impossible to rule out retinoblastoma. This distinction is particularly difficult in the presence of phthisis bulbi. As a result, there is a tendency to overdiagnose retinoblastoma. This tendency is more than acceptable in view of the generally poor visual potential of these eyes with or without retinoblastoma and the dire consequences of its underdiagnosis. A differential diagnosis can be made in many intraocular tumors with great reliability (greater than 96 percent in malignant melanoma and greater than 81 percent in retinoblastoma) with the use of combined A- and B-scan techniques.

REFERENCES

1. Gernet H, Rüther F: Comparative experimental ultrasonic examinations of eye tissues. In Oksala A, Gernet H (eds): Ultrasonics in Ophthalmology. Basel, Karger, 1966, pp 97–102
2. Ossoinig KC: Pre-operative differential diagnosis of tumors with echography: I. Physical principles and morphological background of tissue echograms. In Blodi FC (ed): Current Concepts in Ophthalmology. St. Louis, Mosby, 1974, pp 264–80
3. Ossoinig KC: Tissue diagnosis with ultrasound in ophthalmology. In Limrer M (ed): Proceedings of Tissue Characterization with Ultrasound. Washington DC, NIH, 1975
4. Coleman DJ: An evaluation of diagnostic reliability of 100 ocular ultrasonograms (A- and B-scan). In Massin M, Poujol J (eds): Diagnostica Ultrasonica in Ophthalmologia. Paris, Centre National d'Ophtalmologie des Quinze-Une, 1973
5. Bronson NR: Contact B-scan ultrasonography. Am J Ophthalmol 77:181, 1974
6. Ossoinig KC, Till P: Clinical standardization in ophthalmology I. In Filepczynski L (ed): Ultrasonics in Biology and Medicine. Warsaw, Dun Polish Scientific Publishers, 1972, pp 173–82
7. Ossoinig KC: Pre-operative differential diagnosis of tumors with echography: II. Instrumentation and examination techniques. In Blodi FC (ed): Current Concepts in Ophthalmology, vol 4. St. Louis, Mosby, 1974, pp 280–96
8. Ossoinig KC: Clinical echo-ophthalmography. In Blodi FC (ed): Current Concepts in Ophthalmology, vol 3. St. Louis, Mosby, 1972, pp 101–36
9. Ossoinig KC: Quantitative echography: the basis of tissue differentiation. J Clin Ultrasound 2:33, 1974
10. Ossoinig KC: Quantitative echography: an important aid for tissue differentiation. In Proceedings of the Second World Congress on Ultrasound Diagnostics in Medicine, Rotterdam, Netherlands, 1973. Amsterdam, Excerpta Medica
11. Coleman DJ: Reliability of ocular tumor diagnosis with ultrasound. Trans Am Acad Ophthalmol Otolaryngol 77:OP677, 1973
12. Coleman DJ: Ocular tumor patterns. In Francois J, Goes F (eds): Ultrasonography in Ophthalmology. Basel, Karger, 1975, pp 136–40
13. Coleman DJ, Abramson DH, Jack RL, et al: Ultrasonic diagnosis of tumors of the choroid. Arch Ophthalmol 91:344, 1974
14. Coleman DJ, Abramson DH: Correlation of ultrasonic characteristics and tissue morphology of malignant melanoma. In Massin M, Poujol J (eds): Diagnostica Ultrasonica in Ophthalmologia. Paris, Centre National d'Ophtalmologie des Quinze-Une, 1973, pp 215–18
15. Ossoinig KC, Blodi FC: Pre-operative differential diagnosis of tumors with echography: III. Diagnosis of intraocular tumors. In Blodi FC (ed): Current Concepts in Ophthalmology, vol 4. St. Louis, Mosby, 1974, pp 296–313
16. Gitter KA, Meyer D, White RH: Ultrasonic aid in the evaluation of leukocoria. Am J Ophthalmol 65:190, 1969

Jerry A. Shields

4 The Radioactive Phosphorus Uptake Test in the Diagnosis of Uveal Melanomas

The difficulties in the clinical diagnosis of uveal melanomas are well known to ophthalmologists.[1,2] A recent report indicated that these difficulties may be greatly alleviated by the utilization of certain diagnostic modalities now available.[3] Perhaps the most widely acclaimed diagnostic tool is the ^{32}P uptake test. This procedure was introduced into ophthalmic use several years ago,[4] and the principles, technique, and results have been fully described.[4-10] It involves the injection of ^{32}P, which is incorporated into malignant tumor cells and emits beta radiation that can be quantitated with a Geiger counter. Although this procedure was once widely used, it fell into disfavor for several years because of difficulty in evaluating small tumors in the posterior segment of the eye. A recent report, however, stressed the importance of localization of the lesion with indirect ophthalmoscopy, a conjunctival incision, and an improved probe for counting lesions located in the posterior segment of the globe.[5] Since that time, several articles have stressed the great reliability of this test when carefully performed.[6-13]

When the lesion is located in the anterior segment of the globe, it is not necessary to make an incision to perform the test. If the lesion is located in the posterior segment, however, a surgical approach must be utilized.[8] Although we now have performed more than 400 tests, this report will discuss the accuracy of the ^{32}P test as determined from our initial 300 consecutive tests, which have at least a one-year follow-up as of February 1976. We will first consider the nonsurgical, or transconjunctival, approach and then discuss the surgical, or transscleral, technique.

MATERIALS AND METHODS

A total of 300 ^{32}P tests were performed by the Oncology Unit, Retina Service, Wills Eye Hospital, over a four-year period extending from February 1971 to February 1975. Most tests were performed by or under the supervision of a single investigator (J.A.S.), and all were performed with strict adherence to techniques described in the literature.[5,8] In most instances, both the Geiger-Müller counter and the solid-state semiconductor detector unit were used to perform the procedure

(Fig. 4.1). All transconjunctival (nonsurgical) tests were first analyzed to determine the diagnostic accuracy of the procedure for tumors located in the anterior segment of the globe. A positive test was interpreted as one showing an uptake of greater than 30 percent over the control area at 1 hour after injection, with an increasing uptake during the next 48 hours. The control area was usually the symmetric quadrant of the opposite eye, although the opposite quadrant of the same eye is also a suitable control.

All tests performed by the transscleral (surgical) route were then analyzed in a similar manner to determine the accuracy of the procedure for tumors located in the posterior segment of the globe. A test was considered positive when the uptake was greater than 50 percent over the control area at 48 hours after injection.

The cases were analyzed with regard to accuracy of this test in differentiating benign from malignant lesions. Those cases showing false-negative or false-positive results were selected for closer scrutiny in order to gain insight into reasons for false results.

RESULTS

The data regarding these 300 ^{32}P tests are compiled in Table 4.1. In four cases, the test was performed twice on one lesion several months apart; in five cases, the test was later repeated after a lesion had been treated locally. The 300 tests, therefore, were performed on a total of 291 patients, but this discrepancy does not significantly change any of the statistics.

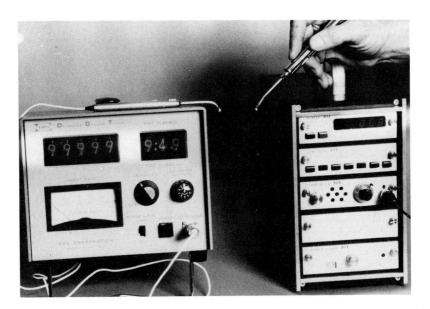

FIG. 4.1. Instruments utilized in performing ^{32}P test. Left: The Detector Ocular Tumor unit (EON Corp.). Right: The solid-state semiconductor detector (Nuclear Associates; Technical Associates). The probes utilized are illustrated above the instruments.

Table 4.1

General Statistics on 300 Consecutive ^{32}P *Tests for Suspected Ocular Tumors*

Tests	No.
Transconjunctival (nonsurgical) route	106
Positive (57)	
Negative (49)	
Transscleral (surgical) route	186
Positive (127)	
Negative (59)	
Both transconjunctival and transscleral route	8
Positive both routes (6)	
Negative both routes (1)	
Positive transconjunctival and	
negative transscleral (1)	
Total	300

Transconjunctival Route

As shown in Table 4.1, 106 procedures were done by the transconjunctival technique and 8 were performed by both the transconjunctival and transscleral routes. A total of 114 procedures, therefore, were performed by the transconjunctival method.

A further breakdown of these 114 cases is presented in Table 4.2. There were 64 positive tests and 50 negative tests. Of the 64 positive tests, 60 were histologically confirmed. These 60 cases all proved to be malignant melanomas, and there were no histologically confirmed false-positive tests. Of the 4 cases that were not confirmed, 3 were clearcut cases of metastatic malignant tumors, which were treated by irradiation and chemotherapy. The only test with positive results for a case that was actually nonmalignant occurred in a patient who had a presumed spontaneous choroidal hemorrhage at the time of cataract surgery, which simulated a malignant melanoma. The transconjunctival test was positive four days after cataract surgery. The test was negative, however, when repeated by the transscleral route six weeks after surgery.

There were 50 negative tests by the transconjunctival technique. Four of these were histologically confirmed as malignant melanomas of the anterior segment and must be classified as false-negative tests. Four other cases were diagnosed clinically as probable iris melanomas, but are being followed conservatively for one reason or another. These should be classified as *possible* false-negative tests. Another false-negative result occurred in the case of a metastatic tumor located in the equatorial region where the probe could not be accurately placed. The diagnoses for the remainder of the negative tests are shown in Table 4.2. Thorough clinical studies and follow-up of from one to four years has clearly shown that these lesions are not malignant. We found no apparent difference between the Geiger-Müller instrument and the solid-state instrument (Fig. 4.1).

For the 114 cases of transconjunctival ^{32}P tests, therefore, there was only 1

Table 4.2

*Distribution and Diagnoses for ^{32}P Tests Performed
by the Transconjunctival Route*

Tests	No.
Positive	64
Histologically confirmed (60)	
Iris and/or ciliary body malignant melanoma (56)	
Metastatic tumor (3)	
Conjunctival malignant melanoma (1)	
Not histologically confirmed (4)	
Metastatic tumors (3)	
Choroidal hemorrhage (1)	
Negative	50
Histologically confirmed (4)	
Iris malignant melanoma (3)	
Ciliary body malignant melanoma (1)	
Not histologically confirmed (46)	
Iris nevus (19)	
Iris malignant melanoma (4)	
Iris or ciliary body cyst (4)	
Vitreous hemorrhage (5)	
Choroidal effusion (2)	
Choroidal hemorrhage (2)	
Heterochromia (2)	
Ectopic disciform degeneration (2)	
Choroidal melanoma (1)	
Hypertrophy, retinal pigment epithelium (1)	
Serous retinal detachment (1)	
Metastatic tumor (1)	
Absolute glaucoma (1)	
Granuloma (1)	
Total	114

possible false-positive test, for an incidence of less than 1 percent; the number of false-negative tests was between 4 and 10, for an incidence between 3.5 and 9 percent. The reasons for false results will be considered shortly.

Transscleral Route

Of the 300 ^{32}P tests in this series, 186 were performed by the transscleral route alone and 8 were performed by both the transconjunctival and transscleral routes, making a total of 194 tests performed by the transscleral technique (Table 4.1). There were 132 positive tests and 62 negative tests (Table 4.3).

Of the 132 positive tests, 107 were histologically confirmed, including 105 cases of malignant melanoma and 2 cases of metastatic tumor. The diagnoses for the 25 positive tests that were not histologically confirmed are listed in Table 4.3. Of these 25 cases, there were 20 small melanomas that were diagnosed by clinical appearance, visual fields, fluorescein angiography, and ultrasonography, in addition to the positive ^{32}P test, leaving no doubt, in our opinion, as to their true diagnosis.

Table 4.3

Distribution and Diagnosis for ^{32}P Tests Performed by the Transscleral Route

Tests	No.
Positive	132
Histologically confirmed (107)	
Malignant melanoma (105)	
Metastatic tumor (2)	
Not histologically confirmed (25)	
Malignant melanoma (20)	
Photocoagulated (8)	
Being followed (6)	
Refused surgery (3)	
Lost to follow-up (2)	
Irradiated (1)	
Metastatic tumor (5)	
Negative	62
Histologically confirmed (5)	
Malignant melanoma (4)	
Choroidal hemangioma (1)	
Not histologically confirmed (57)	
Choroidal nevus (possible small malignant melanoma) (18)	
Choroidal hemangioma (13)	
Malignant melanoma previously treated by photocoagulation (5)	
Serous retinal detachment (4)	
Disciform maculopathy (4)	
Retinal/choroidal hemorrhage (4)	
Chorioretinitis (3)	
Vitreous hemorrhage (3)	
Astrocytoma (2)	
Retinal vein occlusion (1)	
Total	194

Eight were treated with photocoagulation, one with cobalt plaque radiation, and the others were not treated for one reason or another. Five cases were well-documented metastatic tumors, which were treated with external radiation and/or chemotherapy at other institutions. There were no documented false-positive tests.

There were 62 negative tests by the transscleral route, 5 of which were histologically confirmed. Four were malignant melanomas and, therefore, represented false-negative tests. One case was a choroidal hemangioma that was subsequently enucleated despite a negative ^{32}P test. This case has been reported elsewhere.[9]

There were 57 negative cases that were not histologically confirmed. The diagnoses are listed in Table 4.3. Of these 57, 18 were suspicious choroidal nevi which have so far shown no growth during a one- to four-year follow-up period. Thirteen were well-documented cases of choroidal hemangiomas which were referred for the ^{32}P test to rule out an amelanotic melanoma.

Five tests were performed on choroidal melanoma cases in which the tumor had been treated several times with xenon photocoagulation. In every instance, the test converted from positive to negative following presumed eradication of the tumor. These cases are the subject of a separate report.[14] The remaining negative tests included a variety of lesions clinically diagnosed as benign and documented on follow-up studies. For the most part, the readings of the two instruments were consistent, and we found no significant advantage of one unit over the other.

Of the 194 cases on which the transscleral ^{32}P test was performed, there were no documented false-positive tests and only 4 documented false-negative tests. The incidence of false-negative tests, therefore, is about 2 percent.

DISCUSSION

Following the introduction of the ^{32}P test,[4] most of the early investigators utilized primarily the transconjunctival approach for all suspicious lesions regardless of their location in the globe.[15, 16] False-negative results were frequent because the probe could not be placed near enough to the base of the lesion to be evaluated. Our experience has shown that the transconjunctival approach can be reliable only in those cases where the lesion is *anterior* in the globe, involving the

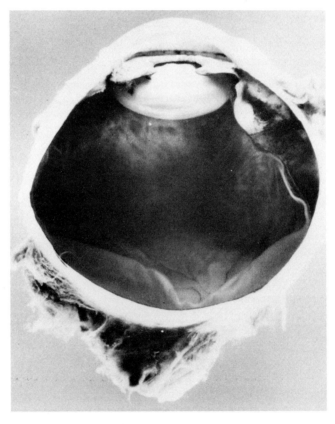

FIG. 4.2. Malignant melanoma arising from ciliary body and extending to iris and choroid. This lesion gave a strongly positive ^{32}P test by the transconjunctival approach.

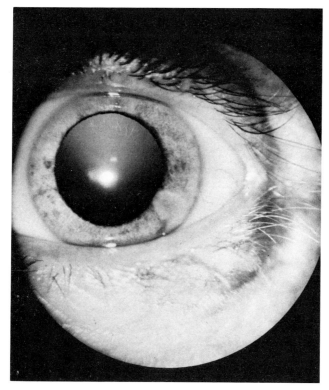

FIG. 4.3. Small, relatively flat iris melanoma that gave a false-negative ^{32}P test.

iris and/or ciliary body (Fig. 4.2). In small, relatively flat iris melanomas, however, false-negative results may occur (Fig. 4.3). In addition, some small peripheral choroidal melanomas may give a false-negative result with the transconjunctival technique. The conjunctiva must be incised in such instances to obtain accurate readings.

Radioactive phosphorus emits beta particles, which travel only an average of 4 mm through tissue; it is feasible that intervening cornea, aqueous, ciliary body, or angle structures might decrease the number of particles reaching the window of the probe. This interference may explain why the ^{32}P test is somewhat less reliable for small iris tumors and why negative results were obtained in four histologically confirmed iris melanomas in this series.

This study tends to support the important role of the transscleral ^{32}P test for *posterior* uveal melanomas. In 194 tests performed by this technique, there were no false-positive results and only four false-negatives. In our experience, most choroidal melanomas greater than 1.5 mm in elevation and 3 mm in diameter will result in a positive test when the procedure is carefully performed[8] (Figs. 4.4, 4.5). The false-negative tests can be explained on the basis of the size and location of the tumor. Two of the false-negative tests were due to small lesions that grew

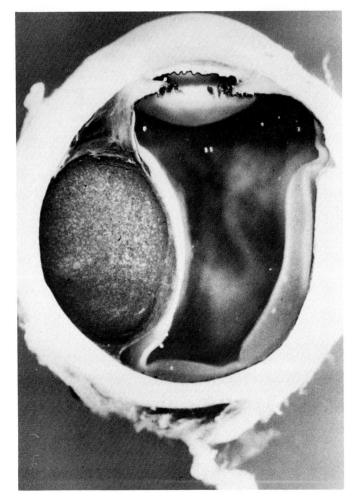

FIG. 4.4. Large equatorial melanoma. This lesion gave a strongly positive result (500 percent) when transscleral ^{32}P test was performed.

around the termination of Bruch's membrane to protrude anteriorly over the optic nervehead. Since the optic nerve is about 3 mm in diameter posterior to the globe and only 1.5 mm in diameter at the optic disk, it becomes technically difficult in such cases to place the window of the probe over the base of the tumor (Fig. 4.6).

In two cases, the false-negative tests were due to small spindle cell melanomas in the posterior choroid. These, however, were borderline false-negative tests. In a large series such as this, it is not surprising that an occasional borderline case is encountered. We must acknowledge that some of the suspicious pigmented lesions that gave a negative test may have been early malignant melanomas of the choroid. This occurrence may not be a matter of great clinical significance, however, since small choroidal melanomas are usually slow growing and offer a relatively good

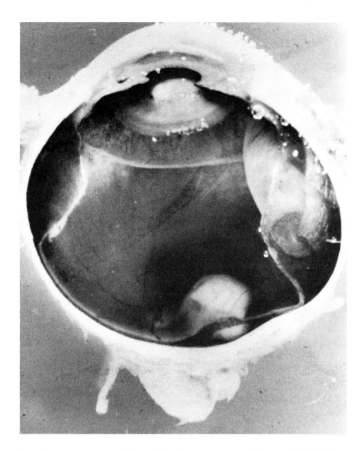

FIG. 4.5. Small melanoma in posterior pole that gave a positive result (200 percent) when transscleral 32P test was performed.

prognosis.[2] In such cases, a period of observation for signs of growth may be an acceptable approach.

Most of the lesions producing negative results were clearcut cases of benign lesions which are known occasionally to simulate melanomas.[1,2] Follow-up studies of from one to four years have thus far substantiated the benign nature of these lesions.

CONCLUSION

Of the 300 consecutive 32P tests performed by the Oncology Unit, Retina Service, Wills Eye Hospital, over a four-year period, 106 were done by the transconjunctival route, 186 by the transscleral route, and 8 by both routes. With the transconjunctival (nonsurgical) technique, the incidence of documented false-positive results was less than 1 percent and the incidence of documented false-negative results was 3.5 percent. With the transscleral (surgical) technique, there were no

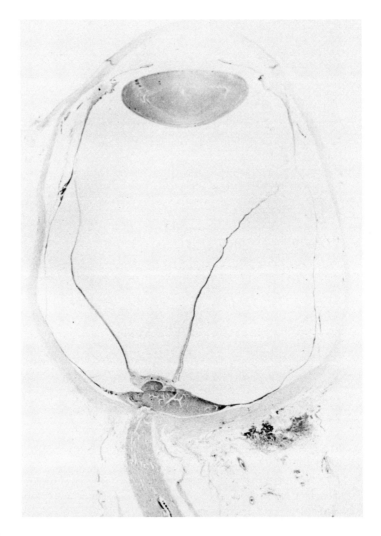

FIG. 4.6. Small choroidal melanoma protruding anteriorly over optic nervehead. It resulted in a false-negative ^{32}P test due to difficulty in placing probe over base of lesion.

false-positive results and an incidence of 2 percent false-negative results. It is concluded that the ^{32}P test, when properly performed, is probably the most accurate ancillary test now available for differentiating benign from malignant intraocular lesions.

REFERENCES

1. Ferry AP: Lesions mistaken for malignant melanomas of the posterior uvea. Arch Ophthalmol 72:463, 1964
2. Shields JA, Zimmerman LE: Lesions simulating malignant melanomas of the posterior uvea. Arch Ophthalmol 89:466, 1973

3. Shields JA, McDonald PR: Improvements in the diagnosis of posterior uveal melanomas. Arch Ophthalmol 91:259, 1974
4. Thomas CI, Krohmer JS, Storaasli JP: Detection of intraocular tumors with radioactive phosphorus: a preliminary report with special reference to differentiation of the cause of retinal separation. Arch Ophthalmol 49:276, 1952
5. Hagler WS, Jarrett WH II, Humphrey WT: The radioactive phosphorus uptake test in the diagnosis of uveal melanomas. Arch Ophthalmol 83:548, 1970
6. Hagler WS, Jarrett WH II, Schnauss RH, et al: The diagnosis of malignant melanoma of the ciliary body or choroid: use of the radioactive phosphorus uptake test. South Med J 65:49, 1972
7. Ruiz RS: New radioactivity detection probe and scaler for phosphorus-32 testing of ocular lesions. Trans Am Acad Ophthalmol Otolaryngol 76:535, 1972
8. Shields JA, Sarin LK, Federman JL, Mensheha-Manhart O, Carmichael PL: Surgical approach to the ^{32}P test for posterior uveal melanomas. Ophthalmic Surg 5:13, 1974
9. Shields JA, Hagler WS, Federman JL, Jarrett WH II, Carmichael PL: The significance of the ^{32}P uptake test in the diagnosis of posterior uveal melanomas. Trans Am Acad Ophthalmol Otolaryngol 79:297, 1975.
10. Shields JA, Carmichael PL, Leonard BC, Federman JL, Sarin LK: The radioactive phosphorus uptake test in the diagnosis of ocular tumors. In Croll M, Brady LW, Carmichael PL, Wallner RJ (eds): Nuclear Ophthalmology. New York, Wiley, 1976, pp 79–88
11. Shields JA, Annesley WH Jr, Totino JA: Nonfluorescent malignant melanoma of the choroid diagnosed with the ^{32}P test. Am J Ophthalmol 79:634, 1975
12. Shields JA, Leonard BC, Sarin LK: Multinodular uveal melanoma masquerading as a postoperative choroidal detachment. Br J Ophthalmol, 60:386, 1976
13. Shields JA, McDonald PR, Leonard BC, Canny CLB: The diagnosis of uveal melanomas in eyes with opaque media. Am J Ophthalmol 82:95, 1977
14. Shields JA, Annesley WH Jr, Sarin LK, Federman JL: Fluorescein and ^{32}P studies in photocoagulated choroidal melanomas. In L'Esperance FA (ed): Current Diagnosis and Management of Chorioretinal Disease. St. Louis, Mosby, in press
15. Carmichael PL, Leopold IH: Radioactive phosphorus test in ophthalmology. Am J Ophthalmol 49:484, 1960
16. Leopold IH, Keates EU, Charkes ID: Role of isotopes in diagnosis of intraocular neoplasm. Trans Am Ophthalmol Soc 42:86, 1964

Lorenz E. Zimmerman
Ian W. McLean

5 Changing Concepts in the Prognosis and Management of Small Malignant Melanomas of the Choroid

During the past several decades much has been learned about malignant melanomas of the uvea, although we still have large informational gaps and our knowledge of the natural history of untreated tumors is negligible. It was once generally assumed that all malignant melanomas of the uvea carry a very poor prognosis and that every effort should be made to enucleate the tumor-containing eye as soon as the diagnosis is strongly suspected. These assumptions were based on the further assumptions that the behavior of uveal melanomas* is comparable to that of cutaneous melanomas, that all these tumors tend to invade blood vessels and to become disseminated hematogenously, and that the ophthalmologist must detect the tumor and remove the eye before such vascular invasion can take place if the patient's life is to be saved.

The following are some of the most important lessons we believe have been learned from many clinicopathologic studies that have been made during recent years—lessons that have significantly altered some of the older views concerning management of uveal melanomas:

1. Uveal melanomas are not identical to cutaneous melanomas. They exhibit greater cytologic variations that can be correlated with prognosis.[1] Pure spindle cell melanomas, which carry a more favorable prognosis, are relatively common among uveal tumors, but are unusual among cutaneous melanomas. In general the mortality is considerably lower from uveal than from cutaneous melanomas.

2. While death from uveal melanomas is almost always the result of hematogenous dissemination, it has become increasingly clear that factors other than vascular invasion are important in determining outcome.[2-8] Patients may remain in excellent health and appear to have been cured only to be found to have metastatic disease 20 to 30 years or more after enucleation. Such cases, which are not

Based on the Mary Louisa Prentice Montgomery Lecture delivered by Dr. Zimmerman at the 1975 meeting of the Irish Ophthalmological Society at Trinity College, Dublin, October 2, 1975. This study was supported in part by training grant EY-00032 from the National Eye Institute, National Institutes of Health.
* In this paper "melanoma" exclusively means malignant melanoma and "nevus" signifies a benign melanocytic tumor.

rare, support the newer concepts that hematogenous spread often occurs early, before the tumor is discovered, and that the body's defense mechanisms are usually effective in either completely eliminating the neoplastic cells that have spread away from the eye or at least keeping them dormant for very long periods.[3, 5, 9-12]

3. Melanomas of the anterior uvea are significantly different from those of the posterior uvea; because of these differences, which include a much more favorable prognosis, they can often be successfully resected by iridectomy or iridocyclectomy with preservation of an eye retaining useful vision.[13-17]

4. Among melanomas of the posterior uvea, there is a striking variation in prognosis between small and large tumors, large tumors carrying a worse prognosis than small tumors.[18-22] Small choroidal melanomas are more likely to be relatively pure spindle cell tumors, whereas large melanomas typically contain a significant component of epithelioid cells.

5. The ophthalmologist's ability to clearly recognize melanomas and to differentiate them accurately from other lesions that should not be treated by enucleation has not been nearly as good as one would have assumed. The error rate, even with clear media permitting direct visualization of the lesions, has been approximately 20 percent.[23-25]

Large intraocular melanomas present the ophthalmologist with a few very difficult decisions concerning management. The affected eye typically has poor vision, attributable to such complications as retinal detachment, opacification of the ocular media, inflammation, and/or secondary glaucoma. Furthermore, these eyes are often painful. It is an easy decision in such cases for the ophthalmologist to recommend enucleation, and it is also comparatively easy for the patient to accept this recommendation.

With small melanomas, the situation is often very different. The tumor may have been discovered incidentally in the course of a routine examination, and the eye typically retains useful vision. Even when the tumor is situated near the macula and visual acuity has been reduced, the remainder of the retina may be unaffected; in addition, there is always the troublesome realization that the lesion observed may be a choroidal nevus or hemangioma, a subretinal hemorrhage, a benign proliferation or detachment of the retinal pigment epithelium, a metastatic carcinoma, or some other process simulating malignant melanoma.

During the past decade increasing efforts have been made to improve differential diagnosis. Binocular indirect ophthalmoscopy, biomicroscopy of the retina, fluorescein angiography, studies of the uptake of radioactive phosphorus, and ultrasonography have made it possible in certain institutions to reduce the error rate to less than 8 percent.[26-29] The clinician is now able to make the correct diagnosis in all but a very few unusual cases. The great remaining problem is what should be done with an eye that is discovered to have a small melanoma of the posterior uvea.

PROGNOSTIC STUDIES

Before discussing the management of small melanomas of the posterior uvea, let us first consider both past and recent studies of their prognosis. Over 20 years ago Flocks et al studied 210 melanomas of the posterior uvea; the three dimensions of the tumors had been measured in each case.[19] They arbitrarily assumed that having information about three dimensions would give the best estimate of size and the best correlation with prognosis. To reduce the number of variables, they eliminated cases in which there was extraocular extension of the tumor. They arranged the 210 tumors into 10 groups of 21 each according to estimates of their respective volumes, and then collected the follow-up data for each group of 21 cases. Only cases with at least five years of postoperative follow-up data were included. In that initial study it was shown that patients with small melanomas had a far better survival rate than patients with large melanomas when the 105 largest tumors were compared with the 105 smallest. Strangely, however, among the individual groups of 21 cases they could not make a direct correlation of size and prognosis for the 105 smallest tumors. Large tumors were found to have a significant component of epithelioid cells, while small tumors were generally pure spindle cell melanomas. When the five groups representing the 105 smallest tumors were analyzed individually, there seemed to be no significant correlation between size and prognosis. This finding has always been a bothersome mystery. Recently, therefore, we have undertaken a much more ambitious study of small melanomas of the posterior uvea.[30]

The criteria for selection of cases for this new study were similar in that only cases in which the tumors had been measured (three dimensions) in the laboratory were included; however, cases in which there was extraocular extension of the tumor were also included. Cases were accepted only if there had been at least six years of follow-up after enucleation. For this study, we also had the services of Dr. W. Foster, a professional biostatistician, and the availability of computer technology. Consequently, it was possible to evaluate multiple variables individually and in various combinations to determine which would give the best possible separation of fatal and nonfatal cases. For each of the 217 small tumors in the study complete information about 14 variables was available, and almost complete information about duration of symptoms before enucleation. Thorough analysis of the data appears elsewhere,[30] but the following points are relevant to the present discussion:

1. In contrast with the earlier study by Flocks et al,[19] and more recent but much more limited studies by others,[18, 22] the new study demonstrated very convincingly that seven factors are closely correlated to outcome within the group of small tumors: cell type (by far the most significant), pigmentation, size, mitotic activity, transscleral extension, optic nerve invasion, and the position of the anterior border of the tumor (the more anterior, the worse the prognosis). In this study size was evaluated in four ways: the single largest diameter of the tumor, the two diameters representing area of scleral contact, the three diameters reflecting volume, and the elevation or height of the tumor. (In the earlier study by Flocks et al[19] only the volume was evaluated.) Contrary to what we had assumed in our earlier study, size, when determined by volume, did not correlate with outcome nearly as well as when determined by the single largest dimension. The main reason for this finding appears to be the fact that small diffuse tumors, which are known to carry a worse prognosis than spheroidal or mushroom-shaped tumors,[31] typically have large linear dimensions but very small volumes. The more complete measurements, the inclusion of small tumors showing extraocular extension, and the larger number of cases in the more recent study are, we believe, the main reasons that we

now find it possible to prognosticate within the groups of small tumors so much better than was possible in the earlier study.

2. Modern, sophisticated methods of statistical analysis have become available through computer technology. Through multivariant discriminant analysis four factors that we routinely evaluate in descriptive pathology (largest diameter of tumor, cell type, mitotic activity, and transscleral extension) provide a mathematical expression of the chances for a fatal outcome. For example, the five hypothetical tumors shown in Table 5.1 provide a range from highly favorable to very poor

Table 5.1

Use of Linear Discriminant Function in Relating Values for Four Most Significant Factors in Predicting Outcome

Case	Prognostic factors				Probability of fatal outcome (%)
	Size (mm)	Cell type	Mitotic activity /40 hpf *	Scleral extension	
1	10	Sp A	1	No	1.6
2	10	Sp B	1	No	9
3	10	Mixed	1	No	39
4	15	Mixed	10	No	71
5	15	Mixed	10	Yes	81

* High power field indicated by hpf.

prognoses, yet all are tumors that would have been judged "small" by the criteria used in the older study.*

3. While the results of this study provide an impressive demonstration of our ability to prognosticate after enucleation, there are some striking exceptions. At one extreme, there were cases in which our estimation of the tumor indicated a highly favorable prognosis, yet the patient died. At the opposite extreme, there were tumors whose characteristics indicated a very poor prognosis, yet the patient was still alive and well. In this connection, it should be realized that each of the seven factors that showed a very high degree of correlation with outcome were characteristics of the tumor. We have not yet found any satisfactory way of evaluating the patient's innate ability to cope with his tumor.

Spontaneous necrosis of melanomas is frequently associated with ocular inflammation,[4] while necrosis produced by photocoagulation is not.[6,7] These facts suggest the possibility that in the former situation necrosis and/or the inflammatory reaction might be causally related to an immunopathologic process. Rahi,[12] who assumed that coagulative necrosis of a tumor might reflect a favorable immunopathologic event, reported increased survival among patients whose tumors had

---

* Our use of the designation "small" has been much less restrictive than its current use in clinical ophthalmology. Warren[22] and Shields[32] consider only tumors measuring less than 10 mm in diameter and 2 mm in elevation to be small. Larger tumors up to 15 mm in diameter and up to 5 mm in elevation they call medium size, and all tumors exceeding these dimensions they consider large. Our group of small melanomas would include all medium-size tumors as defined by Warren and Shields, and even some of their large tumors.

areas of coagulative necrosis. Other workers, however, have found that marked necrosis is associated with increased mortality.[1, 4] Due to the inherent technical difficulties in qualitative and quantitative evaluation of necrosis and inflammatory response, we have not evaluated these potentially significant factors in our studies.

It is possible that psychopersonality studies, such as those used by LeShan,[33] might be useful in predicting which individuals are most likely to succumb to their cancer.[34] It is also possible that the common denominator in such subjects and in those with other forms of chronic stress might be a breakdown in the immunologic defense mechanisms against the neoplastic cells.[33–36] While LeShan suggested that the psychopersonality type he found so dominant among patients with fatal cancer might be indicative of either a special tendency to develop a neoplasm or a weakening of resistance to spread of tumors, current concepts suggest that depression of immunologic surveillance may increase both the development and the spread of cancer cells.

The exceptions noted above may represent extreme variations in the patient's immunologic defense against these tumors. Perhaps the patient who dies of metastatic disease despite the fact that he had a small spindle cell melanoma with little mitotic activity is an individual with an exceptionally poor defense against his tumor, while the patient who survives despite a much larger tumor containing epithelioid cells exhibiting more mitotic activity is an individual with a remarkably effective defense against his tumor and its occult metastases. Melanoma-associated antigens have been demonstrated in uveal melanomas, and there is evidence of both cutaneous delayed hypersensitivity reactions and cell-mediated immunity to these antigens in patients with choroidal melanomas[37–39]; but correlations between these reactions in vitro and in vivo with prognosis have not been established. (See Chapters 7 through 10 for further discussion of the role of immune mechanisms in malignant melanoma.)

MANAGEMENT

Now, with regard to management, how do these considerations affect our judgment and recommendations? First, let us emphasize again that almost all we have learned about the long-term prognosis of tumors of the posterior uvea has been based on studies of patients who have been treated by enucleation. We cannot extrapolate the data derived from such cases to untreated patients or to others treated by different methods. There is no way to predict whether results of other methods of treatment would be as good as, worse than, or better than results obtained by enucleation. The hope, of course, is that by avoiding enucleation one might at least achieve as good results and salvage an eye with some useful vision.

Is it logical to believe that any therapeutic method more conservative than enucleation might be equally or more successful in controlling a choroidal melanoma? Traditional views would lead one to answer in the negative, but some current thinking makes one wonder.

Recently, the possibility has been considered that enucleation and other procedures involving manipulation of and pressure on the globe (such as forceful scleral depression during examination, transillumination, and ^{32}P studies) might be sufficiently traumatic to actually increase intravasation and hasten the spread of tumor cells.[3, 40–42] In general surgery, it has long been appreciated that rough handling of cancerous tissues at the time of surgery may be accompanied by showers of tumor cells in the circulation.[43–46] Fraunfelder and Boozman[41] were so concerned about the possibility that the marked alterations in intraocular pressure occurring during enucleation of the eye might cause a similar release of neoplastic cells into the circulation that they developed an experimental model to test their thesis. Using a transplantable malignant melanoma, they injected tumor cells into the choroid of hamsters. The tumor-containing eyes of one group were enucleated by a procedure similar to the standard enucleation in human subjects, while those of another group were avulsed (a method feasible in the rodent), which is quicker and accompanied by less massaging of the eye than a standard enucleation. Following removal of the tumor-containing eyes, metastasis appeared earlier and deaths were more numerous in the group treated by standard enucleation. Others concerned about this problem have advocated freezing of the eye before proceeding with enucleation.

There is, therefore, some reason for believing that such nonsurgical methods of treatment as photocoagulation and radiation therapy might have the advantage of producing less mechanical trauma to the eye during treatment. It has also been postulated that allowing some devitalized but still antigenic tumor tissue to remain for a while during and after treatment might have a beneficial immunologic effect on any tumor cells that may have already escaped into the circulation.

With these factual and theoretical conditions in mind, let us review some of the alternatives to enucleation.

Surgical Resection

It was only logical that following the notable success that surgeons have had (first with iridectomy and more recently with iridocyclectomy and corneoscleroiridocyclectomy) in controlling melanomas of the anterior uvea (see reviews by Vail[16] and by Zimmerman[17]) they would turn their attention to surgical resection of small melanomas of the choroid. The surgical goals seem to have been achieved by several surgeons who are now following up patients who retain useful vision in a cosmetically fine eye a year or more postoperatively.[32, 47–50]

It will, of course, be a long time before the long-term results of surgical resection of choroidal melanomas can be evaluated. In the meantime, we have some reservations based on the following considerations. First, one cannot equate melanomas of the anterior and posterior uvea. Tumors that have been successfully resected from the iris or anterior ciliary body are typically very different from choroidal melanomas[17]: they are much smaller, usually of pure spindle A cell type, seldom exhibit mitotic activity, and rarely metastasize. Even the smallest of choroidal melanomas tends to be large when compared with iridic tumors, and they are much more likely to contain spindle B or epithelioid cells exhibiting mitotic activity. In our recent study, for example, we found that one-third of our smallest tumors, which measured less than 10 mm in diameter, had a significant component of epithelioid cells. The mortality in these cases was almost 50 percent, whereas the smallest spindle cell tumors showed only a 7 percent mortality. Second, the surgical procedures involved are undoubtedly more traumatic. Often a surgical procedure is necessary to obtain a valid ^{32}P test. Then one or more sessions of photocoagulation about the tumor are required. Subsequently, diathermy and/or cryosurgery over the scleral surface of the tumor is used in an attempt to obliterate all blood supply to the tumor. Several weeks later the tumor is resected. It seems very probable that during these manipulations a tumor containing epithelioid cells would be likely to have cells massaged or otherwise released into the circulation. (See Chapter 13 for a further discussion of sclerochorioretinal resection in the treatment of malignant melanoma.)

Photocoagulation

This procedure has great appeal because it would seem to be the least likely to traumatize the eye mechanically during treatment. The early experience gained with this method showed that it is generally unsuitable for melanomas that are elevated more than 2 mm.[51-53] If the tumor is too thick, only the more superficial layers will be photocoagulated and viable neoplastic cells may remain in the deeper portions. Of course, tumor cells that may have invaded the sclera or penetrated through into the episcleral tissues will also not be affected by this form of therapy. The workers with the greatest experience in this technique have had most success in treating tumors that are not more than 9 to 10 mm in greatest diameter and not more than 2 mm in thickness.[6, 7, 27, 32, 54-56] We know from our own experience that it is exceedingly rare to encounter a lethal tumor of such small size, though we have had two fatalities after enucleation for tumors that measured less than 10 mm in largest diameter and 2 mm in thickness.

In the selection of cases for photocoagulation, the clinical evaluation should be as thorough as possible to make certain that one is indeed treating a melanoma and not a simulating lesion. Shields[32] has reported that in five of his patients treated successfully by photocoagulation, the ^{32}P test changed from a clearcut positive to a clearcut negative. Ultrasonography should be used as an adjunct to ophthalmoscopy in judging the degree of elevation and to ascertain whether there might be any extraocular extension of the tumor. Melanomas with extraocular extension juxtapapillary tumors and those involving the macula are usually considered not suitable for photocoagulation. (See Chapter 12 for a further discussion of photocoagulation in the treatment of malignant melanoma.)

Irradiation

While Lederman, a very experienced radiotherapist, does not recommend radiation as the treatment of choice for uveal melanomas,[57] Stallard, an ophthalmologist who pioneered the surgical application of radioactive devices (mainly cobalt 60 plaques) to the sclera, has found these tumors to be radiosensitive and curable.[58, 59] More recently, several other workers have also reported encouraging results.[49, 60, 61] Radiation therapy has one distinct advantage over photocoagulation: tumor cells deep within scleral canals and those that have extended into the orbital tissues where they may escape photocoagulation are included in the field of radiation. The application procedure, however, requires operative intervention with manipulation of the globe and, therefore, involves the potential for increasing the dissemination of tumor cells. Radiation is not advisable for the more anteriorly located neoplasms, and some workers also question its use for those near the macula or optic disk because of the possibility of producing radiational damage to the lens, cornea, macula, or optic nerve. Stallard, however, prefers radiation to photocoagulation for lesions near the macula or optic disk.

According to Davidorf et al,[60] tumors that are 7 mm or less in diameter and not elevated more than 2 mm are suitable for cobalt radiation therapy. Tumors larger than 12 mm and elevated more than 3 mm are not suitable. Stallard, on the other hand, has successfully treated tumors as large as 16 mm, but most of his success has been with those that measured 5 to 8 mm in diameter.[58, 59] In his series of 72 successfully treated tumors, 3 patients died. If only the successfully treated patients who had been followed up for more than five years are considered, 17 of 20 were five-year survivors (15 percent mortality). These results compare very favorably with results obtained by enucleation in this group of very small tumors. (See Chapter 11 for a further discussion of irradiation in the treatment of malignant melanoma.)

Other Methods of Treatment

Diathermy and cryotherapy[62-64] have also been tried, but they have much less appeal and apparently no serious advocates at the present time. The intensity required to destroy the tumor by these methods might also seriously damage the ocular tissues. Scleral necrosis is a well-known complication of diathermy; in our studies of eyes with unsuspected melanomas that had been treated for retinal detachment with diathermy we have often observed extraocular extension of tumor at the sites of previous diathermy.[65] Cryotherapy has also been suggested as an adjunct to resection or enucleation in an attempt to prevent the dissemination of tumor cells during surgery.

No Treatment

The following facts may influence a decision against treatment: (1) very small tumors have rarely been associated with a fatal outcome; (2) our knowledge of the natural history of uveal melanomas is very meager; (3) the prognosis of small epithelioid cell melanomas treated by enucleation is almost as bad as that of large melanomas and the management of such tumors may have little effect on the outcome; and (4) enucleation might be more harmful than beneficial. In view of the above considerations, currently some clinicians are merely observing patients who have small asymptomatic malignant melanomas in eyes that retain useful vision, particularly when there is no documented evidence of growth or of progressive damage to intraocular structures. In some centers, such patients are being followed up by careful clinical investigation, including repeated fundus photography and fluorescein angiography.[66-68] In these cases it is also very helpful to have periodic evaluation by ultrasonography. Those who are advocating such extremely conservative management point out that there has not yet been a well-documented case in which extraocular extension and/or metastasis has occurred from a small, asymptomatic choroidal melanoma that showed no change by ophthalmoscopy. They feel secure in the belief that truly malignant behavior will become evident to the ophthalmologist long before the tumor affects the patient's chance for survival. From our own voluminous material we cannot produce a case that would refute this assumption, although we have seen a few very small tumors that have pursued a fatal course.

Curtin and Cavender[66] summarized their experience with 14 cases in which the asymptomatic tumor measured 5 to 12 mm in diameter and the patient was followed up five years or longer. They reported that 9 patients were alive and well with no evidence of tumor growth in the untreated eye at the time of their report. In 5 cases, the eye had come to enucleation because of tumor growth and/or complications with deterioration of vision. One of these patients died of metastatic melanoma 26 months after the initial diagnosis and 18 months after enucleation. Another patient died following colectomy for adenocarcinoma 5½ years after initial diagnosis of uveal melanoma; autopsy revealed no evidence of metastasis from the melanoma. The mortality in that small series (one tumor death in 14 cases, or 7 percent) compares favorably with that found in our most recent study. In our group of smallest melanomas (diameters of 4 to 7.9 mm) there were 2 tumor deaths among 13 cases treated by enucleation (15 percent). While these series are small and final judgments cannot be made at this time, the results reported by Curtin and Cavender are encouraging; they support the thesis that retention of an eye containing a small, asymptomatic, untreated melanoma does not jeopardize the patient's chance for survival.

REFERENCES

1. Paul EV, Parnell BL, Fraker M: Prognosis of malignant melanomas of the choroid and ciliary body. Int Ophthalmol Clin 2:387, 1962
2. Everson TC, Cole WH: Spontaneous Regression of Cancer. Philadelphia, Saunders, 1966
3. Hogan MJ: Clinical aspects, management, and progress of melanomas of the uvea and optic nerve. In Boniuk M (ed): Ocular and Adnexal Tumors. St. Louis, Mosby, 1964, p 203
4. Hogan MJ, Zimmerman LE: Ophthalmic Pathology, 2nd ed. Philadelphia, Saunders, 1962
5. Reese AB: Tumors of the Eye, 2nd ed. New York, Hoeber, 1963, p 241
6. Vogel ME: Treatment of malignant choroidal melanoma with photocoagulation: evaluation of ten-year follow-up data. Am J Ophthalmol 74:1, 1972
7. Vogel ME: Histopathologic observations of photocoagulated malignant melanomas of the choroid. Am J Ophthalmol 74:466, 1972
8. Woodruff MW: Cancer—the elusive enemy. Proc R Soc Lond 183:87, 1973
9. Anderson B, O'Neill J: Malignant melanoma of the uvea: observations on growth and behavior, enucleation refused or delayed. Arch Ophthalmol 58:337, 1957
10. Dunphy EG: Management of intraocular malignancy. Am J Ophthalmol 44:313, 1957
11. Newton FH: Malignant melanoma of the choroid: report of a case with clinical history of 36 years and follow-up of 32 years. Arch Ophthalmol 73:198, 1965

12. Rahi AHS: Immunologic aspects of malignant melanoma of the choroid. Trans Ophthalmol Soc UK 93:79, 1973
13. Ashton N: Primary tumors of the iris. Br J Ophthalmol 48:650, 1964
14. Duke JR, Dunn SN: Primary tumors of the iris. Arch Ophthalmol 59:204, 1958
15. Rones B, Zimmerman LE: The prognosis of primary tumors of the iris treated by iridectomy. Arch Ophthalmol 60:193, 1958
16. Vail DT: Iridocyclectomy: a review: gleanings from the literature. Am J Ophthalmol 71:161, 1971
17. Zimmerman LE: Histopathological considerations in the management of tumors of the iris and ciliary body. Ann Inst Barraquer 10:27, 1971–1972
18. Davidorf FH, Lang JR: The natural history of malignant melanoma of the choroid: small vs. large tumors. Trans Am Acad Ophthalmol Otolaryngol 79:310, 1975
19. Flocks M, Gerende JH, Zimmerman LE: The size and shape of malignant melanomas of the choroid and ciliary body in relation to the prognosis and histologic characteristics: a statistical study of 210 tumors. Trans Am Acad Ophthalmol Otolaryngol 59:740, 1955
20. Jensen OA: Malignant melanomas of the choroid in Denmark: extract from the Danish material, 1943–1952. Mod Probl Ophthalmol 7:56, 1968
21. Jensen OA: Malignant melanomas of the human uvea: recent follow-up of cases in Denmark, 1943–1952. Acta Ophthalmol 48:1113, 1970
22. Warren RM: Prognosis of malignant melanomas of the choroid and ciliary body. In Blodi FC (ed): Current Concepts in Ophthalmology, vol 4. St. Louis, Mosby, 1974
23. Ferry AP: Lesions mistaken for malignant melanomas of the posterior uvea. Arch Ophthalmol 73:463, 1964
24. Shields JA, Zimmerman LE: Lesions simulating malignant melanoma of the posterior uvea. Arch Ophthalmol 89:466, 1973
25. Zimmerman LE: Problems in the diagnosis of malignant melanomas of the choroid and ciliary body. Am J Ophthalmol 75:917, 1973
26. Blodi FC, Roy PE: The misdiagnosed choroidal melanoma. Can J Ophthalmol 2:209, 1967
27. Francois J: Treatment of malignant melanoma of the choroid by light coagulation. Mod Probl Ophthalmol 12:550, 1974
28. Howard GM: Erroneous clinical diagnoses of retinoblastoma and uveal melanoma. Trans Am Acad Ophthalmol Otolaryngol 73:199, 1969
29. Shields JA, McDonald PR: Improvements in the diagnosis of posterior uveal melanomas. Arch Ophthalmol 91:259, 1974
30. McLean IW, Foster WD, Zimmerman LE: Prognostic factors in small malignant melanomas of choroid and ciliary body. Arch Ophthalmol 95:48, 1977
31. Font RL, Spaulding AG, Zimmerman LE: Diffuse malignant melanoma of the uveal tract: a clinicopathologic report of 54 cases. Trans Am Acad Ophthalmol Otolaryngol 72:877, 1968
32. Shields JA: In Brockhurst R: Controversies in Ophthalmology, Philadelphia, Saunders, in press
33. LeShan L: An emotional life-history pattern associated with neoplastic disease. Ann NY Acad Sci 125:780, 1966
34. Frank JD: The faith that heals. Johns Hopkins Med J 137:127, 1975
35. Animal study shows intriguing link between chronic stress, cancer. Medical News JAMA 233:757, 1975
36. Riley V: Mouse mammary tumors: alteration of incidence as apparent function of stress. Science 189:465, 1975
37. Char DH, Hollingshead A, Cogan DG, et al: Cutaneous delayed hypersensitivity reactions to soluble melanoma antigen in patients with ocular malignant melanoma. N Engl J Med 291:274, 1974
38. Char DH, Jerome L, McCoy JG, et al: Cell-mediated immunity to melanoma-

associated antigens in patients with ocular malignant melanoma. Am J Ophthalmol 79:812, 1975

39. Federman JL, Lewis MG, Clark WH: Tumor-associated antibodies to ocular and cutaneous malignant melanomas: negative interaction with normal choroidal melanocytes. J Natl Cancer Inst 52:587, 1974

40. Fraunfelder FT: Personal communication, 1975

41. Fraunfelder FT, Boozman F: "No-touch" technique for management of ocular malignant melanomas. Read before the Association for Research in Vision and Ophthalmology annual meeting, Sarasota, Fla, 1974

42. Stanford GB, Reese AB: Malignant cells in the blood of eye patients. Trans Am Acad Ophthalmol Otolaryngol 75:102, 1971

43. Engell HC: Cancer cells in the circulating blood: a clinical study of the occurrence of cancer cells in the peripheral blood and in venous blood draining the tumour area at operation. Acta Chir Scand (Suppl) 201:1, 1955

44. Fisher ER, Fisher BF: Experimental studies of factors influencing hepatic metastasis: I. Effect of a number of tumor cells injected and time of growth. Cancer 12:926, 1959

45. Fisher ER, Turnbull RB Jr: The cytologic demonstration and significance of tumor cells in the mesenteric venous blood in patients with colorectal carcinoma. Surg Gynecol Obstet 100:102, 1955

46. Turnbull RB Jr: The no-touch isolation technique of resection. JAMA 231:1181, 1975

47. Peyman GA, Apple DJ: Local excision of choroidal malignant melanoma: full-thickness eye-wall resection. Arch Ophthalmol 92:216, 1974

48. Malbran E, Dodds R, D'Alessandro C: Conservative treatment of uveal melanomas. Mod Probl Ophthalmol 12:567, 1974

49. Meyer-Schwickerath G: Excision of malignant melanoma of the choroid. Mod Probl Ophthalmol 12:562, 1974

50. Stallard HB: Malignant melanoblastoma of the choroid. Mod Probl Ophthalmol 7:16, 1968

51. Curtin VT, Norton EWD: Pathological changes in malignant melanomas after photocoagulation. Arch Ophthalmol 70:150, 1963

52. Lund OE: Histological studies on light-coagulated melanoblastoma of the choroid. Albrecht von Graefes Arch Klin Ophthalmol 164:433, 1962

53. Meyer-Schwickerath G: The preservation of vision by treatment of intraocular tumors with light photocoagulation. Arch Ophthalmol 66:458, 1961

54. Hopping W, Meyer-Schwickerath G, Lund OE: Light coagulation in intraocular melanomas. In Boniuk M (ed): Ocular and Adnexal Tumors. St. Louis, Mosby, 1964, p 334

55. Lund OE: Lichtcoagulation von malignen Melanoblastomen der Choroidea: klinische und histopathologische Untersuchungen. Mod Probl Ophthalmol 7:45, 1968

56. Meyer-Schwickerath G, Vogel M: Malignant melanoma of the choroid treated with photocoagulation: a 10-year follow-up. Mod Probl Ophthalmol 12:544, 1974

57. Lederman M: Radiotherapy of malignant melanomata of the eye. Br J Radiol 34:21, 1961

58. Stallard HB: Malignant melanoma of the choroid treated with radioactive applicators. In Boniuk M (ed): Ocular and Adnexal Tumors. St. Louis, Mosby, 1964, p 322

59. Stallard HB: Radiotherapy for malignant melanoma of the choroid. Br J Ophthalmol 50:147, 1966

60. Davidorf FH, Makley TA, Lang JR: Conservative management of malignant melanomas of the choroid: follow-up study of patients treated with irradiation. Trans Am Acad Ophthalmol Otolaryngol, in press

61. Long RS, Galin MA, Rotman M: Conservative treatment of intraocular melanomas. Trans Am Acad Ophthalmol Otolaryngol 75:84, 1971

62. Weve HJM: On diathermy in ophthalmic practice. Trans Ophthalmol Soc UK 59:43, 1939

63. Davidorf FH, Newman GH, Havener WH, et al: Conservative management of malignant melanoma: II. Transscleral diathermy. Arch Ophthalmol 83:273, 1970

64. Lincoff H, McLean J, Long RS: The cryosurgical treatment of intraocular tumors. Am J Ophthalmol 63:389, 1967

65. Boniuk M, Zimmerman LE: Occurrence and behavior of choroidal melanomas in eyes subjected to operations for retinal detachment. Trans Am Acad Ophthalmol Otolaryngol 66:642, 1962

66. Curtin VT, Cavender JC: The natural course of selected malignant melanomas of the choroid and ciliary body. Mod Probl Ophthalmol 12:523, 1974

67. Hogan MJ: Intraocular tumors: panel discussion. Mod Probl Ophthalmol 12:591, 1974

68. Rubinstein K, Myska V: Life cycle of choroidal melanoma. Mod Probl Ophthalmol 12:517, 1974

Jerry A. Shields

6 Concepts and Philosophies in the Management of Malignant Melanomas of the Choroid

Until a few years ago, almost all eyes containing malignant melanomas of the uveal tract were treated by enucleation. As the biologic behavior of uveal melanomas became better understood, however, concepts regarding their management became more conservative.[1] Iris melanomas are now known to have a favorable prognosis and may be managed by excisional iridectomy. Choroidal melanomas, however, because of their anatomic location and larger size when diagnosed, are still managed by enucleation in most instances. In the case of small pigmented choroidal tumors, it is often impossible to determine ophthalmoscopically whether the lesion represents a benign nevus or a malignant melanoma. As a result, several philosophies have developed as to the management of such patients.

Some authorities advocate only periodic ophthalmoscopic observation of the lesion and the use of sketches or serial fundus photographs to document enlargement of the tumor before making a therapeutic decision. Others recommend prompt enucleation, believing that this procedure offers the best prognosis. In recent years, some clinicians have stressed the importance of "conservative treatment" of small melanomas. As a result, methods of management by photocoagulation, irradiation, diathermy, cryotherapy, and local surgical excision have been utilized.

A place may exist for each of the approaches noted above. The method chosen, however, depends on the entire clinical situation. In this chapter the approach to the management of small choroidal melanomas will be outlined as practiced by the physicians on the Oncology Unit, Retina Service, Wills Eye Hospital.

For purposes of this discussion, definitions similar to those adopted by Warren are used.[2] A small melanoma is a lesion less than 10 mm in diameter and 2 mm thick. A medium-size melanoma is larger than a small one in either dimension, but not greater than 15 mm in diameter and 5 mm in thickness. Lesions larger than 15 mm in diameter and 5 mm in thickness are considered large melanomas and are most safely managed by enucleation.

This study was supported in part by the Retina Research and Development Foundation, Philadelphia.

It has been shown that small melanomas have a good prognosis after enucleation.[2-5] No one yet has reliable data, however, as to prognosis if such lesions are merely observed or managed by conservative methods. Many of the eyes with small melanomas have relatively good vision, and it is sometimes difficult for an asymptomatic patient to accept enucleation as the treatment of choice. Since the function of the ophthalmologist is to preserve the vision as well as the life of his patient, any method of eradicating a small melanoma without endangering the prognosis for survival seems reasonable.

To justify our approach, it is necessary to review a few basic facts about the biologic behavior of choroidal melanomas. First, choroidal melanomas are potentially lethal, a point often forgotten by ophthalmologists, who are accustomed to seeing healthy patients. It is well documented, however, that between 30 and 45 percent of patients with posterior uveal melanomas die from metastasis within five years, despite enucleation.[2-6]

Second, contrary to the opinion of some clinicians, small choroidal melanomas are not necessarily benign in their biologic behavior. There are reported cases of small melanomas of the spindle cell type that metastasized.[3-5] The prognosis is definitely better, however, if enucleation is performed while a melanoma is small, and the prognosis is considerably worse when the tumor has attained a large size at the time of enucleation.[2-4] It seems reasonable, therefore, to make every effort to make an early, definitive diagnosis before the lesion becomes large.

Third, there is some evidence that most choroidal malignant melanomas arise from preexisting benign nevi.[7] However, there is no reliable way of determining ophthalmoscopically when a benign nevus begins to undergo malignant change. Evidence of enlargement is not always a reliable indication, for we have seen histologically proved benign nevi that apparently enlarged,[8] and histologically proved malignant melanomas that had no evidence of enlargement for several years, even up to the time of enucleation (Fig. 6.1). In most cases, however, clinical enlargement should be considered highly suggestive of malignancy.

Fourth, it is well known that a number of benign lesions may clinically simulate choroidal melanomas. In such cases, advocates of a hasty enucleation assume the risk of enucleating a useful eye containing a benign lesion.[9, 10]

Since small melanomas are potentially lethal, we disagree with those clinicians who continue to periodically observe a choroidal melanoma that is obviously growing. Advocates of this approach may lose the advantage of dealing with a small lesion that has a better prognosis. Because small melanomas have an excellent prognosis compared to larger ones, however, we also disagree with those who advocate prompt enucleation for small asymptomatic tumors. Between these two extremes is the conservative approach to management, in which every effort is made to obtain an early diagnosis and to initiate treatment before the lesion is large enough to threaten the life and vision of the patient.

To make an early accurate diagnosis, we believe that the clinician must use indirect ophthalmoscopy and a number of diagnostic adjuncts. Indirect ophthalmoscopy is perhaps the most important diagnostic procedure. Ophthalmoscopic findings suggestive of early malignant change include elevation of the lesion and presence of subretinal fluid. However, these changes may also occur with benign nevi.[8] Disruption of the overlying retinal pigment epithelium, particularly with the accumulation of lipofuscin pigment over the surface of the tumor, is reported to be highly suggestive of malignancy.[11] It is important, however, that such changes may also occur with benign lesions that simulate malignant melanomas.[12]

In addition to ophthalmoscopy, other ancillary procedures should be used to establish the diagnosis: a complete medical evaluation, visual fields, transillumination, fundus photography, fluorescein angiography, ultrasonography, and circulating antitumor antibody levels.[13-15] If these studies suggest a possible malignant melanoma, a ^{32}P test is performed.[16-21] If all other studies indicate a melanoma and the ^{32}P test is positive, we believe the diagnosis is virtually established.

Once the diagnosis of malignant melanoma is established, any one of several approaches to management may be recommended, depending on the entire clinical situation: simple observation, photocoagulation, irradiation, transscleral diathermy, cryotherapy, sclerochorioretinal resection, and enucleation.

Since no method of management has been unequivocally proved superior, the patient must always be given the choice between observation, conservative treatment, and enucleation. No matter what modality is chosen, it is imperative that the patient be thoroughly informed as to technique, prognosis, and possible complications.

The indications for each approach will be considered. Although we never use transscleral diathermy or cryotherapy, they are included because some clinicians have advocated these techniques.

OBSERVATION

In most cases, we feel that it is unreasonable to merely observe the lesion once the diagnosis of malignant melanoma is unquestionably established. We agree with certain investigators, however, that there are occasional situations where careful periodic observation of a small choroidal melanoma may be justified.[22] Observation is definitely acceptable if diagnostic studies such as fluorescein angiography and the ^{32}P test fail to confirm the diagnosis of melanoma unequivocally. Some small melanomas may be quiescent for many years without clinical evidence of enlargement (Fig. 6.1). It may be safe, therefore, to observe and photograph a small, asymptomatic lesion every two or three months if the involved eye has good vision. Such a patient must not be lost to follow-up, however, because the growth of these tumors is sometimes rather dramatic (Fig. 6.2). Once growth is unequivocally documented, continued observation is usually contraindicated.

The second indication for observation is an asymptomatic melanoma, either small or medium size, in a patient who is more than 60 years old. One study several years ago presented evidence that the prognosis is not improved by performing enucleation in older patients.[23] We believe that it is often justifiable, however, to enucleate the involved eye in an older patient who is in otherwise good health with a choroidal melanoma that has destroyed central vision. A third possible indication for observation is a small or medium-size melanoma in the patient's only remaining

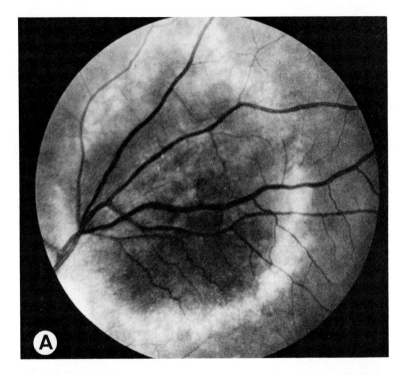

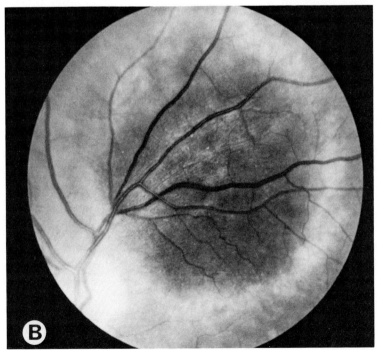

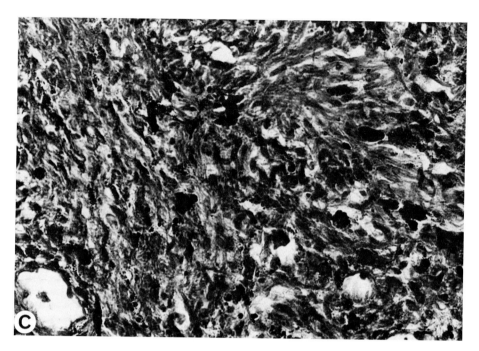

FIG. 6.1 A. Fundus photograph taken in 1967 of minimally elevated, pigmented choroidal lesion superotemporal to optic disk. **B.** The same lesion in 1974, showing no change in the clinical appearance. Eye was enucleated at that time because of concern on part of physician and patient. **C.** Histologic specimen showing malignant melanoma, spindle B cell type.

eye. In such cases, the lesion should be observed closely; if significant growth is detected, the patient should be given the choice of further observation, enucleation, or conservative management.

PHOTOCOAGULATION

With the use of indirect ophthalmoscopy and other diagnostic adjuncts such as the ^{32}P test, it is now possible to diagnose malignant melanomas accurately while they are still small. As a result, some of these lesions are amenable to photocoagulation treatment.[24, 25] On the Oncology Unit, we have used this technique for several years on selected patients with well-documented small choroidal melanomas.

There are certain criteria for selecting patients for photocoagulation treatment[25]: (1) The diagnosis of malignant melanoma should be supported with as many modalities as possible: For example, the lesion in question must have an associated field defect, a melanoma pattern with fluorescein angiography, and a positive ^{32}P test. (2) The lesion must not be elevated more than 2 mm as measured by ultrasonography. (3) Its greatest diameter must not be more than 10 mm. We have photocoagulated a larger lesion on one occasion, but eradication of the tumor was considerably more difficult. (4) The lesion should not have a large amount of

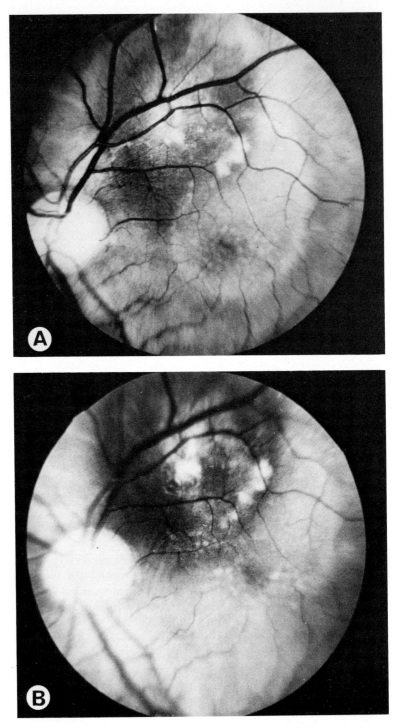

FIG. 6.2 A. Fundus photograph taken in 1967 of pigmented choroidal tumor superotemporal to optic disk with subretinal fluid extending into fovea. **B.** The same lesion in February 1971, showing no change in the size of the lesion.

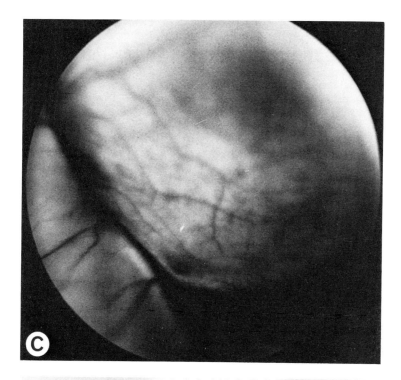

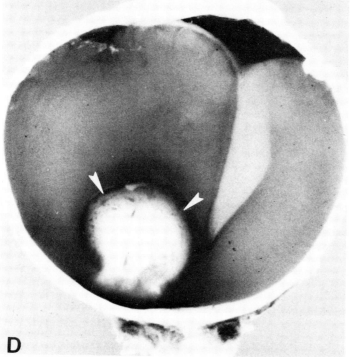

FIG. 6.2 (cont.). **C.** The same lesion in November 1972, when patient returned after being lost to follow-up. **D.** Enucleated globe showing mushroom-shaped choroidal melanoma (arrows).

subretinal fluid, which would prevent adequate photocoagulation. (5) The lesion should be in a location amenable to photocoagulation without destroying central vision. If the tumor is located within 1 disk diameter of the fovea, or within 1 disk diameter of the optic nervehead, photocoagulation may result in significant visual loss; in such cases, enucleation, rather than photocoagulation, should be considered. If the tumor is located anterior to the equator, photocoagulation is also difficult, but successful treatment can often be achieved.

Once these criteria are satisfied, the lesion may be treated with photocoagulation[24, 25] by the technique described in Chapter 12.

For several years we have treated selected patients with this photocoagulation technique. In 5 cases we subsequently repeated the ^{32}P test. In each instance, the test has changed from a clearcut positive to a clearcut negative result after apparent eradication of the tumor by xenon photocoagulation.[26] Among the 12 patients treated by photocoagulation, complications included mild iris atrophy in 1 and a tractional retinal detachment in 2. The 2 retinal detachments were secondary to vitreous alterations possibly due to excess heat. We now believe that such complications may be avoided by keeping exposure time to a minimum.

IRRADIATION

This technique for the treatment of malignant melanomas of the choroid has been available for a number of years. Radon seeds[27, 28] and cobalt plaques[29, 30] have recently been applied as sources of irradiation. This treatment requires a surgical procedure in which the plaque is sutured to the sclera directly over the base of the tumor. The dosage is calculated according to the size of the tumor as measured by ultrasonography. Since most melanomas are not particularly radiosensitive, evidence of tumor regression may take many weeks or months.

Because of the possible complications of radiation,[29] we currently consider this technique only in selected cases. The lesion must be peripheral enough such that the optic nerve or macula are not affected with irradiation, and it must not be elevated more than 3 mm. If significant subretinal fluid is present, irradiation, rather than photocoagulation, should be considered. We currently prefer photocoagulation to irradiation if the lesion is elevated less than 2 mm and has no significant subretinal fluid. Other clinicians, however, believe that radiation is preferable in small lesions and is less effective in medium-size tumors.[28] Irradiation for malignant melanomas requires the assistance of specialists in nuclear medicine.

TRANSSCLERAL DIATHERMY

Although this technique has been advocated by some investigators, they acknowledge that it causes massive destruction of the adjacent sclera.[31] We do not recommend this approach to the management of small choroidal melanomas because extensive weakening and destruction of the adjacent sclera may predispose to extrascleral extension of malignant tumor cells.

CRYOTHERAPY

This technique was used in a few cases, but results were not encouraging.[32] At present, there is probably no role for cryotherapy in the treatment of choroidal melanomas.

SCLEROCHORIORETINAL RESECTION

Sclerochorioretinal resection has been used in a few instances to remove melanomas from the posterior segment of the globe. Local removal of choroidal melanomas had been attempted with limited success in a number of centers, but the experiments of Peyman et al helped refine the technique in the United States.[33,34] During 1975, we used it successfully in two cases on the Oncology Unit of the Retina Service, and we are currently following up the patients.[35] This difficult surgical procedure requires a series of photocoagulation and cryotherapy treatments around the melanoma to create a firm chorioretinal adhesion or an area of bare sclera. The tumor is subsequently removed, along with the adjacent sclera and retina. The eye wall is replaced with a scleral graft from a cadaver eye. The exact technique for this procedure is discussed in the literature.[33,34] (See also Chap. 13.) With further experience, this technique will probably be improved and more frequently used.

ENUCLEATION

In spite of the fact that several conservative methods of management for choroidal melanomas have been developed, enucleation is still performed in many cases. There is some controversy as to whether the removal of an eye containing a malignant melanoma improves the prognosis at all. When the vision is markedly decreased, however, we believe that enucleation is usually justified. As methods of conservative management are further improved, there will probably be fewer enucleations performed for small choroidal melanomas.

REFERENCES

1. Zimmerman LE: Changing concepts concerning the malignancy of ocular tumors. Arch Ophthalmol 78:166, 1967
2. Warren RM: Prognosis of malignant melanomas of the choroid and ciliary body. In Blodi FC (ed): Current Concepts in Ophthalmology, vol 4. St. Louis, Mosby, 1974
3. Flocks M, Gerende JH, Zimmerman LE: The size and shape of malignant melanomas of the choroid and ciliary body in relation to the prognosis and histologic characteristics: a statistical study of 210 tumors. Trans Am Acad Ophthalmol Otolaryngol 59:740, 1955
4. Jensen OA: Malignant melanomas of the human uvea: a recent follow-up of cases in Denmark, 1943–1952. Acta Ophthalmol 48:1113, 1970
5. Davidorf FH, Lang JR: The natural history of malignant melanoma of the choroid: small vs large tumors. Trans Am Acad Ophthalmol Otolaryngol 79:310, 1975

6. Paul E, Parnell BL, Fraker M: Prognosis of malignant melanomas of the choroid and ciliary body. Int Ophthalmol Clin 2:387, 1962
7. Yanoff M, Zimmerman LE: Histogenesis of malignant melanomas of the uvea: II. The relationship of uveal nevi to malignant melanomas. Cancer 20:493, 1967
8. Shields JA, Font RL: Melanocytoma of the choroid clinically simulating a malignant melanoma. Arch Ophthalmol 87:396, 1972
9. Ferry AP: Lesions mistaken for malignant melanomas of the posterior uvea. Arch Ophthalmol 73:463, 1964
10. Shields JA, Zimmerman LE: Lesions simulating malignant melanoma of the posterior uvea. Arch Ophthalmol 89:466, 1973
11. Smith LT, Irvine AR: Diagnostic significance of orange pigment accumulation over choroidal tumors. Am J Ophthalmol 76:212, 1973
12. Shields JA, Rodrigues MM, Sarin LK, Tasman WS, Annesley WH Jr: Lipofuscin pigment over benign and malignant choroidal tumors. Trans Am Acad Ophthalmol Otolaryngol 81:871, 1976
13. Shields JA, McDonald PR: Improvements in the diagnosis of posterior uveal melanomas. Arch Ophthalmol 91:259, 1974
14. Shields JA, McDonald PR, Sarin LK: Problems and improvements in the diagnosis of posterior uveal melanomas. In Croll M, Brady LW, Carmichael PL, Wallner RJ (eds): Nuclear Ophthalmology. New York, Wiley, 1976, pp 37–49
15. Federman JL, Lewis MG, Clark WH, Egerer I, Sarin LK: Tumor-associated antibodies in the serum of ocular melanoma patients. Trans Am Acad Ophthalmol Otolaryngol 78:784, 1974
16. Hagler WS, Jarrett WH II, Humphrey WT: The radioactive phosphorus uptake test in the diagnosis of uveal melanomas. Arch Ophthalmol 85:548, 1970
17. Shields JA, Sarin LK, Federman JL, Mensheha-Manhart O, Carmichael PL: Surgical approach to the ^{32}P test for posterior uveal melanomas. Ophthalmic Surg 5:13, 1974
18. Shields JA, Hagler WS, Federman JL, Jarrett WH II, Carmichael PL: The significance of the ^{32}P test in the diagnosis of posterior uveal melanomas. Trans Am Acad Ophthalmol Otolaryngol 79:297, 1975
19. Shields JA, Carmichael PL, Leonard BC, Sarin LK, Federman JL: The accuracy of the ^{32}P test for ocular melanomas: an analysis of 350 cases. Read before the AMA Section on Ophthalmology, Atlantic City, NJ, 1975
20. Shields JA, Annesley WH Jr, Totino JA: Nonfluorescent malignant melanoma of the choroid diagnosed with the radioactive phosphorus uptake test. Am J Ophthalmol, 79:634, 1975
21. Shields JA, Leonard BC, Sarin LK: Multilobed uveal melanoma masquerading as a postoperative choroidal detachment. Br J Ophthalmol 60:386, 1976
22. Curtin VT, Cavender JC: The natural course of selected malignant melanomas of the choroid and ciliary body. Mod Probl Ophthalmol 12:523, 1974
23. Westerveld-Brandon ER, Zeeman WPC: The prognosis of melanoblastoma of the choroid. Ophthalmologica 134:20, 1957
24. Meyer-Schwickerath G: The preservation of vision by treatment of intraocular tumors with light photocoagulation. Arch Ophthalmol 66:458, 1961
25. Vogel MH: Treatment of malignant choroidal melanoma with photocoagulation: evaluation of ten-year follow-up data. Am J Ophthalmol 74:1, 1972
26. Shields JA, Annesley WH Jr, Federman JL, Sarin LK: Fluorescein and ^{32}P studies in photocoagulated melanomas. In L'Esperance F (ed): Current Diagnosis and Management of Chorioretinal Disease. St. Louis, Mosby, in press
27. Newman GH, Davidorf FH, Havener WH, Makley TA Jr: Conservative management of malignant melanoma: I. Irradiation as a method of treatment for malignant melanoma of the choroid. Arch Ophthalmol 83:21, 1970
28. Davidorf FH, Makley TA, Lang JR: Conservative management of malignant mel-

anomas of the choroid: follow-up study of patients treated with irradiation. Trans Am Acad Ophthalmol Otolaryngol, in press

29. Stallard HB: Radiotherapy for malignant melanoma of the choroid. Br J Ophthalmol 50:147, 1966
30. Long RS, Galin MA, Rotman M: Conservative treatment of intraocular melanomas. Trans Am Acad Ophthalmol Otolaryngol 75:84, 1971
31. Davidorf FH, Newman GH, Havener WH, Makley TA: Conservative management of malignant melanoma: II. Transcleral diathermy. Arch Ophthalmol 83:273, 1970
32. Lincoff H, McLean J, Long RS: The cryosurgical treatment of intraocular tumors. Am J Ophthalmol 63:389, 1967
33. Peyman GA, Ericson ES, Axelrod AJ, May DR: Full-thickness eye-wall resection in primates: an experimental approach to the treatment of choroidal melanoma. Arch Ophthalmol 89:410, 1973
34. Peyman GA, Apple DJ: Local excision of choroidal malignant melanoma: full-thickness eye-wall resection. Arch Ophthalmol 92:216, 1974
35. Shields JA, Sarin LK: Sclerochorioretinal resection for choroidal melanomas. Read before the 1975 Wills Eye Hospital Clinical Conference, Philadelphia, 1975

Devron H. Char

7 Immunologic Aspects and Management of Malignant Intraocular Pigmented Neoplasms

Immunologic factors may play a role in host defense against ocular tumors. Clinical evidence suggesting this possibility is present for both ocular malignant melanoma and retinoblastoma. Spontaneous remissions and regressions in patients with these tumors have been documented when the tumors were in the intraocular stages, and even when there were extraocular extensions of disease.[1-4] Choroidal melanomas have been known to remain stationary for as long as 30 years before increasing in size.[5] Patients with ocular melanoma may have long disease-free intervals after enucleation before developing metastatic disease.[6]

HISTORIC BACKGROUND AND THE IMMUNE SURVEILLANCE HYPOTHESIS

The early investigators of immunology, such as Paul Erhlich, felt that the immune system might be an important surveillance system in host protection against neoplasia. In 1909 Ehrlich wrote that if the self-protection of the immune system did not exist carcinomas would be expected to appear with overwhelming frequency.[7]

The immune surveillance hypothesis provides a good model on which to build a basic understanding of tumor immunology. As postulated by Burnet[8] and amplified by Thomas[9] in the late 1950s, this theory suggests that one of the major roles of the immune system is to detect and eliminate from the body newly mutant cells that have undergone neoplastic transformation, thus providing the host with a primary defense against tumors. For the immune surveillance theory to be valid, at least two conditions must be met. First, when a cell undergoes neoplastic transformation, tumor antigens must be expressed on the surface of the neoplastic cell so that the host's immune system can distinguish it from a normal cell. Second, the host's immune system must be able to destroy it.

In the 1940s the development of syngeneic animal strains allowed researchers to control other histocompatibility parameters and gather experimental evidence

This study was supported in part by Fight for Sight, Inc., New York, and by the Cancer Research Coordinating Committee, University of California, Berkeley.

demonstrating the importance of immunologic factors in host resistance to tumors. An experiment performed in 1943 by Gross,[10] and later repeated by Foley,[11] demonstrated the existence of tumor-associated transplantation antigens and host response to them. Briefly, Gross demonstrated that skin could be successfully transplanted between any members of a colony of syngeneic mice. One group of these mice was immunized with a methylcholanthrene-induced sarcoma. A sublethal dose of tumor was given, and when a small tumor nodule appeared, it was resected. Both the immunized mice and syngeneic control mice were injected with a lethal dose of sarcoma. The control mice developed sarcoma and died. Even though many of the previously immunized mice developed tumor, many had complete spontaneous regressions. Serendipitously, it was observed that this colony of mice had a high incidence of mammary carcinomas and that there was no difference in the incidence between the immunized and nonimmunized mice. This animal tumor model, therefore, demonstrated the existence of a sarcoma tumor-specific transplantation antigen and immunologic reaction to it.

Two broad approaches have been used in tumor immunology which suggest that immune response to tumor antigens, most likely of a cellular nature, is of primary importance in the host defense against neoplasia.[12] Investigators have noted that active immunostimulation of the host can decrease the incidence of many tumors. This decrease has been accomplished in virally induced tumors using immunization with the viral carcinogens, and has also been demonstrated experimentally using nonspecific immunostimulation with adjuvants such as bacillus Calmette-Guerin (BCG), Corynebacterium parvum, and levamisole.[13, 14] Passive immunostimulation of the host by adoptive transfer of immune lymphocytes can prevent tumor development or retard tumor growth.[15, 16] Immunosuppression of the host can result in increased tumor incidence,[17–19] as has been demonstrated with neonatal thymectomy, treatment with antilymphocyte serum, total body radiation, or chemical immunosuppression. Those mice that congenitally lack cell-mediated immunity ("nude mice") generally also seem to have an increased incidence of tumors; however, there are conflicting data on this subject.[20]

In some immunosuppressed human populations there is an increased incidence of cancer. Approximately 10 percent of patients with congenital immunodeficiency diseases develop malignancies, as do nearly 5 percent of patients who undergo immunosuppressive therapy after organ transplantation.[21–23] In some immunosuppressed patients receiving organ transplants, tumors have also been transplanted inadvertently and the malignancies have grown markedly. In a few such patients restoration of immune competence has resulted in total tumor destruction.[24] Many malignancies spontaneously arise in older persons. Immunologic function has been demonstrated to be impaired with aging.[25]

TUMOR ESCAPE FROM IMMUNE SURVEILLANCE

Within the confines of the immune surveillance hypothesis, tumor escape (Fig. 7.1) can occur either as a result of changes in tumor antigenicity or an altered immune response to these antigens. In mouse leukemias, thymic leukemia antigens can undergo antigenic modulation.[26] When cells with the thymic leukemia (T_L)

antigens are exposed to thymic leukemia antibodies in vitro or are injected into mice immunized to these antigens, these cells modulate and the thymic leukemia antigens become undetectable. Similar antigen modulation has also been observed in other tumor-associated antigens.[27] Clones of tumor cells with low density or absent surface tumor antigens may be "selected" for growth over tumor cells with higher antigenic densities.[28] Investigators have noted that some metastatic cells appear to have a lower density of tumor-associated antigens than cells comprising the primary tumor. Some tumor-associated antigens appear to be more deeply imbedded in the cellular membrane. Neuraminidase treatment, a process that disrupts the cell surface membrane by cleaving sialic acid residues, increases the immunogenicity of the tumor cells by exposing these antigens.[29]

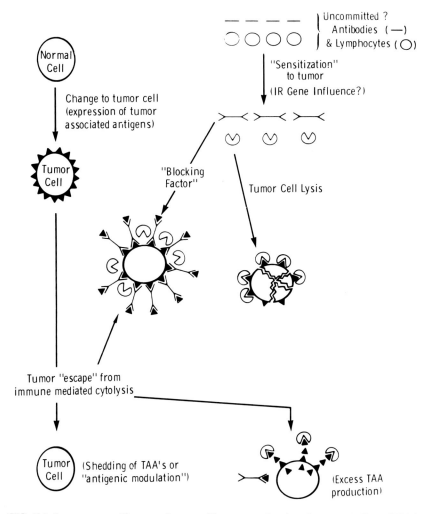

FIG. 7.1. Immune surveillance and escape. Tumor-associated antigens are indicated TAA.

A tumor may also avoid immune attack if it is not recognized as being different from normal tissue. In some animal models, tumor angiogenesis factor can be demonstrated, which induces vessel ingrowth from the surrounding normal tissues.[30, 31] It is conceivable that immune cells recognize these tumor vessels as "self," and therefore the growing neoplasm is not subject to immunologic attack. This is probably not the usual situation, however, since some early primary tumors, on biopsy, are heavily infiltrated with lymphocytes.

The host immune response may be inadequate to destroy tumor even if tumor-associated antigens are present. Immune response genes are believed to be encoded in the same area of the chromosome as the major histocompatibility locus (the H-2 system in mice and the HLA locus in man[30]). These immune response genes appear to be important in determining the host's ability to mount a cell-mediated response to some antigens, and they may play an integral role in the immunologic response to neoplasia.[31] In a cogenic strain of mice that differs only in that small area of the H-2 locus where the immune response genes are thought to be encoded, there is a marked disparity in incidence of leukemia. Mice with the H-2^K are susceptible to the gross leukemia virus, while mice who are H-2^B are resistant.[32] In retinoblastoma and malignant melanoma, the incidence of certain HLA antigens differs significantly from the normal population.[33, 34] Possibly the immune response genes linked to the HLA locus cause an altered response to tumors in these patients. Much work must still be done to delineate the importance of the HLA antigen differences noted in human malignancies.[35] The correlation between some histocompatibility antigen types and malignancy may be accounted for in another manner. The histocompatibility antigens might function as receptors for oncogenic viruses or allow the viruses to go unrecognized because of molecular mimicry of these antigens.[36] At present there is little experimental evidence in support of this concept.

In some chemically induced malignancies the carcinogenic agent can be demonstrated to be immunosuppressive, allowing the tumor to escape immunologically mediated destruction.[37] Immunologic "blocking factors," which can diminish the immune destruction of malignancies, occur. These factors appear to be soluble antigen–antibody complexes. Their presence has usually been demonstrated in hosts with metastatic disease.[38]

EVIDENCE AGAINST THE IMMUNE SURVEILLANCE HYPOTHESIS

The immune surveillance hypothesis has been a part of the conceptual framework of tumor immunology for many years; nevertheless, it does not adequately account for a number of clinical and experimental observations. Most virally induced neoplasms can be demonstrated to have tumor-associated antigens. However, in a number of tumors either produced by chemical carcinogens or arising spontaneously, no tumor antigens can be demonstrated.[39] In at least two experimental settings an intact immunologic system can be deleterious to the host–tumor interaction. In C3H mice the presence of an intact cell-mediated immune system appears to increase the incidence of virally induced mammary carcinoma when compared to mice that have undergone neonatal thymectomy.[40] Immunopotentiation of tumor growth has been demonstrated, and possibly the hypothesized "sneaking through" may occur as a result of it.[41–44] This poorly understood phenomenon occurs when a host is injected with a small number of tumor cells and develops lethal disease. Injection with far greater numbers of tumor cells results in rejection of the neoplasm and host survival.

While some immunosuppressed patient populations have an increased incidence of neoplasia, other immunosuppressed patients, such as those with sarcoidosis, do not. In immunosuppressed patients who develop tumors, the most common malignancies, such as breast and lung carcinoma, do not increase in frequency; instead there is an unusually high incidence of lymphoreticular and epithelial-derived neoplasms.[22]

IMMUNOLOGIC ASPECTS OF OCULAR TUMORS

Immunologic reactions to human tumor-associated antigens have been reviewed elsewhere.[37, 38] Some assays that have been used to detect immune reactions to these antigens are listed in Table 7.1. Most of the data on immune reactions to

Table 7.1

Assays Detecting Immune Reactions to Tumor-Associated Antigens

Indirect immunofluorescent antibody assay
Cutaneous delayed hypersensitivity
Leukocyte migration inhibition
Lymphocyte cytotoxicity (isotope release assay)
Transplantation
Winn adoptive transfer assay
Immunoassay for tumor-related proteins
  (chorioembryonic antigen, alpha fetoglobulin)
Antibody-dependent cellular cytotoxicity
Colony inhibition
Mixed lymphocyte–tumor culture

tumor-associated antigens in ocular malignancies have been obtained using the first four assays listed.[39]

Immunofluorescent Assay

Figure 7.2 depicts the indirect immunofluorescent assay for detecting antibodies to tumor antigens. Fresh tumor material is mounted on microscopic slides. In parallel tests, patients' and control subjects' sera are incubated with the tumor slides. Antitumor antibodies, if present in patient serum, attach to the membrane and cytoplasmic tumor-associated antigens. Since the antibodies in the control subjects' sera are not toward tumor antigens, they do not attach to the tumor cell. When fluorescein-labeled anti-human gamma globulin is incubated with both the patient and control slides, it attaches to all antibodies. Unlike the slides incubated with control sera, in which the fluorescein-labeled antibodies are washed away,

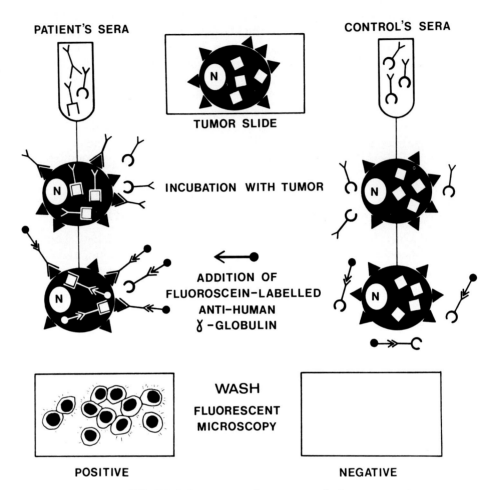

PATIENT'S SERA

CONTROL'S SERA

TUMOR SLIDE

INCUBATION WITH TUMOR

ADDITION OF
FLUOROSCEIN-LABELLED
ANTI-HUMAN
ɣ-GLOBULIN

WASH
FLUORESCENT
MICROSCOPY

POSITIVE

NEGATIVE

FIG. 7.2. Indirect immunofluorescent antibody assay.

when a melanoma patient has antibodies to the tumor-associated antigens, the fluorescein-labeled anti-human gamma globulin is attached to the slides by these antibodies and, under fluorescent microscopy, fluoresces.

Rahi first attempted to demonstrate tumor antibodies in patients with ocular melanoma, but his studies are difficult to evaluate since there were no control subjects.[45] Wong and Oskvig studied anti-melanoma antibodies in patients with ocular melanoma using the technique illustrated in Fig. 7.2.[46] In 19 of 21 patients with choroidal melanoma, allogeneic cytoplasmic staining for IgM antibody was noted. A large number of control subjects were negative in this assay; the exceptions were a few patients with biliary cirrhosis and 4 patients with uveitis. The antibodies measured in the uveitis patients could be absorbed out with normal choroid. Using a similar technique, Federman et al noted the presence of autologous tumor antibodies in 4 patients with ocular melanomas.[47] Negative results were observed when the patients' sera were tested with normal choroidal tissue, thus demonstrating relative specificity. Both of these studies suggest that there are antibodies to melanoma-associated antigens in some patients with ocular melanoma. Unfortunately, patients with lesions simulating choroidal melanomas were not tested in these assays, so that the clinical diagnostic specificity remains to be determined. Although some investigators have noted excellent specificity with the indirect immunofluorescent technique, others have not.[48-50] Similarly, some researchers have observed a correlation between the presence of these antimelanoma antibodies and a good prognosis in systemic melanomas, while others have noted no correlation or a negative one.[48-50] In ocular tumors no immunologic parameters have yet been correlated with prognosis or disease status.

Cell-Mediated Immunity

Cell-mediated immunity to tumor-associated antigens has been studied in ocular tumors. Cellular reactivity to retinoblastoma-associated antigens has been demonstrated in vitro with a ^{125}I-iododeoxyuridine isotope release assay[51] (Fig. 7.3). Viable tissue culture cells derived from retinoblastoma tumor are labeled with the radioactive isotope. Lymphocytes from retinoblastoma patients and from control subjects are separately incubated with these labeled tumor cells and with other control tissue culture cell lines in separate wells. An immunologic reaction occurs between patients with previously sensitized lymphocytes, and retinoblastoma-associated antigens. Lymphokines produced by lymphocytes result in tumor lysis and isotope release. There is no specific immunologic reaction between control lymphocytes and the tumor-associated antigens. Therefore, much less cell lysis and isotope release occurs in the control wells. By counting the percentage of isotope released versus the amount of isotope remaining in the intact control and tumor cells, lymphocytotoxicity can be measured. This is one index of in vitro cell-mediated immunity. Lymphocytes from 14 patients with retinoblastoma and 11 control subjects (consisting of 5 normals, 1 patient with breast carcinoma, and 5 patients with other ocular diseases) were tested for lymphocytotoxicity against the retinoblastoma and other control tissue culture cell lines. Of the 14 patients with retinoblastoma, 11 had significantly increased lymphocytotoxicity against retinoblastoma cell lines as compared to the other tissue culture lines and the cytotoxicity of the control subjects. Some investigators have also noted cellular reactivity to retinoblastoma antigens in retinoblastoma patients by similar techniques,[52] however, others have not (B. Galli, personal communication).

Cell-mediated immunity to tumor-associated antigens has been demonstrated in vitro using a skin-test assay. A skin-test antigen was produced by crude membrane extraction of retinoblastoma cells. Eight patients with retinoblastoma and five control subjects were skin-tested with this antigen. All eight patients with retinoblastoma had positive skin-test responses; none of the five controls had positive responses.[53] All of the control subjects had delayed hypersensitivity reactions with standard recall antigens. Two of the control subjects had pathologically documented ocular melanomas and positive skin-test responses with the soluble melanoma antigen. Two patients had breast carcinoma metastatic to the choroid and gave positive skin responses to breast carcinoma antigens; one had acute leukemia and had a positive reaction to leukemia-associated antigen.

Cellular reactivity to melanoma-associated antigens in vitro has been demon-

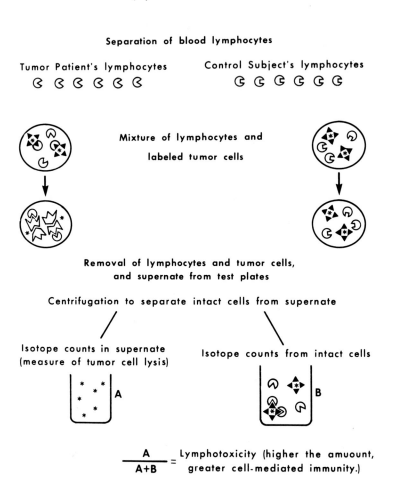

Viable tumor cell
labeled with isotope (*)

Separation of blood lymphocytes

Tumor Patient's lymphocytes   Control Subject's lymphocytes

Mixture of lymphocytes and
labeled tumor cells

Removal of lymphocytes and tumor cells,
and supernate from test plates

Centrifugation to separate intact cells from supernate

Isotope counts in supernate
(measure of tumor cell lysis)

Isotope counts from intact cells

A

B

$$\frac{A}{A+B} = \text{Lymphotoxicity (higher the amuount, greater cell-mediated immunity.)}$$

FIG. 7.3. In vitro cell-mediated immunity isotope release assay.

strated by means of a leukocyte migration inhibition assay[54] (Fig. 7.4). Soluble melanoma-associated antigens are extracted from melanoma tissue. A melanoma patient's white cells are incubated with the melanoma-associated antigens, and if immunologic reactions to these antigens occur, the lymphocytes produce a migration inhibition factor. In contradistinction, the control subjects' lymphocytes are not sensitized to the melanoma-associated antigens and do not elaborate migration inhibition factor. Therefore, the leukocytes migrate out of the capillary tube into the chamber containing the antigens. Migration inhibition is another in vitro correlate of cell-mediated immunity. In a preliminary study it was observed that five of seven patients with ocular melanomas had positive migration inhibition against melanoma-associated antigens, as opposed to no positive responses in a large group

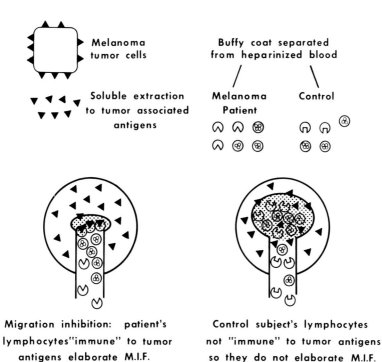

Melanoma tumor cells

Soluble extraction to tumor associated antigens

Buffy coat separated from heparinized blood

Melanoma Patient

Control

Migration inhibition: patient's lymphocytes "immune" to tumor antigens elaborate M.I.F.

Control subject's lymphocytes not "immune" to tumor antigens so they do not elaborate M.I.F.

FIG. 7.4. In vitro cell-mediated immunity leukocyte migration inhibition assay. The immune lymphocytes produce this factor and the white cells do not migrate out of the capillary tube.

of control subjects. Current work in our laboratory continues to show this specificity.[54A] Using a different in vitro technique, Unsgaard and O'Toole have detected cellular reactivity to melanoma-associated antigens in two of five patients with ocular melanoma.[55]

The clinical differentiation of ocular melanoma from simulating lesions can often be difficult. In a previous study of skin-test reactivity to tumor-associated antigens in patients with acute leukemias, excellent specificity was noted and we observed a correlation between the results of skin tests and disease status and prognosis.[56] We have studied a group of patients with ocular melanoma and patients with simulating lesions to determine whether an in vivo response to melanoma-associated antigens would be of diagnostic value.[57] Allogeneic melanomas were obtained under sterile conditions and processed by crude membrane extraction, Sephadex column chromatography, and continuous gel electrophoresis. This material was used to skin-test subjects and a positive skin test was defined as induration greater than 6 mm at 48 hours. In early skin tests with tumor-associated antigens we determined that induration at 48 hours correlated with histologic parameters of cutaneous delayed hypersensitivity. Biopsy specimens of these skin tests demonstrated perivascular round cell infiltration of the upper dermis, a hallmark of delayed hypersensitivity.

Forty-nine patients with pathologically confirmed ocular malignant melanomas were skin-tested before or after enucleation. Forty-three were skin-test positive, and six had false-negative responses. One of the false-negatives had undergone an enucleation 27 years previously for a spindle A cell melanoma and was seen on referral because of a pigmented lesion in the remaining eye. On clinical examination after skin-testing, this lesion was unequivocally a choroidal nevus. Two patients were inadvertently skin-tested during the intraoperative period, a time when delayed hypersensitivity responses are known to be depressed. A fourth patient had initially been skin-test positive; however, on follow-up 1½ years later, he was negative. Of the two other false-negative responses, one had a negative skin test prior to enucleation and the other had a negative skin test when first seen after enucleation. On short clinical follow-up, none has developed metastatic disease.

Twenty-one additional patients with clinical and laboratory evidence of choroidal melanoma had positive skin-test reactions with this antigen. It is conceivable that some of these reactions may prove to be false-positives when these eyes are enucleated and examined histologically. Twenty-four patients who were referred in consultation with the diagnosis of probable ocular melanoma were also skin-tested. On the basis of extensive clinical and laboratory examination (indirect ophthalmoscopy, contact lens examination, visual fields, ultrasonography, fluorescein angiography, ^{32}P test, and fundus photography) these patients were later diagnosed as having simulating lesions. Twenty-one of these patients had negative skin-test reactions with this melanoma antigen. Seven had choroidal nevi, two had choroidal hemangiomas, two had breast carcinomas metastatic to the choroid, and five patients had other systemic malignancies not involving the eye. One patient in each of the following categories was also skin-test negative: choroidal detachment, ciliary body cysts, diffuse uveitis, Jensen's peripapillary chorioretinitis, and precancerous melanosis. All subjects had positive skin tests with standard recall antigens.

Three patients were tested in whom we think false-positive reactions occurred. One we believe had a choroidal hemangioma and had a positive skin test. The second patient had bronchogenic carcinoma and most likely had a choroidal metastatic lesion. To date we do not have histologic confirmation of these diagnoses, and two other patients whom we have tested who had resections of lung carcinomas and presented with choroidal lesions were skin-test positive and had ocular melanomas on histologic examination. The third false-positive response occurred in a patient who was skin-test positive and had previously had fluorescein angiography, ultrasonography, and ^{32}P test results diagnostic of a choroidal melanoma. On pathologic examination, the patient had a benign fibrocytoma of the retina.

Conclusions on Immunologic Assays of Ocular Neoplasms

Our understanding of the biologic importance of the immune system in human tumors is limited. We have demonstrated that tumor-associated antigens exist in ocular tumors and that patients have immune reactions to them. In ocular tumors the clinical diagnosis of a retinoblastoma or an ocular melanoma can sometimes be difficult. These immunologic studies show promise of being useful in this clinical differentiation; however, the specificity and sensitivity of these assays is, as yet, uncertain. While good discrimination between ocular melanoma patients and control subjects has been obtained using the cutaneous delayed hypersensitivity assay with a soluble melanoma antigen, this is still an experimental assay and not a proved diagnostic tool. In some cases the discrimination between the positive and negative response, while present statistically, is small enough to indicate that some nonspecific reactions will occur as more patients are tested. While there are distinct advantages to the in vivo approach, a number of disadvantages have previously been reported.[57] Currently we believe the skin-test assays are an excellent experimental tool for increasing our understanding of the immunobiology of ocular tumors; however, they should be used only in subjects suspected of harboring a malignancy, since it is remotely possible that tumor information could be transmitted. While this transmission is unlikely and has never been observed, it cannot be ruled out.

Some of our work, and the findings of others have suggested that the results of immunologic assays may be of prognostic significance. At present, the follow-up of ocular malignancy patients who have been tested by immunologic means is not long enough to determine the prognostic value of these assays. This area of investigation is being actively pursued.

AREAS OF FURTHER RESEARCH AND IMMUNOTHERAPY

Four basic questions in the immunobiology of tumors need further clarification: (1) What immunologic events occur at the time of oncogenesis? (2) What is the biologic importance of the various immunologic factors in host–tumor interaction? (3) What quality is being measured in the various immunologic assays? (4) Is there a role for immunotherapy in human tumors?

If the immune surveillance hypothesis is correct, there should be immunologic reactivity to tumor-associated antigens in some normal subjects. Our understanding of this phenomenon is limited.[58] Similarly, it is unclear whether the primary event in oncogenesis is suppression of the host immune system, thereby allowing tumor establishment and growth, or whether immunosuppression occurs as an event secondary to tumor growth.[37]

Recent work in immunology has invalidated a dichotomous view of the immune system. Classically, lymphocytes processed in the bursa or bone marrow (B-cells) were thought to be solely responsible for antibody production and lymphocytes processed by the thymus (T-cells) were thought to be solely responsible for delayed hypersensitivity. In tumor immunology, limited data had suggested that these T-cells were responsible for host defense against neoplasia and that antibodies produced by B-cells abrogated this immunologic defense. Recent evidence has suggested that numerous interactions of both a cooperative and a suppressive nature occur between T-cells and B-cells[59] (Fig. 7.5). In tumor immunology antibody and cellular reactions can either be cytotoxic or enhance tumor growth.[38] It has now been demonstrated that in addition to soluble humoral blocking factors, suppressor cells, which can be T-cells, B-cells, or macrophages, are also responsible for inhibition of immunologic tumor defense mechanisms.[60–63] Much current research is

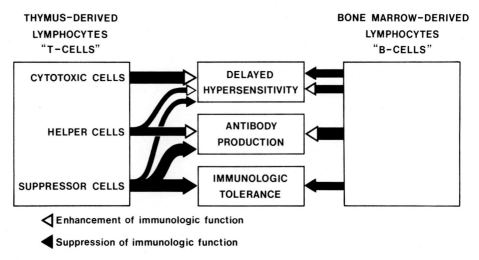

FIG. 7.5. Immunologic cellular interactions.

directed toward understanding what events in vivo lead to either T-cell or B-cell responses that abrogate or enhance tumor growth.

The nature of tumor-associated antigens, the parameters measured in the immunologic assays, and the in vivo correlates of these assays are all areas of ongoing research. The nature of the tumor-associated antigens has not been defined in molecular terms. It is possible that these antigens are of a tissue-associated, viral, or phase-specific nature.[64] This difference may contribute to the disparity of results observed when tumor subjects are simultaneously tested in two different assays.[65, 66] Furthermore, nonspecific reactivity has been a major problem in a number of these assays, and this obstacle mandates numerous types of controls in order to adequately evaluate the data produced.[48-50, 67] It has recently been demonstrated that different T-cell subpopulations (helper cells, cytotoxic cells, and suppressor cells) are distinct prior to antigenic stimulation.[68] In addition to investigating immunologic assays for diagnostic and prognostic purposes in ocular tumors, we are also using ocular tumors as a model for the study of basic tumor immunology; we are attempting to understand which immunologic factors the various assays measure.[69-71]

IMMUNOTHERAPY OF OCULAR TUMORS

As early as the late 1800s investigators were interested in the "immunotherapy" of patients with malignant tumors.[72] Immunologic manipulation as a therapeutic modality has gained popularity since the early work of Mathé et al using immunotherapy in patients with acute lymphocytic leukemia.[73] While that study appeared promising, it was small and uncontrolled, and subsequent reports on the efficacy of human immunotherapy have been conflicting.[74] Table 7.2 presents a number of different approaches to immunotherapy in the prophylaxis and treatment of neoplasms.

Table 7.2

Approaches to Immunotherapy

Prophylaxis
    Specific: causative virus or tumor antigen vaccination (future)
    Nonspecific: immunostimulation—BCG, *parvum*, etc.;? efficacy
Treatment of established neoplasms
    Active specific immunostimulation: autologous or allogeneic tumor material
        Inactivated tumor cells
        Inactivated modified tumor cells (neuraminidase, etc.)
        Purified tumor antigens
    Active nonspecific immunostimulation: BCG, *parvum*, etc.
    Passive immunostimulation: adoptive transfer
        Lymphocytes
        Lymphocyte products, ie, transfer factor, immune RNA, etc.
    In vitro immunization
        Nonspecific: PHA stimulation of lymphocytes, etc.
        Specific: stimulation of lymphocytes with tumor cells or tumor antigens
    Passive transfer with unblocking factor (future)

There have been few prospective, well-controlled, randomized studies using immunotherapy in human tumors.[75] We are currently undertaking such a study of immunotherapy in ocular melanoma. Patients who have recently undergone enucleation and have mixed, necrotic, or epithelioid ocular melanomas are placed in our immunotherapy protocol. These histologic cell types of ocular melanoma have a five-year mortality approaching 50 percent. Nonspecific stimulation of the immune system using adjuvants such as BCG, levamisole, or C. *parvum* have been most commonly used in the immunotherapy of human malignancies. We are treating our patient group with BCG because of its logistic advantage and because results with it have been as good as with any other immunotherapeutic modality.

Ocular melanoma is an excellent model in which to study the immunotherapy of human tumors for a number of reasons. First, tumor-associated antigens and an immunologic response to them have been demonstrated. Second, clinical monitoring of tumor growth can be performed with relative ease both preoperatively and postoperatively. Third, at the time of enucleation, the amount of tumor remaining in the body is quite low. This is a factor which has been demonstrated to be of marked importance in experimental immunotherapy models.[76] Fourth, approximately 90 percent of metastatic disease in ocular melanoma involves the liver primarily; thus the onset of metastatic disease with this tumor is readily detectable,[77] in contradistinction to other tumors with which metastatic disease is often more widespread and more difficult to monitor. For these reasons, ocular melanoma patients may benefit from immunotherapy and provide a good model for its study.

A large number of patients must be studied over a five-year period to determine the value of immunotherapy in ocular melanoma. It is of extreme importance in immunotherapeutic trials that patients' immunologic responses to tumor-associated antigens and to standard antigens be carefully monitored. In some animal studies and a few human case reports, drugs that were used to alter immunologic status have been demonstrated to be immunostimulative or immunosuppressive under different conditions.[75] All patients who are receiving drugs that alter immunologic status should be closely monitored to amend their treatment if the immunotherapy regimen depresses immunologic function.

Since the inception of immunologic research in the late 1800s, investigators have been interested in immunologic techniques for the diagnosis, monitoring, and therapy of human tumors. Much exciting work in tumor immunology has been done in the past few years; it is hoped that further work will provide a basic understanding of the importance of the immune system in the host–tumor interaction.

REFERENCES

1. Reese AB: Tumors of the Eye, 2nd ed. New York, Hoeber, 1964
2. Jensen AO, Andersen SR: Spontaneous regression of a malignant melanoma of the choroid. Acta Ophthalmol 52:173, 1974
3. Ellsworth RM: The practical management of retinoblastoma. Trans Am Ophthalmol Soc 67:462, 1969
4. Everson TC, Cole WH: Spontaneous Regression of Cancer. Philadelphia, Saunders, 1966
5. Newton FH: Malignant melanoma of the choroid. Arch Ophthalmol 73:198, 1965
6. Duke-Elder S, Perkins ES: Diseases of the uveal tract. In Duke-Elder S (ed): System of Ophthalmology, vol 9. St. Louis, Mosby, 1966, p 872
7. Ehrlich P: Uber den jetzigen stand der karzinomforschung. Ned Tijdschr Geneesk 5, 1909
8. Burnet FM: Cancer: a biologic approach. Br Med J 1:779, 841, 1957
9. Thomas L, in Lawrence HS (ed): Cellular and Humoral Aspects of the Hypersensitive State. New York, Hoeber, 1959, p 529
10. Gross L: Intradermal immunization of C3H mice against a sarcoma that originated in an animal of the same line. Cancer Res 3:326, 1943
11. Foley EJ: Antigenic properties of methylcholanthrene-induced tumors in mice of strain origin. Cancer Res 13:835, 1953
12. Klein G: Tumor-specific transplantation antigens: GHA Clowes Memorial Lecture. Cancer Res 28:625, 1968
13. Law LW: Studies of tumor antigens and tumor-specific immune mechanisms in experimental systems. Transplant Proc 2:117, 1970
14. Old LJ, Benacerraf B, Clarke DA, Carswell EA, Stockhert E: The role of the reticuloendothelial system in the host reaction to neoplasia. Cancer Res 21:1281, 1961
15. Old LJ, Boyse EA, Clarke DA, Carswell EA: Antigenic properties of chemically induced tumors. Ann NY Acad Sci 101:80, 1962
16. Wepsic HT, Zbar B, Rapp HP, Borsos T: Systemic transfer of tumor immunity: delayed hypersensitivity and suppression of tumor growth. J Natl Cancer Inst 44:955, 1970
17. Law LW: Studies of thymic function with emphasis on the role of the thymus in oncogenesis. Cancer Res 26:551, 1966
18. Allison AC, Law LW: Effects of antilymphocyte serum on viral oncogenesis. Proc Soc Exp Biol Med 127:207, 1968
19. Payne LN (ed): Symposium on Oncogenesis and Herpes Type Viruses. New York, Cambridge University Press, 1972, p 21
20. DeClercq E: Tumor induction by Maloney sarcoma virus in athymic nude mice. J Natl Cancer Inst 52:473, 1975
21. Gatti RA, Good RA: Occurrence of malignancy in immunodeficiency diseases. Cancer 28:89, 1971
22. Melief CJM, Schwartz RA: A comprehensive treatise. In Becker FF (ed): Cancer, vol 1. New York, Plenum, 1975, p 121

23. Penn I: Occurrence of cancer in immune deficiencies. Cancer 34:858, 1974
24. Zukoski CF, Killen D, Ginn E, et al: Transplanted carcinoma in an immunosuppressed patient. Transplantation 9:71, 1970
25. Weksler ME, Hutteroth TH: Impaired lymphocyte function in aged humans. J Clin Invest 53:99, 1974
26. Old LJ, Stockert E, Boyse EA, Kim JH: Antigenic modulation. J Exp Med 127:523, 1968
27. Ioachim HL, Keller SS, Dorsett BH, Pearse A: Induction of partial immunologic tolerance in rats and progressive loss of cellular antigenicity in gross virus lymphoma. J Exp Med 139:1382, 1974
28. Fenyo EM, Biberfeld P, Klein EJ: Studies on the relations between virus release and cellular immunosensitivity in Maloney lymphomas. J Natl Cancer Inst 42:837, 1969
29. Rios A, Simmons RL: Experimental cancer immunotherapy using a neuraminidase-treated non-viable frozen tumor vaccine. Surgery 75:503, 1974
30. McDevitt HO, Benacerraf B: Genetic control of specific immune responses. Adv Immunol 11:31, 1969
31. Benacerraf B, Katz DH: The histocompatability-linked immune response genes. Adv Cancer Res 21:121, 1975
32. Lily F, Pincus T: Genetic control of murine viral leukomogenesis. Adv Cancer Res 17:231, 1973
33. Betrams J, Schildberg P, Höpping W, Böhme V, Albert E: HL-A antigens in retinoblastoma. Tissue Antigens 3:78, 1973
34. Clark DA, Necheles TF, Nathasson L, et al: Apparent HL-A 5 deficiency in malignant melanoma. Isr J Med Sci 10:836, 1974
35. Takasugi M, Terasaki PI, Henderson B, et al: HL-A antigens in solid tumors. Cancer Res 33:648, 1973
36. Snell GD: The H-2 locus of the mouse. Folia Biol 14:336, 1968
37. Herberman RB: Cell-mediated immunity to tumor cells. Adv Cancer Res 19:207, 1974
38. Hellström KE, Hellström I: Lymphocyte-mediated cytotoxicity and blocking serum activity to tumor antigens. Adv Immunol 18:209, 1974
39. Good RA, Prehn RT, Lawrence HS: Evaluation of the evidence for immune surveillance. In Smith RT, Landy M (eds): Immune Surveillance. New York, Academic, 1970, p 437
40. Yunis EJ, Martinez C, Smith J: Spontaneous mammary adenocarcinoma in mice: influence of thymectomy and reconstitution with thymus grafts or spleen cells. Cancer Res 29:174, 1969
41. Fink MP, Parker CW, Shearer WT: Antibody stimulation of tumor growth in T-cell depleted mice. Nature 255:404, 1975
42. Shearer WT, Atkinson JP, Frank MM, Parker CW: Humoral immunostimulation. J Exp Med 141:736, 1975
43. Prehn RT: The immune reaction as a stimulator of tumor growth. Science 176:170, 1972
44. Yutoku M, Fuji H, Grossberg AL, Pressman D: An experimental model for evaluation of factors in tumor escape from immunologic attack. Cancer Res 35:734, 1975
45. Rahi AHS: Autoimmune reactions in uveal melanoma. Br J Ophthalmol 55:793, 1971
46. Wong IG, Oskvig RM: Immunofluorescent detection of antibodies to ocular melanoma. Arch Ophthalmol 92:98, 1974
47. Federman JL, Lewis MG, Clark WH: Tumor-associated antibodies to ocular and cutaneous malignant melanomas: negative interaction with normal choroidal melanocytes. J Natl Cancer Inst 52:587, 1974
48. Lewis MG, Ikonopisov RL, Nairn RC, et al: Tumor-specific antibodies in human malignant melanoma and their relationship to the extent of the disease. Br Med J 3:547, 1969

49. Whitehead RH: Fluorescent antibody studies in malignant melanoma. Br J Cancer 28:525, 1973
50. Wood GW, Barth RF: Immunofluorescent studies of serologic reactivity of patients with malignant melanoma against tumor-associated cytoplasmic antigens. J Natl Cancer Inst 53:309, 1974
51. Char DH, Ellsworth R, Rabson AS, Albert DM, Herberman RB: Cell-mediated immunity to a retinoblastoma tissue culture line in patients with retinoblastoma. Am J Ophthalmol 78:5, 1974
52. Mosier M, Sulit H: Specific and non-specific cellular cytotoxicity among retinoblastoma patients, abstract. Association for Research in Vision and Ophthalmology, p 94, 1975
53. Char DH, Herberman RB: Cutaneous delayed hypersensitivity responses of patients with retinoblastoma to standard recall antigens and crude membrane extracts of retinoblastoma tissue culture cells. Am J Ophthalmol 78:40, 1974
54. Char DH, Jerome L, McCoy J, Herberman RB: Cell-mediated immunity to melanoma-associated antigens in patients with ocular malignant melanoma. Am J Ophthalmol 79:812, 1975
54A. Char DH: Inhibition of leukocyte migration with melanoma: associated antigens in choroidal tumors. Invest Ophthalmol, in press
55. Unsgaard B, O'Toole C: The influence of tumor burden and therapy on cellular cytotoxicity responses in patients with ocular and skin melanoma. Br J Cancer 31:301, 1975
56. Char DH, Lepourhiet A, Leventhal BG, Herberman RB: Cutaneous delayed hypersensitivity responses to tumor-associated and other antigens in acute leukemia. Int J Cancer 12:409, 1973
57. Char DH, Hollingshead A, Cogan DG, et al: Cutaneous delayed hypersensitivity reactions to soluble melanoma antigen in patients with ocular malignant melanoma. N Engl J Med 291:274, 1974
58. Herberman RB (ed): Conference and Workshop on Cellular Immune Reaction to Tumor-Associated Antigens. Bethesda, Md, National Cancer Institute monograph 37, 1973
59. Katz DH, Benacerraf B: The regulatory influence of activated T cells on B cell responses to antigen. Adv Immunol 15:1, 1972
60. Gershon RK: Regulation of concomitant immunity. Isr J Med Sci 10:1012, 1974
61. Baldwin RW, Embleton MJ, Price MR: Inhibition of lymphocyte cytotoxicity for human colon carcinoma by treatment with solubilized tumor membrane fractions. Int J Cancer 12:84, 1973
62. Gorczynski RM: Immunity to murine sarcoma virus-induced tumors. J Immunol 112:1826, 1974
63. Kurchner H, Chused TM, Herberman RB, Holden HT, Lavrin DH: Evidence of suppressor cell activity in spleens of mice bearing primary tumors induced by Maloney sarcoma virus. J Exp Med 139:1473, 1974
64. Herberman RB: Immunologic reactions of experimental animals to tumor-associated cell surface antigens. In Ioachim H (ed): Pathobiology Annual, vol 3. New York, Appleton 1973, p 291
65. Levanthal BG, Halterman RH, Rosenberg EB, Herberman RB: Immune reactivity of leukemia patients to autologous blast cells. Cancer Res 32:1820, 1972
66. Howell SB, Dean JH, Law LJ: Defects in cell-mediated immunity during growth of a syngeneic simian virus-induced tumor. Int J Cancer 15:152, 1975
67. Takasugi M, Mikey MR, Terasaki PI: Studies on specificity of cell-mediated immunity to human tumors. J Natl Cancer Inst 53:1527, 1974
68. Cantor H, Boyse EA: Functional sub-classes of T lymphocytes bearing different Ly antigens. J Exp Med 141:1376, 1975
69. DeLandazuri MD, Kedar E, Fahey JL: Simultaneous expression of cell-mediated cytotoxicity and antibody-dependent cellular cytotoxicity to a syngeneic rat lym-

phoma: separation and partial characterization of two types of cytotoxic cells. Cell Immunol 14:193, 1974

70. O'Toole C, Stejskal V, Perlmann P, Karlsson M: Lymphoid cells mediating tumor-specific cytotoxicity to carcinoma of the bladder. J Exp Med 139:457, 1974

71. Wybran J, Hellström I, Hellström KE: Cytotoxicity of human rosette-forming blood lymphocytes on cultured human tumor cells. Int J Cancer 13:515, 1974

72. Currie GA: Eighty years of immunotherapy: a review of immunological methods used for the treatment of human cancer. Br J Cancer 26:141, 1972

73. Mathé G, Amiel JL, Schwarzenberg L, et al: Active immunotherapy for acute lymphoblastic leukemia. Lancet 1:697, 1969

74. Borsos T, Rapp HJ (eds): Conference on the Use of BCG in Therapy of Cancer. Bethesda, Md, National Cancer Institute monograph 39, 1974

75. Bast RC, Zbar B, Borsos T, Rapp HJ: BCG and cancer. N Engl J Med 290:1413, 1458, 1974

76. Mathé G: Active immunotherapy. Adv Cancer Res 14:1, 1971

77. Einhorn LH, Burgess MA, Gottlieb JA: Metastatic patterns of choroidal melanoma. Cancer 34:1001, 1974

Jay L. Federman
Wallace H. Clark

8 Circulating Antibodies in Patients with Intraocular Melanomas

The biologic behavior of ocular malignant melanomas is known to be quite variable. Pure spindle cell tumors show a 33 percent ten-year mortality, whereas those tumors with epithelioid cells show an 82 percent mortality.[1-13] In addition to the cell type, the prognosis of uveal melanomas has been associated with tumor size, the presence or absence of extrascleral extension, and the degree of mitotic activity.[1-13]

The mechanisms that are responsible for the control or dissemination of this disease are not clearly understood. Choroidal melanomas may show no evidence of metastasis as late as 32 years after enucleation.[14] The presence of some type of body defense that prevents the uveal melanoma cells from disseminating into the general circulation has been proposed.[8] Reese, in 1963, suggested that metastasis develops only after there is a breakdown in the immunity of the host.[15] The presence of free cells from choroidal melanomas in the peripheral bloodstream has been reported without evidence of metastatic disease.[16-19] In reports on necrosis of malignant melanomas of the choroid, the immunologic role of the lymphocytes has been discussed.[20, 21] There have even been a few reports of malignant melanomas of the choroid, determined by clinical diagnosis, that have spontaneously regressed.[21-23] It has recently been suggested that the presence of lymphocytic–tumor cell reaction in vivo may be deleterious to the host.[24] With this possibility in mind, it is interesting to note that necrotic choroidal melanomas have an extremely poor prognosis. Even though there is the possibility that a cell-mediated immune response in these tumors is operating, these inflammatory cells could also be present secondary to necrosis.

The immune surveillance system, based on the theory that normal tissue does not alert the immune system, has been implicated in tumor control. However, if normal tissue is transformed and is recognized by the immune surveillance system as a new antigen, antibodies are produced. The immune system can respond in two ways—with circulating antibodies or by cell-mediated mechanisms.[25-28]

There has been much work in the past ten years evaluating immune responses in tumor patients. A wealth of material has emerged in an attempt to correlate the biologic behavior of cutaneous melanoma and changes in the immune system in patients with this disease.[22, 29-39] There is good histopathologic–clinical correlation showing cell-mediated immunity to be important in patients with cutaneous melanomas.[40-43] Immune lymphocytes have been shown to cause tumor cell death in vitro.[44] Cellular immune mechanisms have been used to treat secondary disseminated disease in cutaneous melanoma patients.[45, 46] Circulating tumor antibodies may be important in preventing or delaying blood-borne metastatic disease.[39] Thus, both the cell-mediated and humoral systems correlate with the natural history of patients with cutaneous melanomas.

This correlation does not prevail, however, in ocular melanomas. Earlier studies using the material from patients with malignant melanomas of the uveal tract have not consistently demonstrated the presence of humoral cell-mediated antibodies; when such antibodies were observed, there was no definite correlation with the behavior of the malignancy.[31, 47-50] Howard and Spalter, using gel diffusion, hemagglutination, and complement fixation test techniques, were unable to demonstrate antibodies in the sera of patients with uveal melanomas.[48] Hart et al were unable to show evidence of a cell-mediated immunity to uveal melanomas by studying autologous lymphocyte toxicity reactions.[49] Muna et al found positive allogeneic reactions by using immunofluorescent techniques when the sera from 15 patients were tested with allogeneic alcohol-fixed melanoma cells from two patients, one of whom had metastatic disease from an ocular malignant melanoma.[31] They did not state whether the sera were derived from patients with ocular or cutaneous melanomas. Rahi, in immune studies on 21 patients with ocular melanomas, was not able to show cytoplasmic immunofluorescence on sectional paraffin-blocked tissue processed at 4° C.[50] However, he did report evidence of cytoplasmic fluorescence in three positive autologous membrane reactions. Nairn and co-workers reported negative cytoplasmic immunofluorescence on unfixed, dried cell smears of tumor tissue from ten patients with ocular melanoma.[47]

Recently there has been agreement as to the presence of humoral antibodies. Wong and Oskvig tested the sera from 12 patients with choroidal melanomas by indirect immunofluorescence on frozen tissue sections and tumor imprints derived from two allogeneic choroidal melanomas. They reported that 11 had IgM antibodies and 3 had IgG antibodies.[51] We have recently reported two studies on a total of 16 patients with primary intraocular malignant choroidal melanomas.[52] In all patients an autologous circulating tumor-associated antibody to cytoplasmic contents of the tumor cells was detected by indirect immunofluorescence. The specificity of this reaction was demonstrated by negative interaction of the tumor-associated antibodies with normal choroidal melanocytes from the uveal tract.[52] It was also shown that these antibodies were not present at the tumor site in these 16 patients.[52] The patient who had the largest tumor had epithelioid cells in his tumor and by all clinical means would be expected to have the poorest prognosis in the series; he was found to have the lowest serum antibody level to show cross reactivity against allogeneic tumors.

In recent studies using tissue culture cytotoxic techniques, we have been able to show that there appears to be a cytotoxic effect on intraocular choroidal melanoma cells whenever complement is added to the system.[53] By means of indirect and direct immunofluorescent techniques, we now have evidence that there are antibodies to the surface of these melanoma cells that are different than the antibodies to the cytoplasmic contents. These antibodies to the surface of the tumor cells are already present in the primary tumor at the site of the tumor in vivo.[54, 55] It should be kept in mind, however, that there is some cross reactivity between ocular and cutaneous melanomas,[31, 52] and that the studies with cutaneous melanomas are more extensive and clearly suggest that immune mechanisms play a role in the behavior of the disease. Char et al, in 1974, showed that tumor cell membrane antigen injected intradermally in patients with primary choroidal melanomas elicited a cell-mediated skin response.[54]

Inflammatory cells are present at the primary tumor site in less than 20 percent of all uveal melanomas. However, in patients with cutaneous melanomas inflammatory cells are almost routinely found in the primary tumor site and correlate with biologic behavior of the tumor. In patients with disseminated melanoma secondary to an ocular primary growth, the metastatic lesions do not show inflammatory cells. If the immune surveillance system is important in retarding the development and dissemination of the majority of uveal melanomas, the humoral system may play a major role.

The presence of circulating tumor-associated antibodies in patients with primary choroidal melanomas has encouraged the undertaking of experiments to study a possible relationship between the biologic behavior of uveal melanomas and humoral antibodies. Experiments were designed to use immunofluorescent techniques to study the presence or absence of tumor-associated circulating antibodies in patients with uveal melanomas. The primary tumor serves as the source of cells, and that patient's serum serves as the source of human globulin or antibody. Anti-human globulin labeled with fluorescein is used as the marker for a positive reaction.[31] All patients seen at the Oncology Unit of the Retina Service of the Wills Eye Hospital are evaluated. If eyes harboring uveal melanoma are enucleated, the globes are immediately sectioned and the tumor cells are taken for tissue culture studies to provide fresh cells for surface membrane studies; cells are also quick frozen to provide a source for cytoplasmic studies. Both direct and indirect immunofluorescent studies are carried out. Allogeneic studies are done on the serum from all patients, and autologous studies are done in those patients who underwent enucleation.

Indeed, these studies are preliminary, and one cannot be certain whether there is truly any correlation. Further studies to indicate the specificity of these reactions entailed removing the sclera from eye bank eyes and exposing pure beds of normal choroidal melanocytes. With these melanocytes serving as controls, the serum from patients with primary choroidal melanomas did not show any antibody reactions with the normal choroidal melanocytes. There was also no reaction of the serum from normal individuals without melanoma antigens. In another study of serum from 75 patients, it was shown that in the allogeneic situation there was a 77 percent positive reactivity of serum from patients with ocular melanoma to ocular melanoma cells, whereas in patients with cutaneous melanoma there was only a 25 percent positive allogeneic reaction. The serum from patients with breast carcinoma showed a 20 percent positive cross reactivity. While sera from lung, renal, colon, ovarian, and testicular cancer showed varying results, the number of those patients studied was not high enough to allow statistically meaningful results. The studies thus far described involve circulating antibody reactions with the cytoplasmic contents of tumor cells. Studies involving surface membrane antigen–antibody complement-dependent reactions may be more meaningful with regard to the control or dissemination of the disease. Surface membrane studies in this laboratory have been discussed above.

Lewis et al[35] studied surface membrane reactions in melanoma using small tissue culture chambers and serum without complement and demonstrated a slight cytotoxic effect. Elaborating on these findings, we found no cytotoxicity in ocular melanoma cells tested with heat-inactivated serum complement. However, tumor cells incubated with heat-inactivated serum and complement showed a moderate cytotoxicity. These findings seemed confusing at first; then we noticed that only when complement was added did a cytotoxic effect take place. Alternative hypotheses to explain this reaction include the possibilities that (1) the antigen–antibody complex is already present at the primary tumor site and the addition of complement exaggerates the reaction, or (2) this test situation is not adequate and there is some error in the testing and/or findings.

Recently, however, by using the more sophisticated surface membrane immunofluorescent techniques, the direct and indirect immunofluorescent tests were positive for surface membrane antibodies in all patients studied. However, when these cells were trypsinized, which wiped off the antigenic surface, both reactions were negative. After 48 hours, the indirect test remains negative; however, the direct test was consistently positive in the autologous and allogeneic situations. This positive finding indicates that the surface membrane antibodies were already present and coupled to the antigens at the primary tumor site in all patients studied. By removing the antibodies and antigens and allowing the cells to recover for 48 hours, this reaction can be proved specific in the autologous situation; moreover, in all cases studied so far the allogeneic situation is also positive. A cross reactivity to the membrane is present. However, these results do not correlate with findings in skin melanomas.

In another series of experiments, we followed two patients who were treated on several occasions with xenon arc photocoagulation to eradicate their small uveal melanomas. The sera from these patients were tested every week during the course of the treatment over a one-year period. One patient was treated on four occasions, and the other patient was treated five times. Each treatment was considered a separate experiment, and serum was taken before and after treatment. Each serum sample was tested against two different cell lines, and the IgG fraction of the patient's serum showed a significant rise after each treatment. Three patients who received panperipheral xenon arc photocoagulation for diabetic retinopathy were also studied by this technique, and there was no difference in their sera, in regard to tumor-associated antibodies to melanomas, before and after treatment.

CONCLUSION

1. There appears to be a high degree of specificity of tumor-associated antibodies to primary choroidal melanomas, against both the cytoplasmic contents and the cell membrane.
2. The tumor-associated antibodies to the cytoplasmic contents reacted in almost 100 percent of the cases of primary tumors in the autologous situation and approximately 75 percent of the cases in the allogeneic situation. The cell membrane antigens, however, reacted in 100 percent of the cases both in the autologous and the allogeneic situations. Again, we have seen that there are tumor-associated antibodies to the cytoplasmic contents and to the cell membrane surfaces.
3. The cytoplasmic antibodies most probably react in the patient's serum and are only seen with indirect immunofluorescence in vitro.
4. The cell membrane antibodies are already coupled to the antigenic sites at the primary tumor site in the choroid.
5. The cytoplasmic antibody levels in the patient's serum change with tumor cell destruction, as seen in two patients undergoing xenon arc photocoagulation. Therefore, these studies indicate that there is a relationship between tumor-associated circulating antibodies and the primary disease of choroidal melanomas.

How can we use this information in the clinical situation? It is possible to use this test diagnostically since in approximately 75 percent of cases there is an allogeneic positive reaction to the cytoplasmic contents. Therefore, sera from patients with a diagnostic problem can be tested against known melanoma cells. A positive result may be evidence that the patient has a primary melanoma. These studies may also be used as prognostic indicators in patients with melanomas who are being followed up and have or have not undergone enucleation. In patients with primary cutaneous melanomas, the tumor-associated circulating antibody levels fell or disappeared within one month prior to the onset of metastatic disease. If this decrease also occurs with ocular melanomas, the patient may be followed up prognostically with similar studies. If the immunologic surveillance system is important in controlling the dissemination of this disease, perhaps this system can be implemented in the treatment of the disease.

REFERENCES

1. Hogan MJ, Zimmerman LE: Ophthalmic Pathology: An Atlas and Textbook. Philadelphia, Saunders, 1964, p 413
2. Jensen OA: Malignant melanomas of the human uvea. Acta Ophthalmol 48:1113, 1970
3. Zimmerman LE: Intraocular melanomas. Read before the Armed Forces Institute of Pathology course, Ophthalmic Pathology, 1971
4. Callender GR: Malignant melanotic tumor of the eye: a study of histologic types in 111 cases. Trans Am Acad Ophthalmol Otolaryngol 36:131, 1931
5. Callender GR, Wilder HC: Melanomas of the choroid: the prognostic significance of argyrophil fibers. Am J Cancer 25:251, 1935

6. Callender GR, Wilder HC: Malignant melanoma of the choroid. Am J Ophthalmol 22:851, 1939
7. Callender GR, Wilder HC, Ash JE: Five hundred melanomas of the choroid and ciliary body followed five years or longer. Am J Ophthalmol 25:962, 1942
8. Dunphy EB, Forrest AW, Leopold IH, et al: The diagnosis and management of intraocular melanomas. Trans Am Acad Ophthalmol Otolaryngol 62:517, 1958
9. Font RL, Spaulding AG, Zimmerman LE: Diffuse malignant melanomas of the uveal tract: a clinicopathologic report of 54 cases. Trans Am Acad Ophthalmol Otolaryngol 72:877, 1968
10. Sigmund R, Honegger H: Prognosis of melanocytoblastomas of the uvea. Klin Monatsbl Augenheilkd 155:225, 1969
11. Holland G: Pigment tumors of the eye. Tagl Prax 9:431, 1968
12. Benthien H: Clinical course, prognosis and therapy of the malignant melanoma of the uvea: significant correlations between the developmental stage of the tumor and the prognosis could not be established. Klin Monatsbl Augenheilkd 153:4, 1968
13. Kirk HQ, Petty RW: Malignant melanoma of the choroid: a correlation of clinical and histological findings. Arch Ophthalmol 56:843, 1956
14. Newton FH: Malignant melanoma of choroid: report of a case with clinical history of 36 years and follow-up of 32 years. Arch Ophthalmol 73:198, 1965
15. Reese AB: Tumors of the Eye, 2nd ed. New York, Hoeber, 1963, p 241
16. Dobrossy L, Suger J, Toth J: Light and electron microscopic study of malignant melanoma cells, isolated from the peripheral blood. Virchows Arch (Pathol Anat) 345:331, 1968
17. Horodenski J: Investigations on the presence of free cells of malignant melanoma of the uvea in peripheral blood. J Klin Okul 39:407, 1969
18. Gartner J, Nover A: Light and electron microscopic observations in vascular breakthrough of melanoma of the choroid. Ophthalmologica 157:414, 1969
19. Stanford GB, Reese AB: Malignant cells in the blood of eye patients. Trans Am Acad Ophthalmol Otolaryngol 75:102, 1971
20. Reese AB, Archila EA, Jones IS, et al: Necrosis of malignant melanomas of the choroid. Trans Am Ophthalmol Soc 67:31, 1969
21. Reese AB, Archila EA, Jones IS, et al: Necrosis of malignant melanoma of the choroid. Am J Ophthalmol 69:91, 1970
22. Lewis MG: Possible immunological factors in human malignant melanoma in Uganda. Lancet 2:921, 1967
23. McDonald PR: Personal communication, 1973
24. Prehn RT: The immune reaction as a stimulator of tumor growth. Science 176:170, 1972
25. Law LW: Studies of the significance of tumor antigens in induction and repression of neoplastic diseases: presidential address. Cancer Res 29:1, 1969
26. Hellstrom I, Hellstrom KE: Some aspects of the immune defense against cancer: II. In vitro studies of human tumors. Cancer 28:1269, 1971
27. Morton DL, Haskell CM, et al: Recent advances in oncology. Ann Intern Med 77:431, 1972
28. Gleichmann H, Gleichmann E: Immunosuppression and neoplasia: I. A critical review of experimental carcinogenesis and the immune surveillance theory. Klin Wochenschr 51:255, 1973
29. Oettgen HF, Aoki T, Old JL, et al: Suspension culture of a pigment-producing cell line derived from a human malignant melanoma. J Natl Cancer Inst 41:827, 1968
30. Morton DL, Malmgren RA, Holmes EC, et al: Demonstration of antibodies against human malignant melanoma by immunofluorescence. Surgery 64:233, 1968
31. Muna N, Marcus S, Smart C: Detection by immunofluorescence of antibodies specific for human malignant melanoma cells. Cancer 23:88, 1969
32. Romsdahl M, Sebastian I: Human malignant melanoma antibodies demonstrated by immunofluorescence. Arch Surg 100:491, 1970

33. Lewis MG, Ikonopisov RL, Nairn RD: Tumor-specific antibodies in human malignant melanoma and their relationship to the extent of the disease. Br Med J 3:547, 1969

34. Ziegler JL, Lewis MG, Luyombya JMS, et al: Immunologic studies in patients with malignant melanoma in Uganda. Br Med J 23:729, 1969

35. Lewis MG, McCloy E, Blake J: The significance of humoral antibodies in the localization of human malignant melanoma. Br J Surg 60:443, 1973

36. Lewis MG, Phillips TM: The specificity of surface membrane immunofluorescence in human malignant melanoma. Int J Cancer 10:105, 1972

37. Lewis MG, Phillips TM: Separation of two distinct tumor-associated antibodies in the serum of melanoma patients. J Natl Cancer Inst 49:915, 1972

38. Lewis MG, Phillips TM, Cook KB, et al: Possible explanation for loss of detectable antibody in patients with disseminated malignant melanoma. Nature 232:52, 1971

39. Lewis MG, McCloy E, Blake J: The significance of humoral antibodies in the localization of human malignant melanoma. Br J Surg 60:443, 1973

40. Clark WH Jr, From L, Bernardino E, et al: The histogenesis of biologic behavior of primary human malignant melanomas of the skin. Cancer Res 29:705, 1969

41. Clark WH Jr, Mihm MC: Lentigo maligna and lentigo maligna melanoma. Am J Pathol 55:39, 1969

42. Clark WH Jr, Bretton R: A comparative fine structural study of melanogenesis in normal human epidermal melanocytes and in certain human malignant melanoma cells. In Helwig EB (ed): The Skin. Laboratory Investigation International Academy of Pathology monograph, 1971

43. Mihm MC Jr, Clark WH Jr, From L: The clinical diagnosis, classification and histogenetic concepts of the early stages of cutaneous malignant melanomas. N Engl J Med 284:1078, 1971

44. Hellstrom I, Hellstrom KE, Sjogren HO, et al: Demonstration of cell mediated immunity to human neoplasms of various histological types. Int J Cancer 7:1, 1971

45. Jehn UW, Nathanson L, Schwartz RS, et al: In vitro lymphocyte stimulation by a soluble antigen from malignant melanoma. N Engl J Med 283:329, 1970

46. Fossati G, Cognaghi MI, Della Porta G, et al: Cellular and humoral immunity against human malignant melanoma. Int J Cancer 8:344, 1971

47. Nairn RC, Nind APP, Guli EPG, et al: Anti-tumor immunoreactivity in patients with malignant melanomas. Med J Aust 1:397, 1972

48. Howard GM, Spalter HF: Study of autoimmune serologic reactions to ocular melanoma. Arch Ophthalmol 76:399, 1966

49. Hart DRL, Reznikov M, Hughes LE: Cellular resistance to human uveal melanoma. Arch Ophthalmol 79:748, 1968

50. Rahi AHS: Autoimmune reactions in uveal melanoma. Br J Ophthalmol 55:793, 1971

51. Wong IG, Oskvig RM: Identification of antibodies to choroidal melanoma with the indirect immunofluorescent technique, abstract. Association for Research in Vision and Ophthalmology, p 56, 1973

52. Federman JL, Lewis MG, Clark WH: Tumor associated antibodies to ocular and cutaneous malignant melanomas: negative interaction with normal choroidal melanocytes. J Natl Cancer Inst 52:587, 1974

53. Federman JL, Lewis MG, Clark WH, et al: Tumor-associated antibodies in the serum of ocular melanoma patients. Trans Am Acad Ophthalmol Otolaryngol 78: OP784, 1974

54. Char D, Hollingshead A, Cogan D, et al: Cutaneous delayed hypersensitivity reaction to soluble melanoma antigens in patients with ocular malignant melanomas. N Engl J Med 291:274, 1974

55. Federman JL, Clark WH, Lewis MG: Cytotoxicity of choroidal melanoma cells. Read before the Association for Research in Vision and Ophthalmology, 1974

Marcel Frenkel
Jeffrey Rutgard
Anatol Stankevych
Gholam A. Peyman

9 Immunotherapeutic Considerations in Experimental Ocular Tumors

At the University of Illinois Eye and Ear Infirmary, we have initiated a study of the effect of bacillus Calmette-Guerin (BCG) on experimental ocular tumors with a view to possible therapeutic use in human ocular melanomas and retinoblastomas. The current exploratory study deals with the feasibility of using BCG, its tolerance, and its possible toxicity.

BCG is an attenuated live bacillus that has been available since 1921.[1] A variety of strains of varying virulence have been isolated in several countries: in England the Glaxo strain is utilized, and in the United States the Tice vaccine has been more commonly employed. The University of Illinois has developed its own strain of BCG, and it is this strain that we have been using through the courtesy of Dr. Ray G. Crispen.

Over the past 15 years, the possible use of BCG in a number of experimental and human tumors[2,3] has been explored. It has been found that BCG has variable influence in experimental leukemia,[4,5] lymphomas,[6] and sarcomas.[7] It inhibits tumor growth in about 45 percent of instances, while no effect was noted in 45 to 50 percent.[8] It may also reduce immune surveillance and, in fact, enhance tumor growth.[9]

BCG has been found to be effective in the immunotherapy of human cutaneous malignant melanomas by intralesional vaccination; surprisingly, neighboring noninjected lesions have shown regression in 20 percent of instances.[10-13] It has also prolonged survival rates in metastatic melanoma.[14] The vaccine has been reported to be effective in cutaneous metastases of breast carcinoma by direct vaccination and also has been beneficial in the treatment of mycosis fungoides and squamous cell carcinoma.[15,16] The results in lymphatic leukemia and other lymphatic neoplasma are variable and have been the subject of much discussion.[17-19]

The possible antineoplastic effect of BCG relates to tumor size,[20] immune competence of the host,[21] adequate numbers of viable BCG organisms,[22] and proximity of BCG to tumor cells.[23] Experimentally, BCG may be mixed directly with the tumor inoculum.[24] The timing of BCG administration in relation to the induction of tumor is extremely important,[25] as is the relationship of the number of tumor cells and the viability of the tumor prior to the administration of vaccine.[26]

The BCG effect may be due to a stimulation of the immune surveillance system. A systemic, tumor-specific immunity may be enhanced by activation of histiocytes and macrophages.[27] A concentration of thymus-dependent lymphocytes (T-cells) may be released from regional lymph nodes, accumulating within the tumor site. To reduce the tumor load immunotherapy may be combined with chemotherapy clinically.[28, 29] In certain endocrine-dependent tumors hormonal treatment[30] may be useful, and in accessible sites, surgery may reduce the tumor load,[20] as may radiotherapy.[31, 32]

BCG immunotherapy is not an entirely benign procedure. It may cause localized ulceration at the site of injection as well as distant caseating lesions. Fortunately, most of these reactions have been responsive to the usual antituberculous drugs. This local necrotic effect may present an important problem in the eventual therapeutic utilization of this agent in human eyes. Systemic reactions include fever, malaise, erythema nodosum, hepatitis, and anaphylaxis[33] and constitute a considerable problem.

The different strains of BCG vary in their immunotherapeutic capabilities. Cell-mediated immunity appears to be most enhanced by the Pasteur Institute strain and least by the Glaxo series.[34] Studies have also evaluated the effect on tumors of derivatives of BCG vaccine, such as BCG cell walls or cell wall skeletons as opposed to attenuated live organisms.[35, 36] Each modality of treatment introduces a new variable. Integrity of the immune system is most crucial for BCG effect. Tumor patients who are sensitive to dinitrochlorobenzene, a chemical antigen used to demonstrate immune reactivity, have a much better response to BCG inoculation than do those not sensitive to dinitrochlorobenzene.

Our main experimental emphasis has been the determination of BCG tolerance in the animal eye. We have injected BCG subconjunctivally in albino rabbits after scarifying the sclera. In the rabbit's thin sclera, it is not possible to dissect a scleral pouch and vaccinate close to the choroid. This would be an ideal method of administering the vaccine. In order to be effective, an inoculum of 10^6 to 10^8 viable organisms must be delivered. The injections in rabbits have been well tolerated. At 25 days (Fig. 9.1), we have found an accumulation of chronic inflammatory cells in a subconjunctival distribution without penetration through the sclera or involvement of the choroid or ciliary body. The intraocular contents are completely spared. At 25 days, Langhan's giant cells have not yet formed. Animals have received up to three doses of BCG subconjunctivally at weekly intervals without signs of intraocular inflammation or conjunctival necrosis. The anterior and posterior segments have remained perfectly clear of inflammatory reaction. This very fact may present a therapeutic problem since it may not be possible to promote sufficient reaction at the tumor site. Under any circumstance, it is most important to prevent the actual penetration of BCG into the ocular cavity itself, which would create a marked uveitis leading to loss of the eye.

In the human it may be possible to dissect a scleral pouch, vaccinate the sclera close to the choroid, and insert into the pouch a piece of Gelfoam saturated with

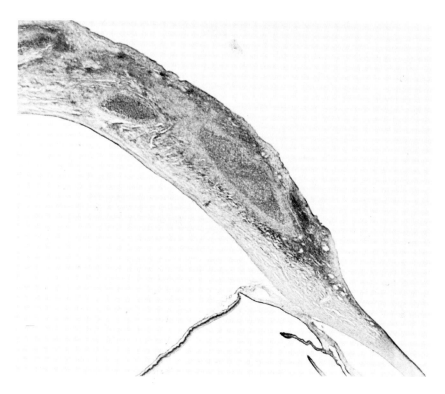

FIG. 9.1. Chronic inflammatory reaction in the subconjunctival space without involvement of intraocular contents at 25 days following subconjunctival injection of BCG. H&E, ×40.

a specific quantity of BCG, thereby delivering vaccine close to the tumor. One of the problems may be the induction of a considerable necrosis of the tumor, which may itself create a marked intraocular reaction leading to loss of the eye due to inflammation.

Another limiting factor in the clinical use of such immunotherapeutic methods may be the large size of the tumor. Conceivably, local therapy by xenon arc photocoagulation or chemotherapy might reduce tumor load and increase the antigenicity of the tumor, thus rendering it amenable to immunotherapy.

Our current experiments involve the inoculation of the V-2 anaplastic tumor in rabbits and the MM 1 melanoma in hamsters directly into the anterior chamber. These tumors infiltrate the iris and then proliferate to fill the globe. They may become grossly hemorrhagic or perforate the sclera. We plan to treat these eyes by subconjunctival injection of BCG at various times in the natural history of the tumor and evaluate any possible differences in tumor growth between treated and control animals.

We hope to show the therapeutic effect of BCG in experimental ocular tumors and subsequently attempt this modality of treatment in humans. The ideal situation would be the treatment of ciliary body melanomas that are proximal to the limbus and may be easily observed.

REFERENCES

1. Guerin C: In Rosenthal SR (ed): The History of BCG: BCG Vaccination Against Tuberculosis. Boston, Little, Brown, 1957, p 48
2. Old LJ, Clarke DA, Benacerraf B: Effect of bacillus Calmette-Guerin infection on transplanted tumours in the mouse. Nature 184:291, 1959
3. Old LJ, Clarke DA, Benacerraf B, et al: Effect of prior splenectomy on the growth of sarcoma 180 in normal and bacillus Calmette-Guerin infected mice. Experientia 18:335, 1962
4. Mathé G, Pouillart P, Lapeyraque F: Active immunotherapy of L1210 leukaemia applied after the graft of tumour cells. Br J Cancer 23:814, 1969
5. Mathé G, Pouillart P, Lapeyraque F: Active immunotherapy of mouse RC 19 and E female K1 leukaemias applied after the intravenous transplantation of the tumour cells. Experientia 27:446, 1971
6. Parr I: Response of syngeneic murine lymphomata to immunotherapy in relation to the antigenicity of the tumour. Br J Cancer 26:174, 1972
7. Rios A, Simmons RL: Comparative effect of Mycobacterium bovis- and neuraminidase-treated tumor cells on the growth of established methyl-cholanthrene fibrosarcomas in syngeneic mice. Cancer Res 32:16, 1972
8. Old LJ, Benacerraf B, Clarke DA, et al: The role of the reticuloendothelial system in the host reaction to neoplasia. Cancer Res 21:1281, 1961
9. Stjernsward J: Immune status of the primary host toward its own methyl-cholanthrene-induced sarcomas. J Natl Cancer Inst 40:13, 1968
10. Morton DL, Eilber FR, Malmgren RA, et al: Immunological factors which influence response to immunotherapy in malignant melanoma. Surgery 68:158, 1970
11. Seigler HF, Shingleton WW, Metzgar RS, et al: Immunotherapy in patients with melanoma. Ann Surg 178:352, 1973
12. Pinsky C, Hirshaut Y, Oettgen H: Treatment of malignant melanoma by intra-tumoral injection of BCG. Proc Am Assoc Cancer Res 13:21, 1972
13. Klein E: Immunotherapy of cancer in man, a reality. Natl Cancer Inst Monogr 39:134, 1973
14. Eilber FR, Morton DL, Carmack Holmes E, Sparks FC, Ramming KP: Immunotherapy with BCG for lymph node metastases from malignant melanoma. N Engl J Med 294:237, 1976
15. Klein E, Holtermann OA: Immunotherapeutic approaches to the management of neoplasms. Natl Cancer Inst Monogr 35:379, 1972
16. Klein E, Holtermann OA, Papermaster B, et al: Immunologic approaches to various types of cancer with the use of BCG and purified protein derivatives. Natl Cancer Inst Monogr 39:229, 1973
17. Mathé G: BCG and cancer immunotherapy. Natl Cancer Inst Monogr 39:107, 1973
18. Treatment of acute lymphoblastic leukaemia: comparison of immunotherapy (BCG), intermittent methotrexate and no therapy after a five-month intensive cytotoxic regimen (Concord trial), preliminary report to the Medical Research Council by the Leukaemia Committee and the Working Party on Leukaemia in Childhood. Br Med J 4:189, 1971
19. Heyn R, Borges W, Joo P, et al: BCG in the treatment of acute lymphocytic leukemia (ALL). Proc Am Assoc Cancer Res 14:45, 1973
20. Zbar B, Bernstein ID, Bartlett GL, et al: Immunotherapy of cancer: regression of intradermal tumors and prevention of growth of lymph node metastases after intra-lesional injection of living Mycobacterium bovis. J Natl Cancer Inst 41:119, 1972
21. Keast D: Immunosurveillance and cancer. Lancet 2:710, 1970
22. Sher NA, Pearson JW, Chaparas SD, et al: Effect of three strains of BCG against a murine leukemia after drug therapy. J Natl Cancer Inst 51:2001. 1973
23. Zbar B, Bernstein ID, Rapp HJ: Suppression of tumor growth at the site of infection with living bacillus Calmette-Guerin. J Natl Cancer Inst 46:831, 1971

24. Tokunaga T, Kataoka T, Nakamura RM, et al: Tumor immunity induced by BCG-tumor cell mixtures in syngeneic mice. Jpn J Med Sci Biol 26:71, 1973
25. Bansal SC, Sjogren HO: Effects of BCG on various facets of the immune response against polyoma tumors in rats. Int J Cancer 11:162, 1973
26. Zbar B, Ribi E, Rapp HJ: An experimental model for immunotherapy of cancer. Natl Cancer Inst Monogr 39:3, 1973
27. Seeger RC, Oppenheim JJ: Macrophage-bound antigens: I. Induction of delayed hypersensitivity and priming for production of serum antibodies in guinea-pigs. J Immunol 109:244, 1972
28. Amiel JL, Berardet M: An experimental model of active immunotherapy preceded by cytoreductive chemotherapy. Eur J Cancer 6:557, 1970
29. Pearson WJ, Pearson GR, Gibson WT, et al: Combined chemoimmunostimulation therapy against murine leukemia. Cancer Res 33:904, 1972
30. Piessens WF, Heimann R, Legros N, et al: Effects of bacillus Calmette-Guerin (BCG) infection on residual disease of the rat mammary tumor after ovariectomy. Eur J Cancer 7:377, 1971
31. Yron J, Weiss DW, Robinson E, et al: Immunotherapeutic studies in mice with MER fraction of BCG: studies with solid tumors. Natl Cancer Inst Monogr 39:33, 1973
32. Haddow A, Alexander P: An immunological method of increasing the sensitivity of primary sarcomas to local irradiation with x-rays. Lancet 1:452, 1964
33. Aungst CW, Sokal JE, Jager BV: Complications of BCG vaccination. Proc Am Assoc Cancer Res 14:108, 1973
34. Mansell PWA, Krementz ET: Reactions to BCG. JAMA 226:1570, 1973
35. Azuma I, Ribi EE, Meyer TJ, et al: Biologically active components from mycobacterial cell walls: I. Isolation and composition of cell wall skeleton and component P3. J Natl Cancer Inst 52:95, 1974
36. Pinsky CM, Harshauf Y, Oettgen HF: Treatment of malignant melanoma by intratumoral injection of BCG. Natl Cancer Inst Monogr 39:225, 1973

Frederick H. Davidorf
Janet R. Lang

10 Immunology and Immunotherapy of Malignant Uveal Melanomas

When counseling a patient with ocular malignant melanoma, the ophthalmologist must be aware of the natural history of this disease. In the course of a recent follow-up study of patients with malignant melanoma of the choroid, we found that 47 percent of the ophthalmologists whose patients had subsequently died of metastases were unaware that their patients had developed metastatic disease.[1] Thus, the prognosis is probably worse than most ophthalmologists realize.

Until recently, treatments for metastatic melanoma offered little more than palliation, and most patients died within one year of the clinical appearance of metastases. However, recent successes with the use of immunotherapy for metastatic cutaneous melanomas indicate that it may be time for serious consideration of this type of adjunctive therapy for ocular melanomas.

The prognosis for any given patient can be fairly accurately determined using the combined criteria of tumor cell type, tumor size, and presence of extrabulbar extension (Figs. 10.1, 10.2). The categories with the poorest prognosis include all large epithelioid and necrotic tumors, large mixed tumors with extrabulbar extensions, and orbital recurrences. Our studies indicate that 90 percent of patients in these categories will probably die of metastases within five years.[1]

The clinician depends on the basic scientist to unravel the mysteries of disease processes, while the practical application of these discoveries lies in the hands of the clinician. In this chapter we examine the rationale for adjunctive therapy in patients with malignant melanoma. We will focus on immunotherapy since previous experience with radiotherapy and chemotherapy has shown that the last two procedures have little curative effect on metastatic melanoma. The following essential questions will be considered: What is the evidence that immune mechanisms influence the natural course of uveal melanoma? What have clinical and laboratory studies revealed about the interactions of host immunity and ocular

This project was supported in part by the Medical Research Service, Veterans Administration, and by USPHS Grant 5-PO1-CA-16058-02 from the National Cancer Institute.

119

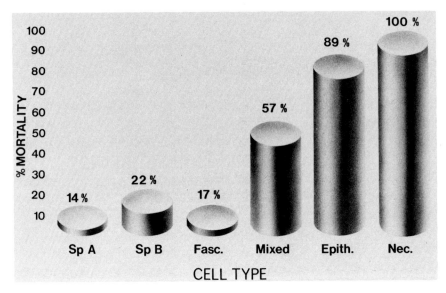

FIG. 10.1. Five-year mortality for patients with choroidal melanomas larger than 10 mm in diameter and 3 mm in elevation. Patients who died during the five-year follow-up period of causes other than metastatic melanoma were excluded from the percentages.

melanoma? What immunotherapeutic regimens have been used in the treatment of cutaneous melanomas, how effective are they, and are they also applicable to ocular melanoma patients?

IMMUNOLOGY AND NEOPLASIA

A rapidly growing body of knowledge correlates the immunologic competence of the host with the growth of a tumor and its ability to metastasize. Not only are malignant cells different from normal cells morphologically, they also contain antigens, some of which are tumor associated. While tumor immunology is still in its infancy, it has been shown that some tumors are antigenic and capable of inducing an immune response. This response involves both antibody production and immune cell proliferation.

Antibody production is induced by the growth of an antigenic tumor, and there are many techniques for detecting these antibodies in vitro. Antibodies are complex protein molecules produced by plasma cells and B-lymphocytes. Antibody-mediated mechanisms are referred to as the humoral branch of the immune system. These antibodies probably operate via the bloodstream by destroying circulating antigens (Fig. 10.3A).

The second type of immune response is mediated by sensitized lymphocytes and is referred to as cell-mediated immunity. Cellular immunity is probably active at the site of solid tumors, rather than in the general circulation. In the presence of antigen, T-lymphocytes develop receptor sites on their surfaces that are specific for the antigen. The antigen binds to the receptor sites on a sensitized T-lymphocyte,

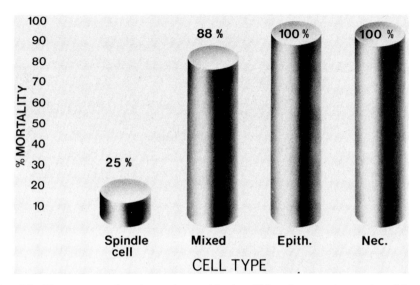

FIG. 10.2. Five-year mortality for patients with choroidal melanomas larger than 10 mm in diameter and 3 mm in elevation that also showed extrabulbar extension.

and the lymphocyte is stimulated to secrete products collectively called lymphokines. These products include: migration inhibition factor, which prevents leukocytes from leaving the area surrounding the antigen; blastogenic factor, which stimulates more lymphocytes to become sensitized; and lymphotoxin, which lyses cells (Fig. 10.3B).

IMMUNOLOGY AND OCULAR MALIGNANT MELANOMA

The spontaneous regression of malignant melanoma[2-4] and the appearance of metastases many years after excision of the primary tumor[5] have often been cited as indirect evidence that immune mechanisms play an important role in the course of both cutaneous and ocular melanomas. In recent years a number of techniques have been developed for the study of specific phases of host immunity to neoplasia. Cutaneous melanomas have been intensively studied, perhaps more than any other human malignancy, with regard to both humoral and cellular immunity. Some of these techniques have also been applied to the study of ocular melanomas. Results of investigations on ocular melanomas thus far parallel results obtained in investigations of cutaneous melanomas, and most investigators agree that the tumors are closely related in their ability to evoke an immune response.

Humoral Immunity

The sera of patients with both ocular and cutaneous melanomas contain melanoma-associated antibodies.[6-12] Tumor-specific antibodies can be formed in response to tumor-associated antigens, both in the cytoplasm of the neoplastic cell and on the cell surface (Fig. 10.4). Antibodies can bind to tumor antigens and

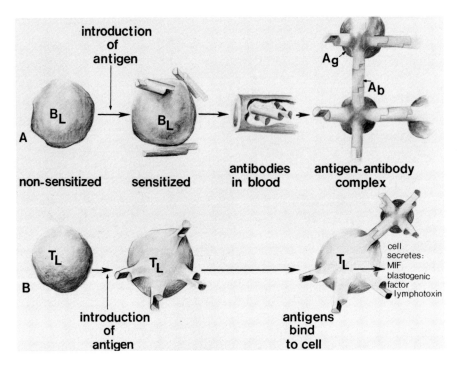

FIG. 10.3. Mechanisms of humoral and cellular immunity. **A.** Humoral immunity. Following the introduction of antigen, B-lymphocytes and plasma cells produce antibodies specific to the given antigen. These antibodies are secreted into the bloodstream and are capable of complexing with the specific antigen. **B.** Cellular immunity. T-lymphocytes form specific surface receptor sites in the presence of antigen. The sensitized lymphocytes can attach to antigen and are stimulated to secrete various soluble factors that lead to destruction of antigen.

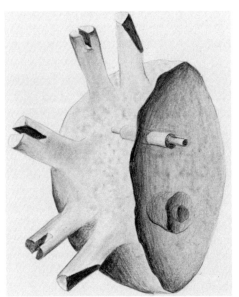

FIG. 10.4. Melanoma cells are characterized by tumor-associated antigens both in the cytoplasm and on the cell membrane.

lysis may occur in the presence of complement (Fig. 10.5A). There is cross reactivity (indicating common antigens) between patients with ocular and cutaneous melanoma,[6, 8] but not between melanoma patients and patients with most other neoplasms.[6, 13]

Cellular Immunity

Experimental work indicates that cellular immunity is a host's major defense against solid tumors, and that it acts primarily at the tumor site. Like humoral immunity, cellular immunity depends on the recognition of tumor-associated antigens, but in the case of cellular immunity the cytotoxic response is mediated by the sensitized lymphocyte. The lymphocytes sensitized to a specific tumor antigen attach to the neoplastic cell at the site of the antigen. This action stimulates the lymphocytes to secrete lymphokines, resulting in the death of the tumor cell (Fig. 10.5B).

TESTS OF CELLULAR IMMUNITY. Delayed hypersensitivity (skin testing) is the only in vivo test of specific cellular immunity. It involves intradermal injection of antigen and observation of the induration at a specified interval (usually 48 hours) following inoculation. Patients tested with a given antigen must also be tested with standard recall antigens to determine whether anergy, if it exists, is general or selective.

There are a variety of in vitro tests of cellular immunity, the most important and widely used of which are (1) lymphocyte-mediated cytotoxicity, (2) lympho-

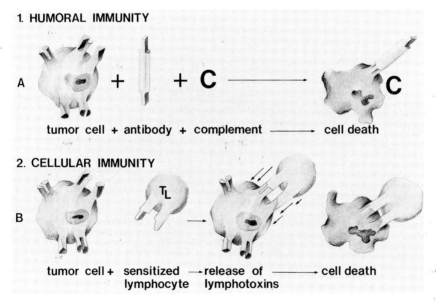

1. HUMORAL IMMUNITY

A

tumor cell + antibody + complement ———→ cell death

2. CELLULAR IMMUNITY

B

tumor cell + sensitized ——→ release of ————→ cell death
              lymphocyte   lymphotoxins

FIG. 10.5. Mechanisms of immunity to neoplastic cells. **A.** Humoral immunity. Tumor-specific antibodies complex with tumor antigen, and lysis occurs in the presence of complement. **B.** Cellular immunity. T-lymphocytes sensitized to tumor-associated antigens attach to the tumor cells, resulting in the release of soluble factors that lead to the death of the tumor cell.

blast transformation, and (3) leukocyte migration inhibition. Numerous technical variations of each are employed.

Lymphocyte-mediated cytotoxicity measures the ability of a patient's lymphocytes to destroy target tumor cells in culture. A known number of lymphocytes is added to a known number of target cells. After a specified incubation interval, the lymphocytes are washed off and the remaining live tumor cells are counted with the use of supravital stains or radioactive markers.

Lymphoblast transformation measures the ability of patient lymphocytes to transform into blast cells (thought to be precursors of cytotoxic "killer" lymphocytes) in the presence of tumor antigen. Blast cells are counted by measuring the uptake of radioactive-labeled thymidine, uridine, or amino acids.

Leukocyte migration inhibition results from the release of migration inhibition factor from sensitized lymphocytes in the presence of tumor antigen. This cell product prevents leukocytes from leaving the area surrounding the antigen. The degree of migration inhibition is assayed either by migration from capillary tubes or by migration from cell suspensions in semisolid media.

All of these tests have been used to demonstrate cell-mediated immunity in cutaneous melanoma patents. Only delayed hypersensitivity testing and leukocyte migration inhibition have demonstrated cell-mediated immunity in ocular melanoma patients.

INDICATIONS OF CELLULAR IMMUNITY TO OCULAR MELANOMA. *Delayed Hypersensitivity and Leukocyte Migration Inhibition.* The available information on results of delayed hypersensitivity in ocular melanoma patients was reviewed in Chapter 7. The study of cellular immunity using a leukocyte migration inhibition assay was also discussed.

Lymphocyte-Mediated Cytotoxicity. The cytotoxic action of immune cells on neoplastic cells in culture is thought to be somewhat analogous to the immune response to malignancy in vivo. From observations with phase microscopy and transmission electron microscopy, it seems likely that the attacking immune cells become adherent to the target neoplastic cells, secreting toxins that kill the target cells. We have used the scanning electron microscope (SEM) to study the interaction between choroidal melanoma cells in culture and cytotoxic immune cells.

Melanoma cells were cultured on plastic culture plates. Peripheral blood samples were collected from patients with various stages of melanoma and from normal subjects. The blood was defibrinated and lymphocytes and monocytes were collected. Lymphocytes and monocytes were added to target melanoma culture plates in the ratio of 150 immune cells to each target melanoma cell. Control melanoma plates were maintained to which no immune cells were added. Following periods of incubation of 12 to 72 hours, the medium was poured off and the plates were fixed for scanning electron microscopy. Morphologic changes induced by immune cells were correlated with the degree of cell-mediated cytotoxicity measured quantitatively by means of a radioactive uptake assay.

Malignant melanoma cells in culture have characteristically smooth surfaces with elongated cytoplasmic processes extending two to five times the diameter of the main body of the cell. The nuclear area can be identified as an elevated region in the center of the cell body (Fig. 10.6, large arrow). The cells are attached to the

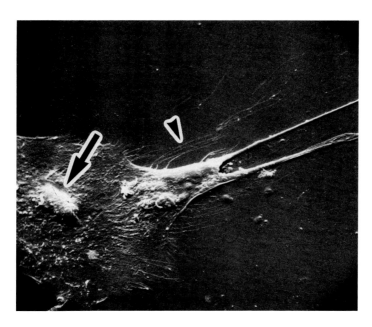

FIG. 10.6. Morphologic composition of ocular melanoma cells in culture. The cytoplasmic surface is fairly smooth, and long cytoplasmic extensions are common. A central raised area (large arrows) marks the nuclear area. The cell is anchored to the plate by means of minute pseudopodia (arrowhead). SEM, ×1050.

plate by numerous minute pseudopodia (Fig. 10.6, arrowhead). Dying melanoma cells withdraw their cytoplasmic extensions, lose their pseudopodia, and detach from the plate.

Viewed with the scanning electron microscope, lymphocytes are spherical cells with villous surfaces. Various lymphocyte morphologies can be seen on the same specimen and on the same target cell (Figs. 10.7–10.9). It is unlikely that morphologic differences in these specimens are due to preparation artifacts; various mitotic stages of lymphocytes may be represented. Monocytes are characteristically less spherical, and their surfaces are ruffled (Fig. 10.10). Melanoma cells with adherent lymphocytes and monocytes develop numerous microvilli on their surfaces (Fig. 10.11, arrow); this effect may be a reaction of the target cell to cytotoxic substances secreted by the immune cells. The degree of cytotoxicity (measured by a radioactive assay) demonstrated by various patients correlates well with both the presence of adherent lymphocytes and the occurrence of degenerative changes in the target melanoma cells observed with scanning electron microscopy.

Lymphocytic Infiltration. It is generally held that cellular immunity is the most important aspect of the host's response when considering the immunology of solid tumors. Lymphocytic infiltration in a tumor may be a measure of the host's cellular immune response to this tumor. Lymphocytic infiltration at a tumor site has been associated with an improved prognosis in many neoplasms.[14–20] Tritsch[21] has found that intense lymphocytic infiltration at the periphery of a cutaneous melanoma is a favorable prognostic sign. Spontaneous regression of cutaneous mel-

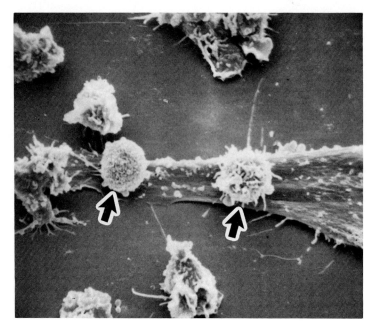

FIG. 10.7. Lymphocytes and monocytes are adherent to melanoma cells. Two distinct morphologic forms of lymphocytes are adherent to the central melanoma cell (arrows). SEM, ×1900. (From Lang et al: Scanning Electron Microscopy, vol 2. Chicago, ITT Research Institute, 1976)

anomas and regression induced by immunotherapy are associated with intense round cell infiltration.[22, 23] Reese et al[3] and Rahi[10] advanced the theory that inflammation surrounding a choroidal melanoma is an indication of the host's attempt to destroy the tumor.

In reviewing the histopathologic characteristics of ocular melanomas, lymphocytic infiltration was observed in 18.6 percent (54 of 291) of the cases examined (Figs. 10.12–10.14). We attempted to determine whether the presence of intense or moderate lymphocytic infiltration had any effect on the prognosis. Cases demonstrating both necrosis and lymphocytic infiltration were counted as a separate group since it could not be determined whether the necrosis had preceded the lymphocytic infiltration or vice versa.

In evaluating the effect of lymphocytic infiltration on prognosis, other factors known to influence prognosis must also be taken into consideration. Since the tumors with infiltration were primarily large mixed and epithelioid tumors without extrabulbar extension, these must be compared to a similar group of tumors not showing lymphocytic infiltration. Of 15 patients with large mixed or epithelioid tumors with lymphocytic infiltration, 5 (33.3 percent) died of metastatic melanoma within five years. Of 25 comparable patients not demonstrating lymphocytic infiltration, 15 (60 percent) died of metastatic melanoma. Although these data suggest that lymphocytic infiltration is a favorable prognostic sign, the difference is not statistically significant ($0.10 < p < 0.20$).

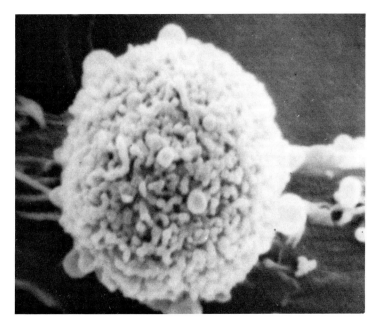

FIG. 10.8. High-power view of lymphocyte on the left in Figure 10.7. Villi are short and convoluted. SEM, ×95000. (From Lang et al: Scanning Electron Microscopy, vol 2. Chicago, ITT Research Institute, 1976)

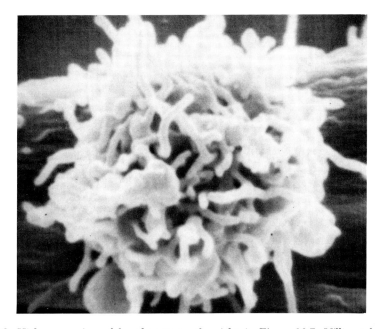

FIG. 10.9. High-power view of lymphocyte on the right in Figure 10.7. Villi are longer and straighter. SEM, ×9500. (From Lang et al: Scanning Electron Microscopy, vol 2. Chicago, ITT Research Institute, 1976)

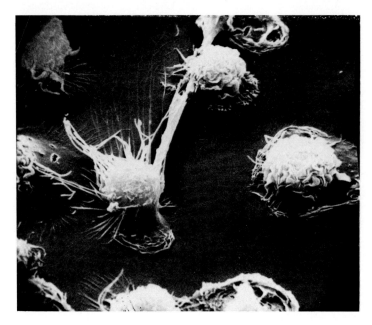

FIG. 10.10. Monocytes are characterized by surface ruffles rather than villi. In this photograph, the monocytes are adherent to the culture plate. SEM, ×2100.

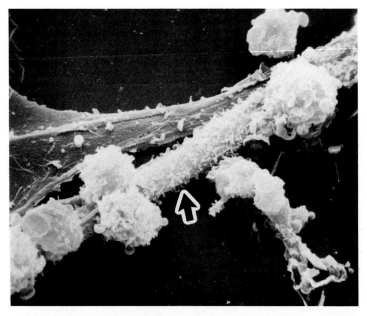

FIG. 10.11. Two adjacent melanoma cells exhibit different cytoplasmic characteristics. The melanoma cell with adherent lymphocytes has developed numerous microvilli on the cytoplasmic surface (arrow). The adjacent cell is comparatively smooth. SEM, ×2000.

IMMUNOTHERAPY OF MALIGNANT MELANOMA

Malignant melanomas are among a group of human tumors demonstrating convincing evidence of interaction with immune mechanisms. The documentation of spontaneous regression, the appearance of metastatic disease 15 or more years after complete resection of the tumor, and the observation of lymphocytic infiltration surrounding some melanomas provide indirect evidence of immunologic factors. Direct evidence of immunologic effects in melanoma patients has recently been demonstrated with the identification of melanoma-associated antibodies and the demonstration of cellular immunity in vivo and in vitro.

Experimental models have demonstrated that immunologic mechanisms are likely to be more effective with a small tumor cell population. The clinical application of this finding is to combine immunotherapy with surgical resection of the tumor for maximum effectiveness. A useful clinical situation for evaluating the immune response to a given neoplasm is one in which the immune mechanisms are known to be operative in response to the neoplasm in question and the primary tumor can be completely resected, thus reducing tumor cell burden. Ocular melanomas fulfill these two criteria admirably; they provide a human system that may yield information that can later be generalized to other neoplasms. A consideration of the various methods of immunotherapy used in the treatment of cutaneous melanoma will provide a starting point for possible modes of immunotherapy useful in the treatment of ocular melanomas.

A variety of melanoma-specific immunotherapeutic approaches have been tried in the treatment of cutaneous malignant melanoma. Currie et al[24] immunized 12 patients, all of whom had some degree of metastatic spread, with their own cobalt-60-irradiated melanoma cells. The patients were subcutaneously injected with 3 to 5×10^8 autologous melanoma cells in at least five sites involving all limbs. There was no evidence that this procedure altered the course of the disease other than effecting a transient (one- to two-week) increase in cytotoxic lymphocytes.

Other tumor-specific methods that have been tried with varying degrees of success include cross transplantation of melanoma cells and sensitized lymphocytes,[25] blood transfusions from melanoma patients who have had spontaneous remissions, [2, 26] and injections of transfer factor from patients who recovered from malignant melanoma, close relatives, and black persons.[27]

Nonspecific augmentation of cellular immunity has proved more effective in the treatment of cutaneous melanoma. Roenigh et al[28] injected vaccinia virus into cutaneous metastatic melanoma nodules. Increased survival time was observed in eight patients with stage II metastatic melanomas. Complete remissions occurred in three patients. Favorable responses to vaccinia virus were associated with increased levels of cytotoxicity to melanoma target cells.

Seigler et al[29] have treated 142 patients with a combination of BCG intratumor injection and inoculation with their own irradiated neuraminidase-treated tumor cells. There were complete remissions (as long as 3½ years) in 23 percent of the patients. Those patients who were helped by immunotherapy were those with metastases confined to the skin, subcutaneous tissue, and lymph nodes.

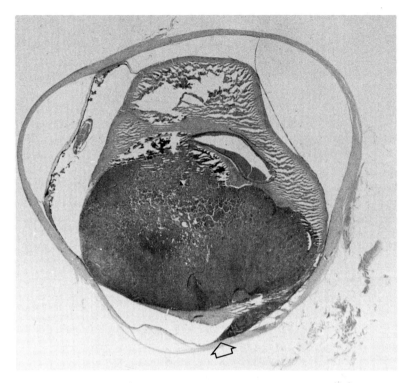

FIG. 10.12. Tumors with lymphocytic infiltration usually show a dense infiltration at the tumor base, especially at the periphery of the lesion (arrow). H&E, ×4.3.

For nonspecific stimulation of the cellular immune system in patients with cutaneous malignant melanoma, BCG alone has been the most successful method of immunotherapy to date. Injection of BCG into melanoma nodules has produced regression of the injected nodules.[22] The view that this regression results from nonspecific stimulation of cellular immunity, rather than a direct BCG antitumor effect, is supported by the following evidence. First, regression of noninjected nodules was observed in many cases. Second, histopathologic examination of completely regressed nodules revealed an intense lymphocytic and mononuclear infiltration and no remaining tumor cells. This inflammatory infiltrate was also observed in biopsies of regressed noninjected nodules. Third, BCG had no beneficial effect in patients who were generally anergic.

Gutterman et al[30] have reported a series of patients with unresectable disseminated metastatic melanoma treated with intravenous dimethyl triazeno imidazole carboxamide and BCG by scarification. There were partial or complete remissions in 27 percent of the patients, including 6 percent complete remissions. Improved immunocompetence, as measured by skin tests to standard recall antigens, was correlated with improved clinical status. Thus far, there have been no reported studies on immunotherapy of ocular melanoma.

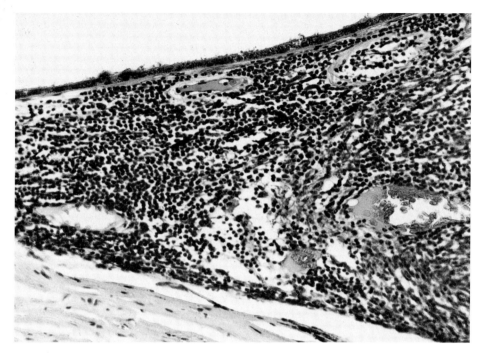

FIG. 10.13. Area located by arrow in Figure 10.12. There is an intense infiltration of lymphocytes at the tumor periphery. H&E, ×344. (From Lang et al: The prognostic significance of lymphocytic infiltration in malignant melanoma of the choroid. Cancer, in press)

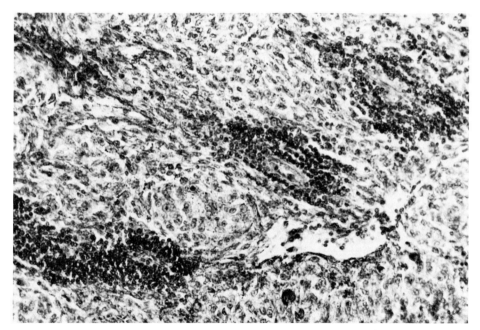

FIG. 10.14. Another common pattern of lymphocytic infiltration occurs surrounding the tumor vessels. H&E, ×344. (From Lang et al: The prognostic significance of lymphocytic infiltration in malignant melanoma of the choroid. Cancer, in press)

131

CONCLUSION

The mechanisms by which the host immune system affects the growth of a tumor are currently defined. A number of immunologic factors are functioning in a patient with a choroidal melanoma, and as knowledge increases there are greater opportunities for manipulation of the immune response. Many laboratory studies are now available that can measure the changing aspects of antibody and cellular immunity during the course of therapy. At the present time, nonspecific stimulation of cellular immunity using BCG has been the most effective treatment for cutaneous melanoma. However, there is little information concerning this therapy in ocular melanomas.

Through the study of the natural course of malignant melanoma of the choroid treated with enucleation, several categories can be identified that have especially grave prognoses. To date little attention has been directed to adjunctive treatment of ocular melanomas following removal of the primary tumor. Perhaps it is time for the ophthalmologist to initiate consultation with the oncologist concerning adjunctive therapy, especially in those patients harboring the highly malignant types of ocular melanomas.

ACKNOWLEDGMENT

We thank Judith I. Willis, Ph.D., for the design of the in vitro SEM experiments, Donald A. Keller for providing the illustrations, and Douglas D. Sharpnack for providing technical assistance.

REFERENCES

1. Davidorf FH, Lang JR: The natural history of malignant melanoma of the choroid: small vs. large tumors. Trans Am Acad Ophthalmol Otolaryngol 79:310, 1975
2. Sumner WC, Foraker AC: Spontaneous regression of human melanoma: clinical and experimental studies. Cancer 13:79, 1960
3. Reese AB, Archila EA, Jones IS, et al: Necrosis of malignant melanoma of the choroid. Am J Ophthalmol 69:91, 1970
4. Jensen OA, Andersen SR: Spontaneous regression of a malignant melanoma of the choroid. Acta Ophthalmol 52:173, 1974
5. Wilber DL, Hartman HR: Malignant melanoma with delayed metastatic growths. Ann Intern Med 5:201, 1931
6. Muna NM, Marcus S, Smart C: Detection by immunofluorescence of antibodies specific for human malignant melanoma cells. Cancer 23:88, 1969
7. Nairn RC, Nind APP, Guli EPG, et al: Antitumor immunoreactivity in patients with malignant melanoma. Med J Aust 1:397, 1972
8. Wong IG, Oskvig RM: Immunofluorescent detection of antibodies to ocular melanoma. Arch Ophthalmol 92:98, 1974
9. Rahi AHS: Autoimmune reactions in uveal melanoma. Br J Ophthalmol 55:793, 1971
10. Rahi AHS: Immunologic aspects of malignant melanoma of the choroid. Trans Ophthalmol Soc UK 93:79, 1973
11. Federman JL, Lewis MG, Clark WH, et al: Tumor-associated antibodies in the serum of ocular melanoma patients. Trans Am Acad Ophthalmol Otolaryngol 78:784, 1974

12. Bodurtha AJ, Chee DO, Laucius JF, et al: Clinical and immunologic significance of human melanoma cytotoxic antibody. Cancer Res 35:189, 1975
13. Wood GW, Barth RF: Immunofluorescent studies of serologic reactivity of patients with malignant melanoma against tumor-associated cytoplasmic antigens. J Natl Cancer Inst 53:309, 1974
14. Black MM, Opler SR, Speer FD: Microscopic structure of gastric carcinomas and their regional lymph nodes in relation to survival. Surg Gynecol Obstet 98:725, 1954
15. Zamcheck N, Doos WG, Prudente R, et al: Prognostic factors in colon carcinoma: correlation of serum carcinoembryonic antigen levels and tumor histopathology. Human Pathol 6:31, 1975
16. DiPaola M, Angelini L, Berolotti A, et al: Host resistance in relation to survival in breast cancer. Br Med J 4:268, 1974
17. Akazaki K: Some problems in the pathologic histology of carcinoma of the cervix, with special consideration of its relationship to prognosis. Gann 44:401, 1953
18. Martin RF, Beckwith JB: Lymphoid infiltrates in neuroblastomas: their occurrence and prognostic significance. J Pediatr Surg 3:161, 1968
19. Mancini RE, Andrada JA, Saraceni D, et al: Immunological and testicular response in man sensitized with human testicular homogenate. J Clin Endocrinol 25:859, 1965
20. Lukes RJ, Butler JJ, Hicks EB: Natural history of Hodgkin's disease as related to its pathologic picture. Cancer 19:317, 1966
21. Tritsch H: Studies on relation between inflammatory infiltration, cell type, and prognosis in malignant melanoma. Arch Dermatol Forsch 244·222, 1972
22. Morton DL, Eilber FR, Malmgren RA, et al: Immunological factors which influence response to immunotherapy in malignant melanoma. Surgery 68:158, 1970
23. Lloyd OC: Regression of malignant melanoma as a manifestation of a cellular immunity response. Proc R Soc Med 62:9, 1969
24. Currie GA, LeJeune F, Hamilton-Fairley G: Immunization with irradiated tumor cells and specific lymphocyte cytotoxicity in malignant melanoma. Br Med J 2:305, 1971
25. Brandes LJ, Galton DAG, Wiltshaw E: New approach to immunotherapy of melanoma. Lancet 2:293, 1971
26. Symes MO, Riddell AG, Immelman EJ, et al: Immunologically competent cells in the treatment of malignant disease. Lancet 1:1054, 1968
27. Price FB, Hewlett JS, Deodhar SD, et al: The therapy of malignant melanoma with transfer factor: a preliminary report. Cleve Clin Q 41:1, 1974
28. Roenigh HH, Deodhar S, St. Jacques R, et al: Immunotherapy of malignant melanoma with vaccinia virus. Arch Dermatol 109:668, 1974
29. Seigler HF, Shingleton WW, Metzgar RS, et al: Immunotherapy in patients with melanoma. Ann Surg 178:352, 1973
30. Gutterman JU, Mavligit G, Gottlieb JA, et al: Chemoimmunotherapy of disseminated malignant melanoma with dimethyl triazeno imidazole carboxamide and bacillus Calmette-Guerin. N Engl J Med 291:592, 1974

Frederick H. Davidorf

11 Radiotherapy and Diathermy of Malignant Melanoma of the Choroid

In spite of the fact that 95 percent of all choroidal melanomas are completely resected with enucleation,[1] about one-third of the patients with tumors localized within the eye die of metastases within five years. Thus, removal of the tumor with enucleation does not prevent metastases in many cases, and a less traumatic treatment would be beneficial so long as it did not result in increased mortality. It was this thought that stimulated our interest in conservative treatment of choroidal melanomas.[2-5] Initially, conservative treatment was considered only in patients who refused enucleation or in individuals who were blind in the fellow eye.

Conservative management of malignant melanoma of the choroid remains a controversial topic due to the elusiveness of the factors governing metastatic spread and the difficulty of assessing the efficacy of conservative treatment. Numerous types of conservative treatment have been used in the management of choroidal melanomas, including radiotherapy, diathermy, photocoagulation, and en bloc excision. In this report, we will examine the clinical results of 22 patients treated with radon rings and 4 patients treated with diathermy. We will also discuss the histologic changes seen in 9 radon-treated eyes that were subsequently enucleated.

RADIOTHERAPY OF CHOROIDAL MELANOMAS

Radiotherapy has been used since 1939 in the treatment of choroidal melanomas.[6] Radon seed explants, cobalt plaques, and ^{106}Ru/^{106}Rh beta-ray applicators have all been used to deliver the radiation to the tumor, and nearly 200 cases have been reported to date.[6-11]

Method

Patients are carefully evaluated prior to the initiation of any conservative therapy. The recommended preoperative evaluation includes fundus drawings, fundus photographs, fluorescein angiography, B-scan ultrasonography, and a complete medical work-up. In this series of 22 patients treated with radon rings,

This project was supported in part by the Medical Research Service, Veterans Administration, and by USPHS Grant 5-PO1-CA-16058-02 from the National Cancer Institute.

135

the ages of the patients at insertion ranged from 22 to 75 years, with a mean age of 52.7 years. Six patients had refused enucleation. One patient had counting-fingers vision in the fellow eye due to macular degeneration, and one patient had 20/100 vision in the fellow eye due to a macular cyst. The remaining 14 patients were treated conservatively because their tumors were small and the vision was normal in the affected eye.

Radiation from an external port is of little use in the treatment of ocular tumors since the doses necessary are too damaging to adjacent structures. Thus, the method of choice has been to suture a radioactive applicator to the sclera overlying the tumor (Fig. 11.1). We use radon gas encapsulated in gold seeds as the source of radiation. Radon gas undergoes radioactive decay, producing alpha, beta, and gamma radiation. The wall of the gold seed absorbs alpha and beta radiation, allowing gamma rays to pass (Fig. 11.2). The calculations of dose are concerned only with gamma radiation in relation to the diameter and height of the lesion to be treated.[12] These calculations are done preoperatively by the radiotherapist, who is given an accurate estimate of tumor diameter and elevation. The radiation dose delivered is 8,000 to 10,000 rads to the tumor apex and 20,000 to 25,000 rads to the tumor base (Fig. 11.3).

The radiotherapist designs an applicator that will overlap the edges of the tumor by 1 to 2 mm when sutured to the sclera, thus providing a margin of safety around the tumor. Radon seeds are uniformly distributed around the circumference of an applicator ring fashioned of 20-gauge polyethylene tubing. An empty mold of the same dimensions is also made. Both molds are gas sterilized and delivered in a lead container to the operating room.

With the patient under either local or general anesthesia, a conjunctival and Tenon's capsule incision is made in the quadrant overlying the tumor. Extraocular muscles are tenotomized as necessary, and bare sclera is exposed. Using indirect

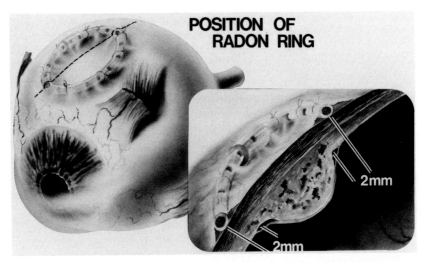

FIG. 11.1. The radon ring is sutured to the sclera overlying the tumor. (From Davidorf et al: Trans Am Acad Ophthalmol Otolaryngol, 81:849, 1976)

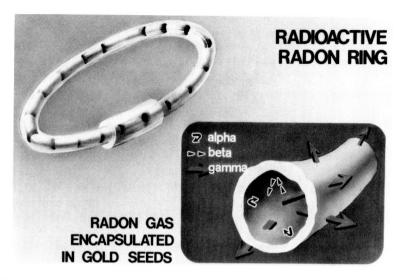

FIG. 11.2. Radon gas emits alpha, beta, and gamma radiation. Only gamma rays are able to penetrate the wall of the gold seed, and dosimetry calculations are concerned only with gamma radiation. (From Davidorf et al: Trans Am Acad Ophthalmol Otolaryngol, 81:849, 1976)

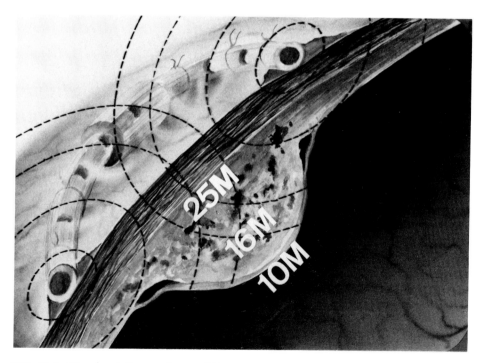

FIG. 11.3. The ring delivers a dose of 8000 to 10,000 rads to the tumor apex and 20,000 to 25,000 rads to the tumor base. (From Davidorf et al: Trans Am Acad Ophthalmol Otolaryngol, 81:849, 1976)

ophthalmoscopy and forceps localization, the tumor margins are located and marked on the sclera (Fig. 11.4). Three 4-0 Dacron anchoring sutures are placed in the sclera. The "dummy" polyethylene tube is loosely sutured to the sclera to ensure that no problems will arise when the active ring is put into place (Fig. 11.5). The active unit is then removed from its lead shield and firmly sutured to the sclera (Fig. 11.6). Tenotomized muscles are reattached to their insertions, and Tenon's capsule and the conjunctiva are closed in two layers.

Using radiation monitors attached to the surgeon's index fingers, we have measured the irradiation received during the surgical procedure. Dosimetry reports indicate that 80 milliroentgens are delivered to each hand. This amount is well within the permissible dose range for an occasional exposure.[13]

Postoperatively, the patient is not restricted to his bed, but radiation health authorities do recommend a private room and hospitalization for seven days following surgery. In the first seven days, 72 percent of the irradiation is delivered to the tumor. The remaining 28 percent of the irradiation is delivered to infinity and is considered to be biologically ineffective. As such, it does not represent a radiation hazard to the patient or his family.[14] The polyethylene rings are left in place as long as they are tolerated by the patient, thus avoiding a second operation in most cases.

Candidates for radon rings must have useful vision in the affected eye, and the tumors must be located at least 2 mm away from the macula and optic nerve to

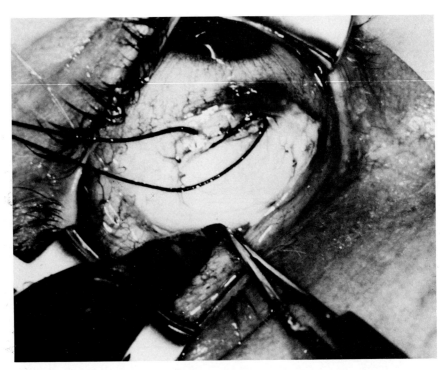

FIG. 11.4. Indirect ophthalmoscopy and forceps localization are used to locate the tumor, and the limits of the tumor are marked on the sclera with a marking pencil.

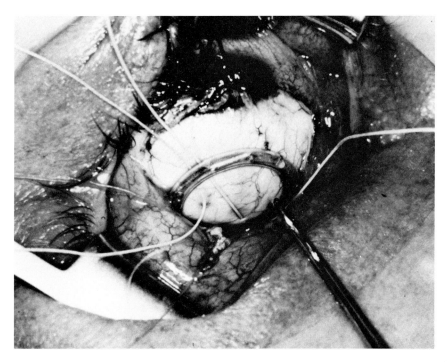

FIG. 11.5. The "dummy" polyethylene tube is loosely sutured to the sclera to ensure that no problems will arise when the active ring is put into place.

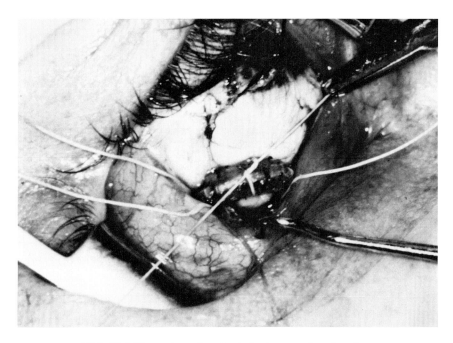

FIG. 11.6. The active radon ring is firmly sutured to the sclera.

avoid damage to these structures. Fundus photography, fluorescein angiography, and B-scan ultrasonography are repeated at three- to six-month intervals to monitor the response of the tumor. In most cases, no change is evident for six months or more. Initially, we felt that a radiation response should be evident within a year if it was to occur. However, several cases that failed to show significant regression within one year have regressed dramatically after two to three years. We now advise enucleation if the tumor shows evidence of growth or if it fails to shrink substantially within two years.

Results

Follow-up data for the 22 patients are given in Fig. 11.7 and Table 11.1. The follow-up periods range from 11 to 84 months, with a mean follow-up of 43 months. Clinically, there was successful tumor regression in 14 of 22 patients (64 percent) in the series. Objective signs of tumor regression included improvement of visual acuity, marked decrease in size and elevation of the tumor, pigment clumping surrounding the lesion, reduction of sinusoids, resolution of dependent retinal detachments, and decrease in staining with fluorescein angiography. All the patients with successfully treated tumors retained their pretreatment visual acuity.

CLINICAL COURSE. The response of a malignant melanoma of the choroid to radiation therapy varies considerably from patient to patient. Generally, the clinical course of an irradiated melanoma can be summarized as follows. There is a lag between the delivery of the radiation to the tumor and a visible response, even though almost 90 percent of the total radiation dose is delivered within the first 10 days. One begins to see pigment changes at the base of the tumor after 2 to 3 months. Initially, there is pigment clumping with a gradual loss of adjacent pigment epithelium and obliteration of the choriocapillaris. It takes 6 to 12 months for the tumor mass itself to regress. Frequently, in larger tumors, one may see hard exudates at the tumor base. We feel this finding is an indication of cell death. The next change

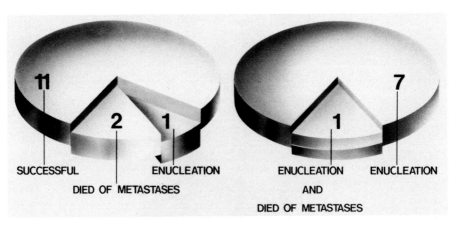

FIG. 11.7. Follow-up data for 22 patients with malignant melanoma of the choroid treated with radon rings showing incidence of successful and unsuccessful tumor regression respectively. (From Davidorf et al: Trans Am Acad Ophthalmol Otolaryngol, 81:849, 1976)

Table 11.1

Radiotherapy of Malignant Melanoma of the Choroid

Case	Treatment Date	Complications	Present Status	Follow-up (mo)
Successful tumor regression, alive and well				
1	11/19/68	None	Alive, no metastases	75
2	1/24/73	None	Alive, no mestastases	30
3	10/16/68	None	Alive, no metastases	80
4	5/1/72	None	Alive, no metastases; patient has had one photocoagulation treatment since radon ring placement	39
5	10/23/70	None	Alive, no metastases	57
6	11/17/71	Intraocular hemorrhage	Alive, no metastases	44
7	4/23/71	None	Alive, no metastases	51
8	10/4/72	None	Alive, no metastases	33
9	7/31/70	Intraocular hemorrhage extrusion of ring, removal 8/71	Alive, no metastases	60
10	5/17/74	None	Alive, no metastases	13
11	8/23/74	None	Alive, no metastases	11
Enucleation				
12	9/1/71	Extrusion of ring, removal 12/71	Enucleation 1/11/72 Alive, no metastases	39
13	8/3/72	None	Enucleation 3/73; alive, no metastases	29
14	4/18/73	None	Enucleation 4/74; alive, no metastases	17
15	6/11/71	Intraocular hemorrhage	Enucleation 1/74; alive, no metastases	48
16	6/4/71	None	Enucleation 9/72; alive, no metastases	49
17	4/30/68	Extrusion of ring, removal 5/68	Enucleation 9/68; alive, no metastases	84
18	4/26/72	None	Enucleation 5/73; alive, no metastases	39
19	6/6/73	Extrusion of ring, removal 7/73, globe rupture 3/74	Enucleation 3/74; alive, no metastases	33
Died of metastatic melanoma				
20	4/26/68	Intraocular hemorrhage	Died metastases 11/3/73	
21	9/4/68	Intraocular hemorrhage	Died metastases 7/71	
22	6/21/71	None	Enucleation 3/72; died metastases 3/74	

occurs in the tumor itself. As the tumor shrinks, one can see convolutions on the tumor surface, indicative of a reduction in tumor mass. There is progressive shrinkage, and ultimately the choroidal tumor completely flattens (Figs. 11.8, 11.9). The amount of pigmentation varies greatly. In most eyes, even with apparent total tumor atrophy, some of the larger choroidal vessels persist. At this stage, there is complete atrophy of the retinal pigment epithelium and choriocapillaris, as well as marked attenuation of the overlying retinal vessels.

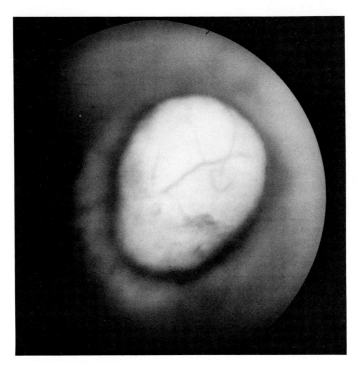

FIG. 11.8. Initial fundus photograph prior to treatment of case 6. The tumor has broken through Bruch's membrane, and sinusoids are readily visible. (From Davidorf et al: Trans Am Acad Ophthalmol Otolaryngol, 81:849, 1976)

COMPLICATIONS. Complications secondary to the placement of the ring include intraocular hemorrhage (five patients), extrusion of the polyethylene ring necessitating its removal after the course of therapy (four patients), and scleral atrophy and rupture of the globe (one patient). All cases of intraocular hemorrhage cleared with no resultant decrease in visual acuity. Complications made enucleation mandatory in only one eye in the series. One patient developed optic atrophy secondary to the radiation. The tumor was located adjacent to the disk, but conservative therapy was attempted because the patient had counting-fingers vision in the fellow eye. The eye was enucleated because the vision in the treated eye declined to light perception, and the tumor had not regressed completely.

Excluding the tumors of patients who had died of metastases, tumors that showed successful regression had diameters of 4.5 to 15 mm (mean 7.9 mm) and elevations of 1.5 to 3 mm (mean 2 mm). In contrast, those tumors requiring enucleations due to unsuccessful regression had diameters of 7.5 to 16 mm (mean 12 mm) and elevations of 2.5 to 6 mm (mean 4 mm). The mean age of patients whose tumors regressed was 59 years, compared to 42 years in the patients treated unsuccessfully.

FOLLOW-UP. Five-year follow-up data are available for seven patients. Two of these (29 percent) have subsequently died of metastases. The time elapsed between placement of the ring and death was three and five years. Both of the patients who

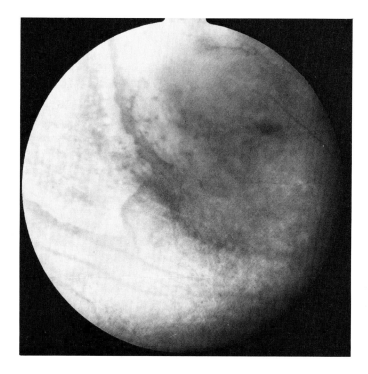

FIG. 11.9. Case 6, 35 months following radon ring placement. The tumor is completely flat, with pigment changes and chorioretinal atrophy. (From Davidorf et al: Trans Am Acad Ophthalmol Otolaryngol, 81:849, 1976)

died of metastases had shown successful tumor regression clinically. Unfortunately, the eyes could not be obtained for pathologic examination. One additional patient died of metastases who cannot yet be counted in the five-year follow-up data since less than five years has elapsed since his enucleation. It is difficult to draw conclusions from these data since follow-up is less than five years in the majority of the patients in this series.

HISTOPATHOLOGIC FINDINGS. Of the 22 cases of malignant melanoma treated by irradiation, 8 were enucleated because of tumor size and inadequate regression (Table 11.2). In one additional patient, there was a scleral rupture necessitating enucleation. Of patients requiring enucleation, one died of metastases two years after enucleation. The others are living and well two to seven years after treatment.

The histologic changes varied.[5] In a few eyes there was marked evidence of necrosis. In others the changes were minimal. Viable tumor cells were observed in all cases examined. Several eyes removed 4 to 9 months after irradiation showed extensive areas of pigment dissolution and necrosis (Figs. 11.10, 11.11). In the eye that remained the longest (31 months), little tumor necrosis was noted, although the tumor had decreased considerably in elevation.

In several tumors there were large areas of hemorrhage, and near the base, islands of hyalinization were present. Some of the larger tumor vessels had thickened walls, but most of the vessels were little different from those seen in any untreated malignant melanoma. In the heavily pigmented tumors there was marked dissolution of pigment granules and islands of pigment-laden macrophages. In other cases there were large areas where tumor cells became extremely attenuated, with only a few cytoplasmic processes remaining and fibrinous exudate filling the spaces (Fig. 11.11).

In all cases, the retina overlying the tumor showed marked changes. Cystic degeneration was almost always present. In some cases there was marked gliosis,

Table 11.2

Histologic Findings in Eyes Irradiated for Malignant Melanoma of the Choroid

Case	Age (yr)	Tumor Location	Cell Type	Tumor Size Prior to Treatment (mm)	Time Elapsed Since Ring Placement (mo)	Histologic Findings
12	48	Between posterior pole and equator	Sp. B	$15 \times 15 \times 4$	4	Central tumor necrosis, pigment-laden macrophages
13	56	Posterior pole	Mixed	$6 \times 7 \times 4$	7	Tumor unaffected
14	28	Between posterior pole and equator	Mixed	$7.5 \times 7.5 \times 2.5$	12	Some scarring in deep areas of tumor; pigment dissolution
15	55	Posterior pole	Sp. B	$7.5 \times 9 \times 4$	31	Tumor elevation greatly decreased, tumor surface convoluted
16	38	Equator	Sp. B	$15 \times 18 \times 6$	15	Hemorrhage, hyalinization at tumor base, vacuolization of tumor cells
17	22	Equator and periphery	Sp. A	$15 \times 15 \times 5$	4	Little necrosis, some tumor cells lack nuclear detail, marked hyalinization of base of tumor, scleral thinning
18	54	Between posterior pole and equator	Sp. B	$9 \times 10 \times 2.5$	11	Some pigment dispersion, very little effect noted
19	66	Periphery	Sp. B	$10 \times 10 \times 3$	9	Large area of necrosis, pigment-laden macrophages, scleral thinning
22	37	Between posterior pole and equator	Fasc.	$16 \times 16 \times 4$	9	Vacuolization of cells and liberation of pigment from tumor cells

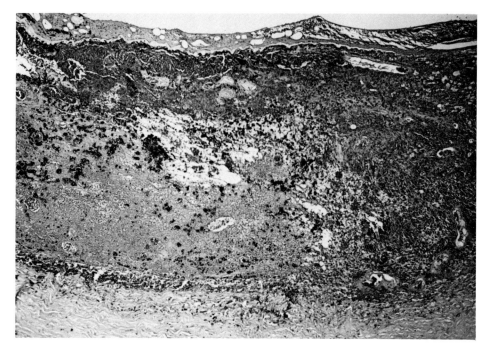

FIG. 11.10. Extensive areas of pigment dissolution and necrosis in a tumor enucleated nine months after radon ring placement (case 19). H&E, ×172. (From Davidorf et al: Trans Am Acad Ophthalmol Otolaryngol, 81:849, 1976)

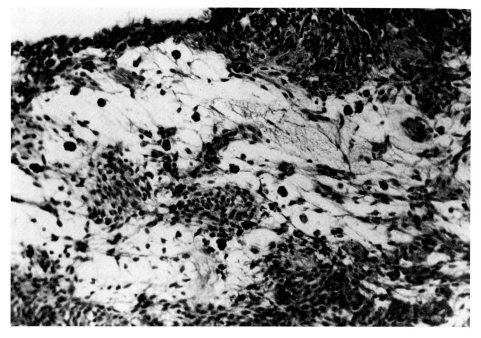

FIG. 11.11 Area near the apex of a tumor removed 15 months after radon ring placement, showing an absence of tumor cells with cytoplasmic processes and fibrinous exudate filling the spaces (case 16). H&E, ×344. (From Davidorf et al: Trans Am Acad Ophthalmol Otolaryngol, 81:849, 1976)

145

the retina being represented by a thin gliotic band. Away from the tumor, however, the retina appeared normal.

It is interesting that the necrotic changes secondary to radiation took place deep in the tumor rather than near the base, where the greatest dose of radiation was received. This observation and the fact that tumor regression is so slow has led Stallard[6] to speculate that the necrosis is secondary to ischemia rather than the direct effect of radiation. Although occasional vessels showed a degree of sclerosis, for the most part, the vessels of the tumors in eyes enucleated appeared normal and were engorged with red blood cells.

An alternative hypothesis is that the radiation damages the tumor cells and prevents replication, although the cells remain intact. Eventual regression of the tumor may thus relate to the life span of individual tumor cells. In our unsuccessfully treated cases, there were many cells that, by light microscopy, appeared to be viable. It is conceivable that these cells, although they appeared viable, were actually incapable of replication. Stallard showed histologic evidence of complete tumor destruction five years after placement of a cobalt plaque.[6] The eyes that we have been able to examine histologically unfortunately represent those patients whose tumors were too large and treated with too low a radiation dose; however, there is definite evidence of tumor necrosis in many of the eyes that we studied. It is very interesting to note that two of our patients and five of Stallard's patients who had complete tumor regression died of metastatic disease.

The experience we have had with radiotherapy over the past seven years can be summarized as follows. Relatively large doses of radiation (at least 8000 rads to the tumor apex) must be used if the tumor is to be effectively obliterated. Second, large tumors (over 12 mm in diameter and 3 mm in elevation) simply do not respond, and therefore size of tumor is a major criterion in selecting patients for radiation therapy. Failure to destroy the tumor may be due to either too large a tumor or too low a radiation dose. We feel that radiation can effectively destroy a small choroidal melanoma.

Radiation therapy is likely to be effective in patients with very small tumors no more than 7 mm in diameter and 2 mm in elevation. There were no cases effectively treated in which the tumor was larger than 12 mm in diameter and 3 mm in elevation. The response of tumors that fall between these extremes is variable, and it is difficult to predict the clinical course following radon ring placement. Treatment of tumors in this category may be justified in special cases such as monocular patients or patients who refuse enucleation.

DIATHERMY OF CHOROIDAL MELANOMAS

The use of diathermy in the treatment of malignant melanoma of the choroid was first introduced by Weve[15, 16] in 1935. Approximately 25 cases have been reported in the world literature,[15-21] but the use of diathermy for melanomas has not been generally accepted in this country. Most of the adverse reports on the use of diathermy for malignant melanomas were based on cases that were operated on for apparent rhegmatogenous retinal detachment.[22] In reality, the detachment was secondary to an unsuspected malignant melanoma, and the diathermy accentuated the spread of the tumor. The use of transscleral diathermy in the treatment of retinal detachment is a completely different procedure than its use in the treatment of malignant melanoma.

Method

We have used transsceral diathermy in the treatment of four cases of choroidal melanoma. The ages of the patients ranged from 45 to 65 years, with a mean age of 56.7 years. One of these patients had a retinal detachment in the fellow eye, one patient had bilateral melanomas (enucleation was performed on the left eye and diathermy on the right), and the remaining patients had small melanomas and normal vision in the affected eyes. The tumors measured between 5 and 9 mm in diameter and 1 to 2 mm in elevation.

The sclera is exposed in the area of the melanoma with a routine conjunctival and Tenon's incision. If necessary, the insertions of the muscles are tenotomized to achieve the proper exposure. Fixation sutures are placed in the muscle insertions to allow adequate rotation of the globe during the procedure. The exact location of the tumor is then identified using binocular indirect ophthalmoscopy and forceps indentation (Fig. 11.12). A single diathermy mark is made at the edge of the tumor. The electrode tip is used to apply sufficient current to the dried scleral surface so that subsequent ophthalmoscopic inspection shows a heavy, dead white coagulation of the retina (Fig. 11.13). If inadequate retinal destruction has resulted, more diathermy is applied to the same spot until the desired dead white snowball is achieved. Next, comparable diathermy is applied to each side of the original spot; the aim is to position this application along the periphery of the melanoma. Ophthalmoscopic inspection should now confirm the presence of three dense retinal burns, confluent along the edge of the tumor and extending at least 2 mm beyond it (Fig. 11.14). Additional burns are now placed on each side of the original three, appropriately curved to circle the melanoma. Internal inspection after each new pair of burns is necessary to confirm their exact location and their adequate intensity. This process is repeated until the melanoma is completely encircled. Placing multiple burns without ophthalmoscopic inspection does not save time and leads to incomplete and poorly placed burns.

A solid ring of diathermy will now exist on the scleral surface. The electrical current is now considerably increased and applied just inside the ring. The time and intensity of this application is enough to cause visible internal coagulation extending through the inner surface of the melanoma and destroying the retina internal to the melanoma.

Repeated applications to the same spot are usually necessary before the retina is adequately burned. Similar applications, one or, at most, two at a time are made and inspected until the entire area of the melanoma has been totally destroyed by coagulation (Fig. 11.15). A surprising amount of time is expended in this repeated diathermy–inspection procedure. Destruction of a small melanoma may take as long as an hour or more.

Following diathermy, the scleral surface will be shrunken flat and will be horribly burned. The inner surface of the melanoma will be entirely white. The vitreous may be hazy and recognizably condensed just internal to the tumor.

The patient should be kept in bed with binocular patches and with the treated

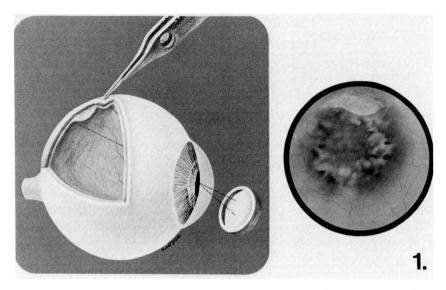

FIG. 11.12. The exact location of the tumor is identified using binocular indirect ophthalmoscopy and forceps indentation.

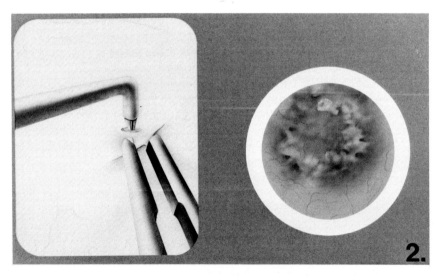

FIG. 11.13. The electrode tip is used to apply sufficient current to the dried scleral surface so that subsequent ophthalmoscopic inspection shows a heavy, dead white coagulation of the retina.

site lowest. At the first dressing change, the eye will be red, moderate iritis and vitreous inflammation will be present, and an alarming amount of transudative detachment may be found. Since the burned retina is very fragile and movement can easily cause a retinal tear, the eye should be kept quiet until the detachment has completely subsided and the chorioretinal adhesions have had at least an

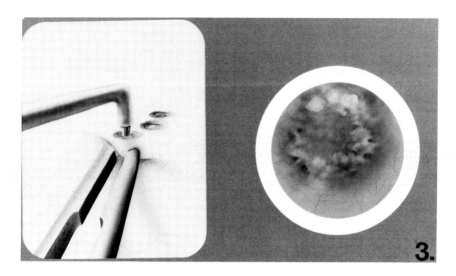

FIG. 11.14. Additional diathermy burns are placed along the edge of the tumor.

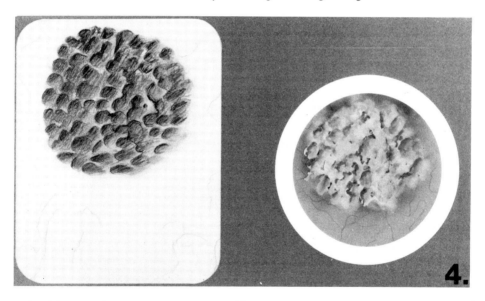

FIG. 11.15. The electrical current is considerably increased and diathermy burns are made until the entire area of the melanoma has been destroyed.

additional day to become snugly apposed and securely adherent. Probably, the patient will need to stay in bed for at least a week before these healing changes are complete. Activity should be limited for the following several weeks.

The use of diathermy is indicated only when there is adequate exposure. Posterior tumors near the disk cannot be treated with diathermy because of inadequate exposure. Tumors located in the area of the macula cannot be treated with diathermy because of secondary damage to the macula caused by shrinking and retinal traction.

The tumor elevation will persist for many months, perhaps even as long as a year. Ultimately, an almost flat, pigmented atrophic scar will result (Fig. 11.16).

Results

Follow-up data for the patients treated with diathermy are given in Table 11.3. The follow-up periods vary from 2 to 11 years, with a mean follow-up of 79 months. There was successful tumor regression in all four patients, and all patients retained their pretreatment visual acuity. There were no significant complications noted in the patients in this series. One patient died of a coronary thrombosis 21 months after treatment. The other patients are alive and well 11, 7, and 6 years after treatment.

Table 11.3

Diathermy of Malignant Melanoma of the Choroid

Case	Treatment Date	Present Status	Follow-up (mo)
23	7/10/64	Alive, no mestastases	129
24	6/16/65	Died coronary thrombosis 3/67	21
25	2/26/68	Alive, no metastases	81
26	11/14/68	Alive, no metastases	84

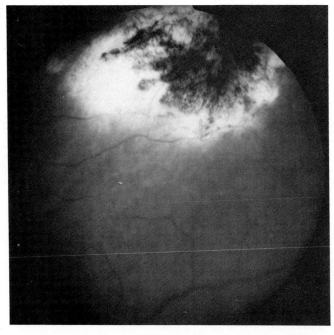

FIG. 11.16. Fundus photograph of case 26, taken six years after diathermy treatment.

DISCUSSION

Diathermy and radiotherapy are likely to be effective in patients with tumors no more than 7 mm in diameter and 2 mm in elevation. Tumors larger than 12 mm in diameter and 3 mm in elevation do not respond adequately to either form of therapy. Tumors between these two extremes may in some cases respond to radiotherapy but probably will not be destroyed by diathermy. We feel that both radiation and diathermy can effectively destroy small choroidal melanomas.

The advantages of radiotherapy over diathermy include the general lack of scleral destruction, the greater ease and shorter duration of the operative procedure, and the possibility of successfully treating tumors greater than 2 mm in elevation. The chief disadvantage is the lag time required for the tumor to respond to the radiation.

The major advantage of diathermy over radiotherapy and photocoagulation is the ability to observe full-thickness tumor response intraoperatively. Tumor destruction following diathermy occurs more quickly than when radiotherapy is employed. Optic atrophy is not a complication of diathermy, although it may result from radiotherapy if the tumor is located near the optic nerve. The major disadvantage of diathermy is extensive scleral destruction with the possibility of extraocular spread of tumor. Should this spread occur, it would be nearly impossible to detect clinically during the postoperative period. This danger has led us to discontinue the use of this procedure.

Fifteen percent of choroidal melanomas exhibit extraocular extension,[1] and both radiotherapy and diathermy offer the opportunity of intraoperative examination of the sclera for extraocular tumor growth. This observation is not possible with photocoagulation. Neither radiotherapy nor diathermy is effective in the treatment of tumors of the posterior pole, although photocoagulation may be useful in the treatment of these tumors.

In considering new therapies for neoplastic diseases, it is important that the newer treatments be continually reevaluated through analysis of the effect of the treatment on the natural course of the disease. The three primary prognostic criteria in malignant melanoma of the choroid are tumor size, tumor cell type, and the presence or absence of extrachoroidal extension. Available information indicates that enucleation is a relatively effective procedure in the treatment of small malignant melanomas of the choroid that are less than 10 mm in diameter and 3 mm in elevation.[1] The five-year survival rate is about 94 percent in this group, and the ten-year survival rate is about 77 percent. Patients with larger tumors do not fare so well: five-year survival is about 64 percent and ten-year survival drops to 54 percent.

When we consider these alternative methods for treatment of malignant melanoma of the choroid, we must compare these statistics to survival rates of comparable patients treated with enucleation. The treatment of malignant melanoma of the choroid with radiotherapy and diathermy remains a controversial topic. Of the 195 reported cases treated with radiotherapy, five-year follow-up data are available on 54 successfully treated cases; the survival rate was 87 percent. In the largest reported diathermy series[17] (18 patients) no proved metastatic deaths occurred. In general, conservatively treated patients are those with smaller tumors who would normally have a five-year survival of about 94 percent. We are not aware of any report of death from a melanoma smaller than 7 mm in diameter and 2 mm in elevation treated with enucleation. This size coincides fairly closely with that which may respond to conservative therapy.

While there is a great deal of interest in the conservative management of malignant melanoma of the choroid, this form of therapy is still in its trial period. There have been a limited number of patients treated and follow-up periods are not long enough to make any definitive judgments as to the role of conservative therapy in the management of this malignant disease.

ACKNOWLEDGMENT

I appreciate the participation of the Radiology Department in this project. Gunther Ehlers, M.D., Frank Batley, M.D., and Mukund Kartha, Ph.D., were responsible for the design and preparation of the radon rings and the dosimetry calculations. I also thank Torrence A. Makley, M.D., for pathologic examination of enucleated eyes, Janet R. Lang for data compilation and help in the preparation of the manuscript, and Donald A. Keller for preparation of the illustrations.

REFERENCES

1. Davidorf FH, Lang JR: The natural history of malignant melanoma of the choroid: small vs. large tumors. Trans Am Acad Ophthalmol Otolaryngol 79:310, 1975
2. Newman GH, Davidorf FH, Havener WH, Makley TA: Conservative management of malignant melanoma: I. Irradiation as a method of treatment for malignant melanoma of the choroid. Arch Ophthalmol 83:21, 1970
3. Davidorf FH, Newman GH, Havener WH, Makley TA: Conservative management of malignant melanoma: II. Transscleral diathermy as a method of treatment for malignant melanomas of the choroid. Arch Ophthalmol 83:273, 1970
4. Ehlers G, Batley F, Kartha M: Radiotherapeutic management of malignant melanoma of the eye. Am J Roentgenol Radium Ther Nucl Med 123:486, 1975
5. Davidorf FH, Makley TA, Lang JR: Radiotherapy of malignant melanoma of the choroid. Trans Am Acad Ophthalmol Otolaryngol 81:849, 1976
6. Stallard HB: Radiotherapy for malignant melanoma of the choroid. Br J Ophthalmol 50:147, 1966
7. Stallard HB: Malignant melanoblastoma of the choroid. Mod Probl Ophthalmol 7:16, 1968
8. Long RS, Galin MA, Rotman M: Conservative treatment of intraocular melanomas. Trans Am Acad Ophthalmol Otolaryngol 75:84, 1971
9. Lommatzsch PK: Experiences in the treatment of malignant melanoma of the choroid with [106]Ru/[106]Rh beta-ray applicators. Trans Ophthalmol Soc UK 93:119, 1973
10. Bedford MA: The use and abuse of cobalt plaques in the treatment of choroidal malignant melanomata. Trans Ophthalmol Soc UK 93:139, 1973
11. Boniuk M, Girard LJ: Malignant melanoma of the choroid: treated with photocoagulation, transscleral diathermy, and implanted radon seeds. Am J Ophthalmol 59:212, 1965
12. Meredith WJ: Radium Dosage: The Manchester System. Edinburgh, Williams & Wilkins, 1967
13. Recommendations of the International Commission on Radiologic Protection: Report of Committee IV. Oxford, Pergamon, 1964, p 37

14. The Prescription Service for the Radiotherapist. Kenilworth, Ill, Radium Service Corp of America, 1960, p 48
15. Weve HJM: Ueber operative Behandlung von intraokularen Tumoren mit Erhaltung des Bulbus. Arch Augenheilkd 110:482, 1937
16. Weve HJM: Diathermy in ophthalmic practice. Trans Ophthalmol Soc UK 59:61, 1939
17. Melchers MJ: Diathermy Treatment of Intraocular Tumors. Utrecht, The Netherlands, Schotanusan Jens, 1953
18. Lauber H: Zur Diathermischen Behandlung beginnender Geschwulsts an der Haut. Ber Dtsch Ophthalmol Ges 52:119, 1938
19. Savin LH, Pritchard GC: Choroidal melanoma treated by surgical diathermy. Br J Ophthalmol 26:551, 1942
20. Dunphy EB: Management of intraocular malignancy. Am J Ophthalmol 44:313, 1957
21. Lund OE: Changes in choroidal tumors after light coagulation (and diathermy coagulation): a histologic investigation of 43 cases. Arch Ophthalmol 75:458, 1966
22. Reese AB: Tumors of the Eye. New York, Harper & Row, 1963

Martin H. Vogel

12 Xenon Arc Photocoagulation of Small Malignant Melanomas of the Choroid

In the past many clinicians have been dissatisfied with the results of enucleation as a treatment of choroidal melanoma. Published reports indicate an average ten-year mortality of between 40 and 97 percent after enucleation to treat choroidal malignant melanoma.[1-3] Moreover, the problem of monocular patients with choroidal melanoma in their remaining eye stimulated the search for an effective sight-retaining form of therapy. Weve[4, 5] explored diathermy, Stallard[6-8] investigated irradiation, and in 1952 Meyer-Schwickerath introduced photocoagulation of these choroidal tumors.[9-12] Photocoagulation has the advantage of being the least traumatic procedure since no surgery is performed and it can be done on an outpatient basis.

DIAGNOSIS

It has been suggested that some of the choroidal melanomas that we coagulated might have been benign nevi. In order to diagnose malignant melanoma correctly, we use the following diagnostic methods: indirect ophthalmoscopy, fluorescein angiography, infrared photography, transillumination, ^{32}P uptake test, and ultrasonography. If any one of these tests is not suggestive of melanoma, we prefer to observe the patient, particularly since we are trying to treat only small tumors. With infrared photography we can exactly monitor the size of the tumor and its growth. Color photography, while being helpful, can lead to errors since photographic quality depends on the processing, film quality, and photographer's skill.

Fluorescein angiography may be of additional help. The pattern of the choroidal and tumor circulation can sometimes give an accurate assessment of the size of a lesion. We believe that tumor growth is the most important criterion for the diagnosis of a malignant melanoma, and we believe that nevi can be excluded from our series with great certainty. In our clinic cases histopathologic examination of 325 clinically diagnosed malignant melanomas requiring enucleation demonstrated a 1.8 percent rate of misdiagnosis.

INDICATIONS

Our present indications for photocoagulation as a treatment for choroidal malignant melanoma require that all of the following criteria be met:

1. The diagnosis of malignant melanoma must be made with certainty. If there is any doubt, the tumor is observed until unequivocal growth is documented.
2. We obtain informed consent from the patient. We inform the patient thoroughly about the prognosis of malignant melanoma and this type of therapeutic modality. However, I do not think that we as physicians should lay the responsibility of therapeutic choice entirely in the hands of the patients, since they cannot always judge the pros and cons of each available treatment modality.
3. The tumor must not be elevated more than 5 diopters or 2 mm, because the rate of success decreases with increase in the height of the tumor. This is very close to the maximum tumor elevation allowable for treatment with diathermy or radon seeds as described by Dr. Davidorf (Chapter 11).
4. The lateral extent of the tumor should be equal to or less than 5 to 6 disk diameters or 7 to 8 mm. This size corresponds to approximately 30° of field if we look at the tumor with a 14-diopter lens using an indirect ophthalmoscope. Again, these are approximately the same size tumors treated with other conservative forms of treatment.
5. The retina must be attached over the tumor. If the retina is detached we cannot get sufficient photocoagulation effects around the tumor or on the tumor surface to occlude the choroidal vasculature, which is one of our main goals of therapy.
6. The localization of the tumor must be such that it can easily be surrounded with photocoagulation, ie, not too far in the periphery. The ideal location for such a lesion is the midperiphery.
7. The tumor must not be located at the optic disk margin. If it is, it is impossible to surround the tumor with coagulation in order to shut off the tumor's blood supply. In addition, a tumor close to the disk margin may already have penetrated into the optic nerve.

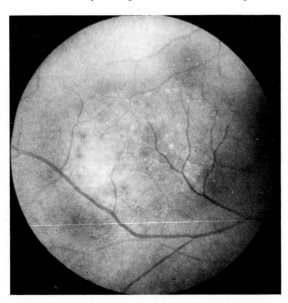

FIG. 12.1. Untreated tumor with drusen and lipofuscin (orange pigment) on the surface.

8. The tumor must not be located within the circle of the central retinal vessels since approximately 12 short ciliary arteries enter the choroid through the sclera in this area and it would not be possible to shut off the blood supply to the tumor. In addition, there is a great risk of extraocular extension through one of these emissarial channels.
9. The ocular media must be clear, otherwise photocoagulation treatment is impossible.
10. Maximum dilatation of the pupil must be possible. Photocoagulation through a partially dilated pupil will heat the iris, which will become necrotic and form posterior synechias, making further photocoagulation impossible.
11. Large retinal vessels must not cross the tumor because their obliteration may lead to new vessel formation and its subsequent complications.
12. In the case of a monocular patient, these criteria may be liberalized somewhat.

These criteria are based on our experience with 54 malignant melanomas treated by photocoagulation with a follow-up of ten years or more.[13]

TREATMENT TECHNIQUE

Initially we apply a circular double row of photocoagulation around the tumor (Figs. 12.1, 12.2). At the second sitting, performed approximately three weeks later, the area of previous photocoagulation has developed a pigmented chorioretinal scar and the circular barrage is repeated over the same area (Fig. 12.3). The procedure is repeated three weeks later; the final result of these treatments is a well-pigmented scar (Fig. 12.4).

At the fourth sitting we begin to treat the tumor mass itself by creating an

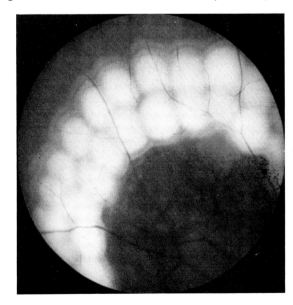

FIG. 12.2. First circular photocoagulation barrage. A double row of strong effects with green 2, field diaphragm 6, and completely open iris diaphragm is placed around the tumor.

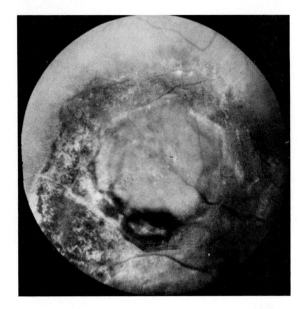

FIG. 12.3. The same case as Figure 12.2. After the second circular barrage, a well-pigmented scar has formed surrounding the tumor. As a result of photocoagulation of retinal vessels an intraretinal hemorrhage has occurred.

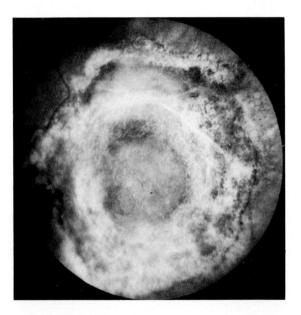

FIG. 12.4. The circular barrages have been applied three times with each barrage a little closer to the tumor center. The retinal vessels have disappeared.

atrophic choroidal scar (Fig. 12.5). Finally, we try to break up the tumor by causing repeated explosive reactions on its surface to destroy the tumor tissue (Fig. 12.6). This process may require three or four more sittings. Following this treatment there is practically no vascular supply to the tumor, and bare sclera and proliferations of retinal pigment epithelium can be seen at the edges of the scar (Fig. 12.7). The tumor is considered ophthalmoscopically eradicated when this scar has remained unchanged for at least two years.

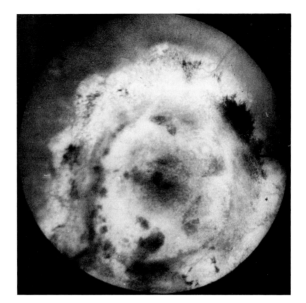

FIG. 12.5. The tumor surface has been treated. The retina overlying the tumor reveals a gray discoloration.

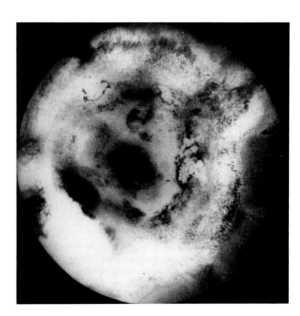

FIG. 12.6. The tumor surface has been coagulated with red 1, field diaphragm 6, and open iris diaphragm. Explosions have occurred, resulting in a crater at the base of which pigmented tumor tissue becomes visible.

The central pigmentation within the scar may make the ophthalmologist uneasy because it may indicate the presence of viable tumor cells. I believe that the absence of a vascular supply reaching this area is good presumptive evidence that there is no viable tissue within the scar. When we studied some of these tumors histopathologically,[14-16] when we were still inexperienced with them, I thought that we had caused viable tumor cells to explode into the vitreous. However, bleached sections of these photocoagulated tumors revealed that the vitreous cells were

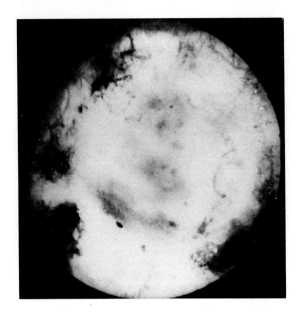

FIG. 12.7. There have been three or four sittings with repeated explosions. Five months after the last treatment, bare sclera is visible surrounded by proliferations of the retinal pigment epithelium. No choroidal vessels are present. Fluorescein angiography confirmed avascularity of this scar. Ophthalmoscopically the tumor is considered destroyed.

macrophages that engulf pigment and other tumor debris. The pigment in these macrophages is not the fine, dusty, uveal pigment found in intact malignant melanoma cells, but rather a rough, scaly material. In addition, the tumor cells at the base of the tumor are replaced by a loose fibrovascular tissue with an occasional pigment-laden macrophage (Figs. 12.8, 12.9).

I think there is no question that it is possible to destroy a malignant melanoma with photocoagulation and the follow-up data that we have collected provide substantial evidence for this stand.[13, 16]

COMPLICATIONS

Photocoagulation therapy of malignant melanomas is not without its complications. As discussed previously, if the pupil is not maximally dilated there is a good chance of producing iris burns (Figs. 12.10, 12.11).

If explosions of the tumor are performed prematurely, before the tumor has been surrounded three times with barrages of photocoagulation, vitreous hemorrhage may develop from the tumor tissue and thus make further treatment impossible. Vitreous hemorrhages rarely occur if the circular barrage has been done properly and if the first coagulation of the tumor mass has not been too intensive. Dispersion of pigment into the vitreous is another possible complication. In a few cases a dense cloud of pigment in the vitreous has hung over the scar tissue, making further treatment impossible. This problem occurs when the tumor is initially coagulated too intensely and extensive tumor debris erupts into the vitreous.

If large retinal vessels crossing a tumor are coagulated, new vessels can proliferate from the stumps of the obliterated vessels several months later (Figs. 12.12, 12.13), causing repeated vitreous hemorrhage. As soon as the scar cannot be seen clearly, we recommend enucleation because a recurrence can be hidden behind vitreous blood or pigment.

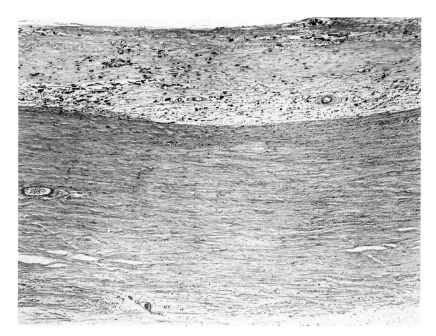

FIG. 12.8. Histopathologic specimen of a completely eradicated malignant melanoma of the choroid 2 mm in elevation and 5 disk diameters in lateral extent. Tumor, retina, and choroid have been replaced by scar tissue. Numerous pigmented cells are scattered throughout the scar tissue. A small vessel is visible in the deep, loose layer of the scar. The sclera is unaffected by the treatment.

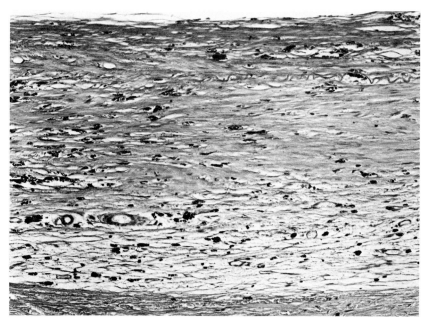

FIG. 12.9. Higher magnification of Figure 12.8. The pigmented cells contain coarse pigment granules. Some of the pigment is dispersed extracellularly. In some cases remnants of Bruch's membrane can be demonstrated. This photograph shows the center of a scar that clinically revealed a grayish center. This finding was interpreted as tumor residue and the eye was therefore enucleated.

161

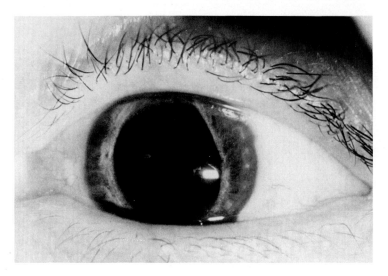

FIG. 12.10. As a result of insufficient dilatation of the pupil during photocoagulation, burns of the iris were produced with subsequent posterior synechias.

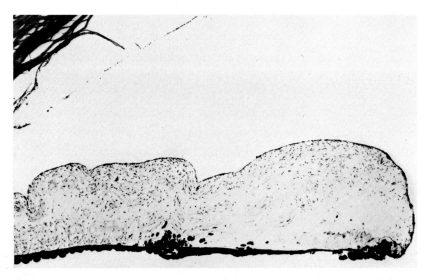

FIG. 12.11. Histopathologic specimen of a coagulated iris. The dilator and sphincter muscles have atrophied. There is atrophy as well as proliferation of the iris pigment epithelium.

The main argument against photocoagulation of choroidal malignant melanomas is that even if we are destroying the tumor within the eye, we cannot see if the patient is developing extraocular extension. Among 130 malignant melanomas treated, this complication has occurred twice. One of these tumors was coagulated in the mid-1950s, and today we would regard it as unsuitable for photocoagulation treatment. The tumor demonstrated 22 diopters of elevation, and we now know that it would be impossible to destroy this tumor. The second case of extraocular

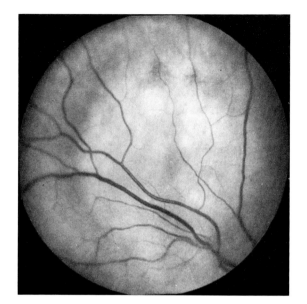

FIG. 12.12. This malignant melanoma was covered by the temporal superior branches of the central retinal vessels.

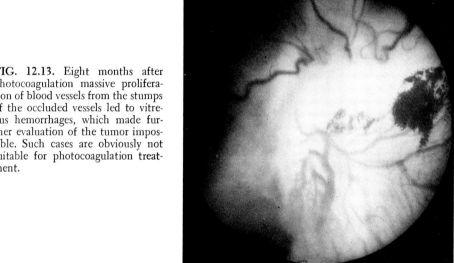

FIG. 12.13. Eight months after photocoagulation massive proliferation of blood vessels from the stumps of the occluded vessels led to vitreous hemorrhages, which made further evaluation of the tumor impossible. Such cases are obviously not suitable for photocoagulation treatment.

extension occurred in a monocular patient who previously had a cobalt plaque sutured over his tumor, and it looked as if this therapy had been successful. Approximately two years later, however, a recurrence developed at the edge of the scar. Photocoagulation failed to destroy the tumor, and we recommended enucleation, at which time extraocular extension was noted. It is likely that the small number of cases of extraocular extension in our series is due to the rare occurrence of this complication in the small tumors we usually treat.

RESULTS

Results of our ten-year follow-up study on the photocoagulation treatment of choroidal malignant melanomas have been published previously.[13] This group of tumors included many which today we consider too large for photocoagulation therapy.

We established a new series in which only cases fulfilling our present criteria were included.[17] From January 1969 to April 1973, we photocoagulated 32 melanomas. Of these, a total of 21 (66 percent) of the tumors were destroyed and the remaining 11 (34 percent) eyes were enucleated. In 2 of the enucleated globes the tumor was eradicated as demonstrated by histologic examination. Thus the rate of tumor destruction in this series is 72 percent. The causes of enucleation in those 11 cases are shown in Table 12.1. In one case the patient was monocular and the

Table 12.1

**Causes of Enucleation
in 11 Cases**

Vitreous opacities	3
Retinal detachment	3
Fast growth; tumor too large	3
Vascular proliferation	1
Recurrence	1
Total	11

tumor was too large for photocoagulation. It is not our purpose to show the prognosis in this small series of 32 melanomas observed for only slightly over two years, but rather to show the early ophthalmoscopic cure rate. None of the patients, so far, has died either of metastatic disease or any other cause. The number of treatments has varied from four to ten, with an average of six sittings at three-week intervals.

DISCUSSION

The initial study of photocoagulation to treat malignant melanoma was conducted in 1968.[18] The controversy surrounding this use of photocoagulation[19-25] is understandable because photocoagulation treatment was performed in an ineffective way. Producing a few burns on a tumor surface with a photocoagulator or laser will not destroy the tumor at all. It is mandatory to surround it first with a photocoagulation barrage, shut off its blood supply, and then start to photocoagulate the tumor mass with higher intensities. Results comparable to ours were published in 1963 by Francois,[26] and in 1968 by Dufour and co-workers[27] and Pischel.[28] Francois reported two recurrences after seven and eight years,[29, 30] but both tumors were located adjacent to the disk margin; in other words, they were tumors we do not consider suitable for photocoagulation treatment at all.

Finally, photocoagulation of malignant melanomas is no routine procedure. It should be limited to those tumors that fulfill all of the criteria outlined above. This type of therapy should be done only in large centers where numerous tumor patients are seen, where the necessary equipment is available to make the right diagnosis, and where physicians are skilled in the use of the xenon arc photocoagulator.

REFERENCES

1. Von Hippel E: Fortsetzung meiner Sarkomstatistik II. Albrecht von Graefes Arch Klin Exp Ophthalmol 135:76, 1936
2. Thiel R, Otto J, Toppel L: Statistische Untersuchungen über das intraoculare Melanoblastom und Retinoblastom. Klin Monatsbl Augenheilkd 138:682, 1961
3. Paul EV, Parnell BL, Fraker M: Prognosis of malignant melanomas of the choroid and ciliary body. Int Ophthalmol Clin 2:387, 1962
4. Weve HJM: Über die operative Behandlung von intraocularen Tumoren mit Erhaltung des Bulbus. Arch Augenheilkd 110:482, 1937
5. Weve HJM: Die Möglichkeiten zur Behandlung intraocularen Tumoren unter Erhaltung des Sehvermogens. Ber Dtsch Ophthalmol Ges 63:176, 1960
6. Stallard HB: Malignant melanoma of the choroid treated with radioactive applicators. Trans Ophthalmol Soc UK 79:373, 1959.
7. Stallard HB: Malignant melanoma of the choroid treated with radio-applicators. Ann Coll Surg Engl 29:170, 1961
8. Stallard HB: Malignant melanoma of the choroid. Mod Probl Ophthalmol 7:16, 1968
9. Meyer-Schwickerath G: New indications for coagulation by light. Trans Ophthalmol Soc UK 77:421, 1957
10. Meyer-Schwickerath G: Indications and limitations of light coagulation. Trans Am Acad Ophthalmol Otolaryngol 63:725, 1959
11. Meyer-Schwickerath G: Lichtkoagulation: Bücherei des Augenarztes. Stuttgart, Enke, 1959
12. Meyer-Schwickerath G: Die Möglichkeiten zur Behandlung intraocularer Tumoren unter Erhaltung des Sehvermögens. Ber Dtsch Ophthalmol Ges 63:178, 1960
13. Vogel MH: Treatment of malignant melanomas with photocoagulation. Am J Ophthalmol 74:1, 1972
14. Lund OE: Changes in choroidal tumors after light coagulation (and diathermy coagulation): a histopathological investigation of 43 cases. Arch Ophthalmol 75:458, 1966
15. Lund OE: Konsequenzen aus histologischen Untersuchungen an lichtkoagulierten Melanoblastomen. Mod Probl Ophthalmol 5:352, 1967
16. Vogel MH: Histopathologic observations of photocoagulated malignant melanomas of the choroid. Am J Ophthalmol 74:466, 1972
17. Vogel MH, Schmitz-Valckenberg P: Photocoagulation of small malignant melanomas of the choroid. Read before the International Congress of Photocoagulation, New York, 1975
18. Lund OE: Lichtkoagulation von malignen Malanoblastomen der Chorioidea: klinische und histopathologische Untersuchungen. Mod Probl Ophthalmol 7:45, 1968
19. Curtin V, Norton EWD: Pathological changes in malignant melanomas after photocoagulation. Arch Ophthalmol 70:150, 1963
20. Boniuk M, Girard LJ: Malignant melanoma of the choroid treated with photocoagulation, transscleral diathermy and implanted radon seeds. Am J Ophthalmol 59:212, 1965
21. Frezzotto R, Guerra R: Considerazioni sulla fotocoagulazione nel melanoma maligno della coroide. Minerva Oftalmol 8:201, 1966

22. Davidorf FH, Newman GH, Havener WH, et al: Conservative management of malignant melanoma. Arch Ophthalmol 83:273, 1970
23. Manschot W: Therapie van melanoma chorioideae. Ned Tijdschr Geneeskd 116: 297, 1972
24. Apple DJ, Goldberg MF, Wyhinny G, et al: Argon laser photocoagulation of choroidal malignant melanoma. Arch Ophthalmol 90:97, 1973
25. Gerhard JP, Brini A, Risse JF: Tumeur de la choroide traitee par photocoagulation. Bull Soc Ophtalmol Fr 5:433, 1974
26. Francois J: Malignant melanomata of the choroid. Br J Ophthalmol 47:736, 1963
27. Dufour R, Leuenberger A, Brückner R, et al: Traitement conservateur des melanoblastomes de la choroide dans les cliniques ophthalmologiques de Bâles, Lausanne et Zurich. Mod Probl Ophthalmol 7:38, 1968
28. Pischel DK: Malignant melanomas of the choroid. Mod Probl Ophthalmol 7:84, 1968
29. Francois J, Hanssens M: Recidive d'un melanome malin de la choroide apres photocoagulation: examen histopathologique. Bull Soc Belge Ophtalmol 128:292, 1961
30. Francois J: Recurrence of malignant melanoma of the choroid seven and eight years after light coagulation. Ophthalmologica 162:188, 1971

Gholam A. Peyman
Donald R. Sanders
Donald R. May

13 Local Excision of Malignant Melanoma of the Choroid

We have studied extensively the feasibility of full-thickness eye wall resection.[7-10] The technique has been modified several times on the basis of experimental studies that used various graft materials[1,2] and tested the importance of preoperative photocoagulation, cryotherapy, and diathermy.[4,5] The technique has been tested in various animal species[9] and in humans,[6,10] and the tumor size limitations of the surgical procedure have been determined experimentally.[8] Somewhat surprisingly, most of these experiments were successful. The operation was well tolerated and the feared complications, such as retinal detachment and bleeding from the choroidal and retinal vessels, were easily controlled. Our current indications and technique have evolved from these studies. It should be emphasized that the procedure is still experimental and the technique is still undergoing change.

INDICATIONS FOR EYE WALL RESECTION

The most suitable candidates are patients with tumors fulfilling all of the following criteria:

1. The base diameter of the mass does not exceed 10 mm.
2. An exudative detachment of the retina covers no more than one-third of the fundus.
3. The tumor is not within 4.5 mm (3 disk diameters) of the disk margin. The best tumors for resection are located near the equator.
4. The media are clear.
5. The patient has no evidence of metastatic disease after a complete work-up to detect metastases.
6. The patient is able to tolerate general anesthesia for three to four hours.

PREOPERATIVE EVALUATION AND TREATMENT

The patient should have a complete ocular examination. Special studies such as fluorescein angiography, ultrasonography (A- and B-scan), ^{32}P uptake test, and transillumination are considered mandatory to localize the mass and estimate the size of the lesion properly.

Preoperatively, xenon arc photocoagulation with Zeiss green 1 to red 1, 6-degree spot size is applied in three concentric rows around the tumor in attached retina (Fig. 13.1). In four to five weeks, photocoagulation can be repeated, usually closer to the tumor since the initial photocoagulation promotes reabsorption of subretinal fluid around the mass. Preoperative photocoagulation diminishes the choroidal and retinal vascular bed, thus diminishing the chance for intraocular hemorrhage during and after resection. In addition, it helps prevent postoperative retinal detachment and helps delineate the tumor when transillumination is used during the resection.

Cryopexy ($-60°C$) is applied for 30 seconds four to five weeks after the second photocoagulation, 360° around the tumor directly onto the previously photocoagulated area. Cryopexy accentuates the effects of photocoagulation on diminishing the vascular bed. Photocoagulation must precede cryocoagulation because the pigment dispersal caused by cryopexy makes subsequent photocoagulation less effective.

Aminocaproic acid (4 g) is given orally every six hours one day before and for five days after each photocoagulation and cryopexy treatment. The drug acts principally via competitive inhibition of plasminogen-activator substances, that is, by blocking conversion of plasminogen to plasmin. By blocking fibrinolysis, theoretically aminocaproic acid can prevent recanalization of photocoagulated or cryocoagulated vessels. It also is used for five days postoperatively to prevent dissolution of the clot and subsequent recanalization of the blood vessels cut at the time of resection.

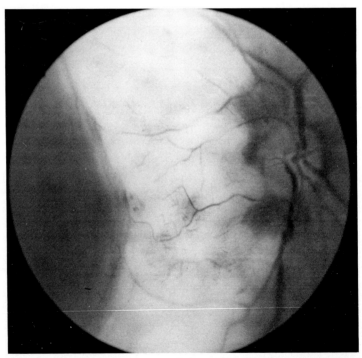

FIG. 13.1. Preoperative xenon arc photocoagulation performed in a centrally located, successfully resected malignant melanoma. With our present criteria, this tumor would be considered too close to the optic nerve for resection. Figure 13.10H shows histologic section of the resected area.

SURGICAL TECHNIQUE

General anesthesia is preferred. A 360° conjunctival peritomy with muscle isolation exposes the area of sclera subtending the tumor. The conjunctiva is pushed down into the orbit to avoid exposure of the inner conjunctival surface and postoperative adhesions. If necessary, one of the extraocular muscles is severed to provide adequate scleral exposure and is resutured at the end of the procedure. If a vortex vein is noted in the operative area, it is closed with a silk suture and cut away. A long posterior ciliary artery and nerve may also be cut without any significant problem. Transillumination is then carried out through the pupil, while the borders of the tumor are marked on the scleral surface with diathermy. The tumor appears as an easily discernible dark area surrounded by a translucent halo caused by the photocoagulation burns (Fig. 13.2).

The tumor border, as outlined by diathermy, is centered in the ring of the Peyman eye basket[10] (Figs. 13.3, 13.4), which is sutured into place with 5-0 Dacron. The eye basket stabilizes the eye to minimize distortion of the globe and vitreous loss at the time of resection. The suturing of the homograft under these conditions becomes a minor task.

A partial-thickness (two-thirds) scleral groove is made with a No. 64 Beaver blade outside of the diathermy marks outlining the tumor but within the ring of photocoagulation (Fig. 13.5). Heavy diathermy applications are made to the scleral groove (Fig. 13.6). The operative assistant then performs penetrating diathermy for marking in the scleral groove with simultaneous indirect ophthalmoscopy by the surgeon, who monitors accurate placement of the probe outside the margins of the tumor.

The intraocular pressure is frequently checked by palpation because it can increase secondary to the heat and scleral shrinkage. Vitreous aspiration through the pars plana is usually required. (After photocoagulation and cryocoagulation, the vitreous is frequently liquid and can be aspirated easily.)

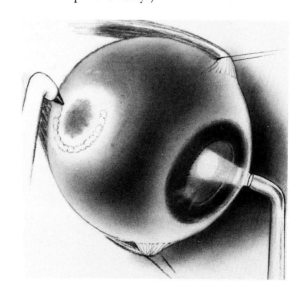

FIG. 13.2. Tumor borders outlined by transillumination and diathermy marking.

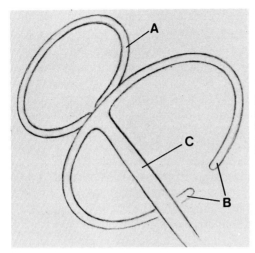

FIG. 13.3. Peyman eye basket. A, ring for stabilization of the operative area. B, Side arms for stabilization around the limbus. C, Arm for controlled movement of the eye during the operative procedure.

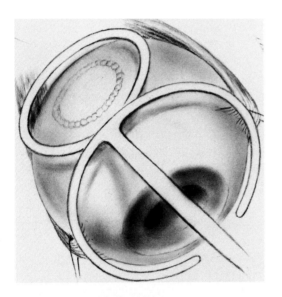

FIG. 13.4. The eye basket is placed with the tumor centered within the ring prior to being sutured to the sclera around the tumor with running 5-0 Dacron.

Fresh homograft donor sclera, presoaked for 12 to 24 hours in 40 μg of gentamicin per milliliter of saline solution, is cut and molded to fit the area to be resected. Preserved tissue can be used, but its toughness and lack of pliability make attachment more difficult.

Preplacement of a 5-0 Dacron suture from the host through the graft allows the graft to be slid in place after the resection (the more posterior the resection, the more sutures are desirable). Usually four or five 5-0 Dacron sutures are preplaced in the external lip of the scleral groove at the posterior aspect of the site of resection and through the posterior aspect of the donor graft sclera. One suture is preplaced through the anterior lip of the scleral groove and donor graft.

The final scleral fibers are cut with the diathermy, and the choroid and retina

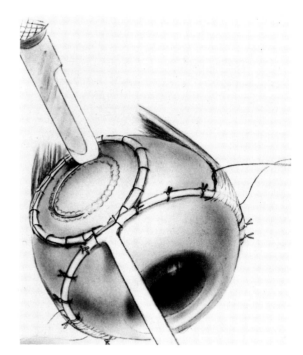

FIG. 13.5. A partial-thickness scleral groove is made around the borders of the tumor within the ring of photocoagulation.

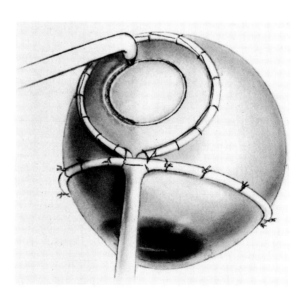

FIG. 13.6. Diathermy applications to the scleral groove.

are diathermized. The vitreous cavity is entered with a sharp scissors at the most anterior aspect of the wound, and the excision is completed with corneoscleral scissors (Fig. 13.7). Vitrectomy with the vitrophage or Weck sponge and scissors excision of vitreous through the resection site are now being done routinely in all cases.

The graft is then secured with the preplaced interrupted sutures and closed

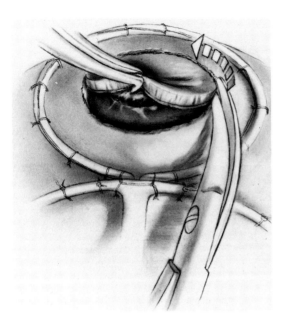

FIG. 13.7. Full-thickness scissors excision of the eye wall containing the tumor.

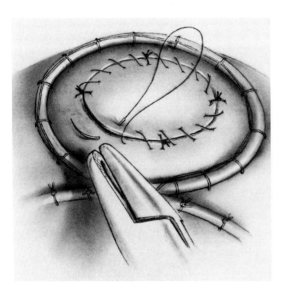

FIG. 13.8. Scleral homograft is sutured into place with running 5-0 Dacron over the resected area.

with a running 5-0 Dacron suture (Fig. 13.8). Air is injected through the graft edge to reestablish the intraocular pressure (Fig. 13.9), the conjunctiva is closed, 10 mg of gentamicin is given subconjunctivally, and a patch and shield are applied.

Postoperative medications include oral prednisone, 60 mg every morning for one week and then tapered; atropine, two drops twice a day; Neo-Cortef 1.5 percent, two drops four times a day; and oral aminocaproic acid, 4 g every six hours for five days.

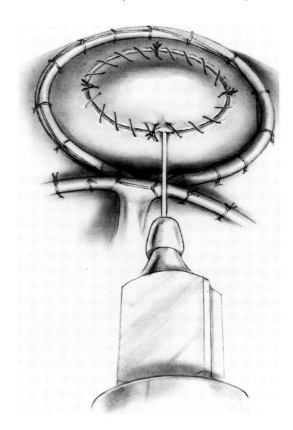

FIG. 13.9. Air injection through the graft edge reestablishes intraocular pressure.

If histologic examination reveals tumor involvement of the borders of resection, the eye should be enucleated as soon as possible. This approach has the obvious advantage of histologic confirmation of malignancy prior to enucleation.

RESULTS AND DISCUSSION

The described procedure or a modification of it has been performed on a total of 16 patients who were given the option of eye wall resection as an alternative to enucleation by their referring physicians. Three patients required enucleation because of intraoperative hemorrhage. In the first two eyes, this complication was due to the use of an electrocautery knife rather than corneoscleral scissors to perform the resection. In the third eye, preoperative photocoagulation was not feasible due to the presence of a cataract; thus we were unable to diminish the choroidal vascular bed prior to resection and massive hemorrhage ensued. In such a situation we now recommend a cataract extraction to be performed, followed in four to six weeks by photocoagulation and cryotherapy around the tumor as previously described, and finally the resection procedure.

A fourth eye was enucleated because the resection edge demonstrated tumor involvement (Fig. 13.10N). This tumor was centrally located within 1½ disk diam-

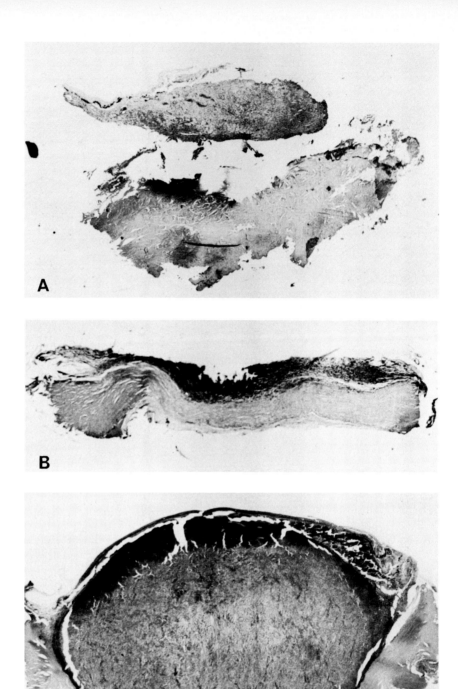

FIG. 13.10. Low-power photomicrographs of resected choroidal malignant melanomas. H&E, ×20. See legend on p. 178.

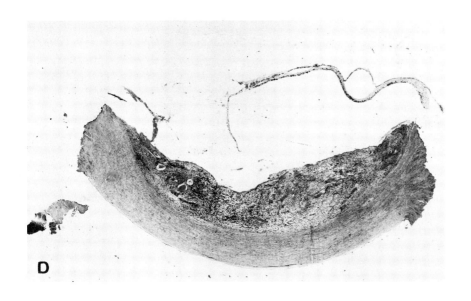

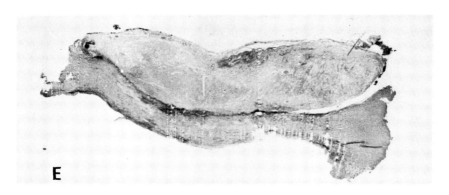

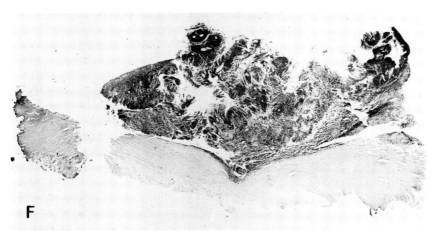

FIG. 13.10 (cont.).

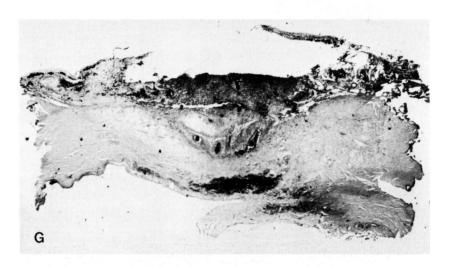

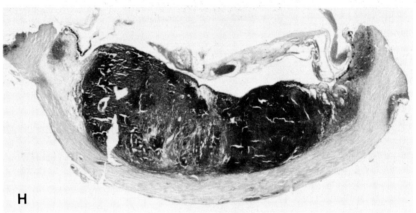

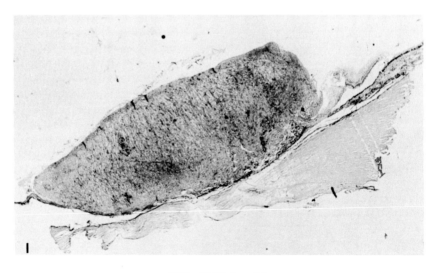

FIG. 13.10 (cont.).

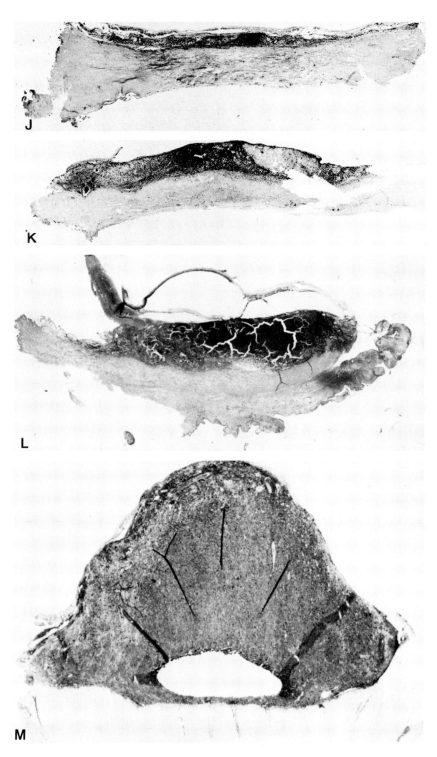

FIG. 13.10 (cont.).

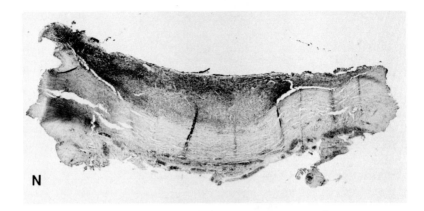

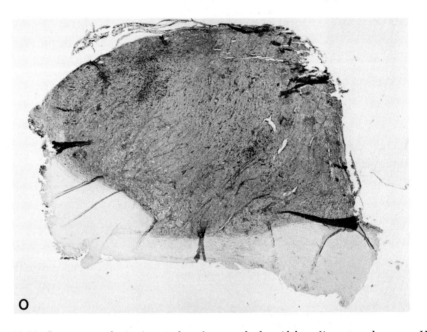

FIG. 13.10. Low-power photomicrographs of resected choroidal malignant melanomas. H&E, ×20. **A.** Melanoma composed predominantly of spindle A with scattered spindle B cells. **B.** Spindle B melanoma. **C.** Spindle B melanoma. **D.** Spindle A and spindle B melanoma. **E.** Necrotic-appearing melanoma (see also Fig. 13.14). **F.** Spindle B melanoma. **G.** Spindle A melanoma. **H.** Spindle B melanoma. **I.** Mixed cell melanoma. **J.** Spindle A melanoma. **K.** Spindle A melanoma. Moderate necrosis is due to preoperative photocoagulation. **L.** Mixed cell melanoma. **M.** Spindle B melanoma. **N.** Incompletely resected spindle A and spindle B melanoma. **O.** Epitheliod melanoma.

eters (2.5 mm) of the disk margin. After operating this case, we established the indication criteria that the tumor be at least 3 disk diameters (4.5 mm) from the disk margin; this operation was an example of poor patient selection. This patient reveals no evidence of metastatic disease after six-month postoperative follow-up.

Two other cases must be considered treatment failures (a total of 6 of 16 cases) because of the development of inoperable tractional retinal detachment. In these cases the time intervals between each coagulation treatment and surgery were too short (three weeks), the eyes were still inflamed at the time of surgery, and massive vitreous retraction ensued. We now feel that it is imperative that the eye be given sufficient time to recover from each preoperative step before subjecting it to further insults.

The postoperative fundus appearance of the successfully resected cases (10 of 16) was quite striking (compare preoperative views in Fig. 13.11 to postoperative views in Fig. 13.12). In five cases, a centrally located tumor necessitated loss of macular vision (Fig. 13.12A, E, F, and G). In some of these cases preoperative photocoagulation encompassed the macular region. In others the burns were adjacent to this region and wrinkling of the internal limiting membrane occurred. In all of these cases involving the macula, the patients were informed prior to treatment that they would lose central visual acuity and that the procedure was meant to remove the tumor while retaining peripheral vision and good cosmesis. Cosmesis in all successful cases was excellent (Fig. 13.13). In one case a large resection caused postoperative enophthalmos although the final visual acuity was 20/80 (Fig. 13.13F).

There has been no local or systemic metastasis in any of our patients with follow-up ranging from six months to four years. Photocoagulation has been shown to increase tumor antibody production. It is possible, though certainly not proved, that our preoperative preparation with photocoagulation and cryotherapy diminishes the tumor vasculature and induces necrosis and release of tumor antigen, thereby

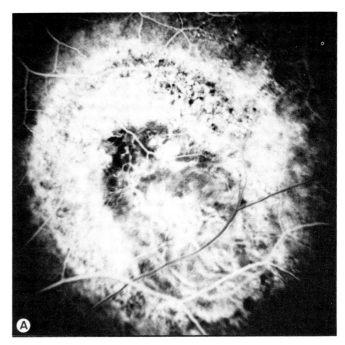

FIG. 13.11. Preoperative fluorescein angiographic appearance of suspected malignant melanomas that were successfully resected. For histology, postoperative fundus appearance, and postoperative cosmesis, see Figures 13.10, 13.12, and 13.13 respectively.

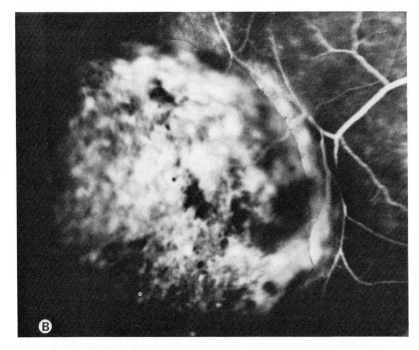

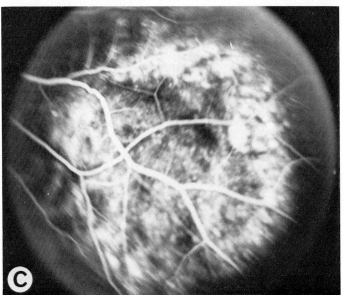

FIG. 13.11 (cont.).

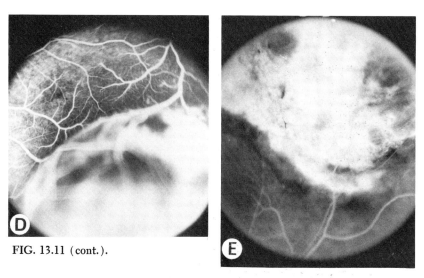

FIG. 13.11 (cont.).

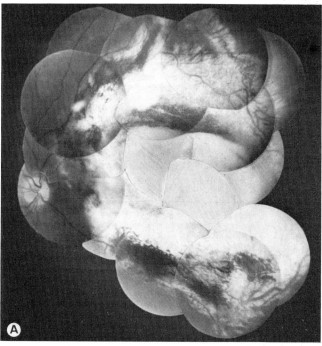

FIG. 13.12. Postoperative fundus montages of successfully resected malignant melanomas. **A.** Resection size 7 × 5 mm. Visual acuity, counting fingers due to resection of macular area. **B.** Resection size 10 × 7 mm. Note traction lines through macular region. Visual acuity, 20/40. **C.** Resection size 10 × 10 mm. Visual acuity, 20/100. **D.** Resection size 12.5 × 11 mm. Visual acuity, 20/50. **E.** Resection size 9 × 11 mm. Visual acuity, finger counting due to resection of macular area. **F.** Resection size 13 × 13 mm. Visual acuity, 20/200 due to resection of macular area. **G.** Resection size 12 × 10 mm. Visual acuity, 20/200 due to macular involvement. For histology preoperative fluorescein angiographic appearance, and postoperative cosmesis, see Figures 13.10, 13.11, and 13.13 respectively.

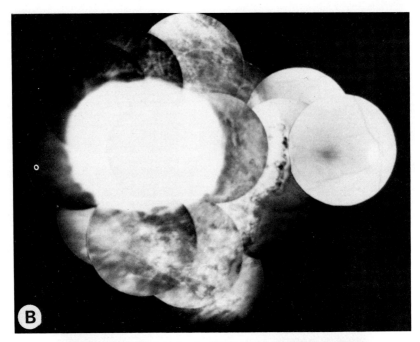

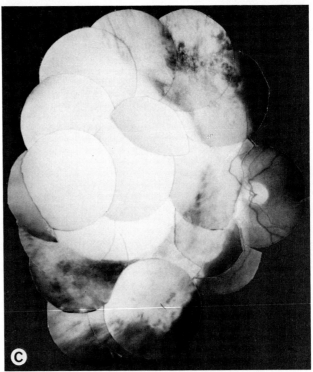

FIG. 13.12 (cont.).

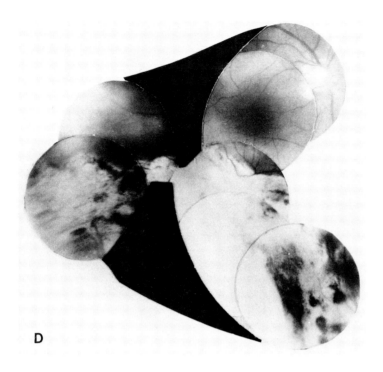

D

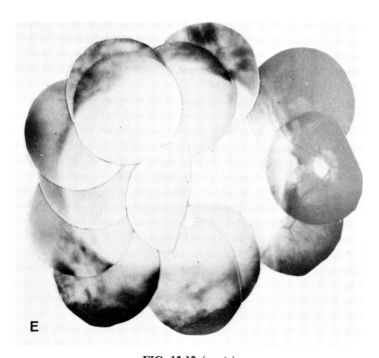

E

FIG. 13.12 (cont.).

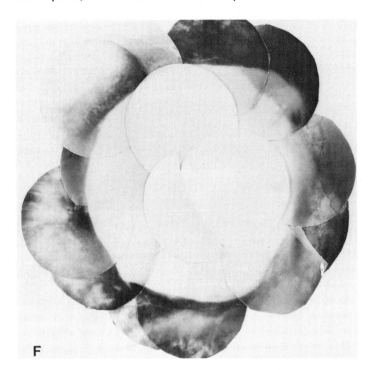

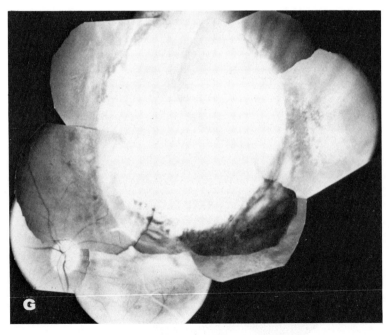

FIG. 13.12 (cont.).

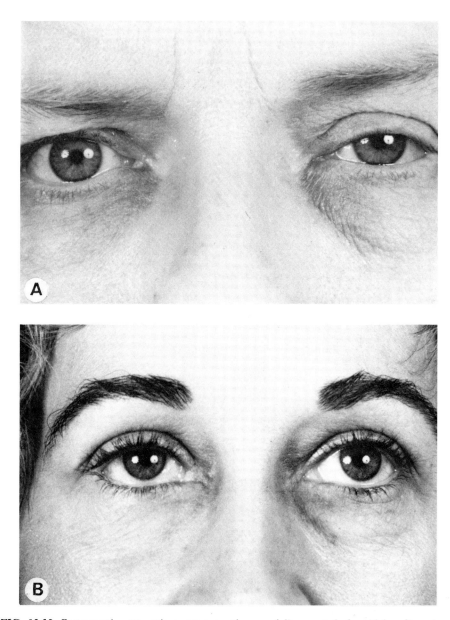

FIG. 13.13. Postoperative cosmetic appearance of successfully resected choroidal malignant melanomas. **A.** Six months after resection of left eye. **B.** Six months after resection of right eye. **C.** Twelve months after resection of left eye. **D.** Eight months after resection of right eye. Pupil dilatation due to mydriatic administration; pupils are equal at other times. **E.** Eight months after resection of right eye. **F.** Twelve months after resection of right eye. Enophthalmus is due to large resection size (13 × 13 mm). For histology preoperative fluorescein angiographic appearance, and postoperative fundus appearance, see Figures 13.10, 13.11, and 13.12 respectively.

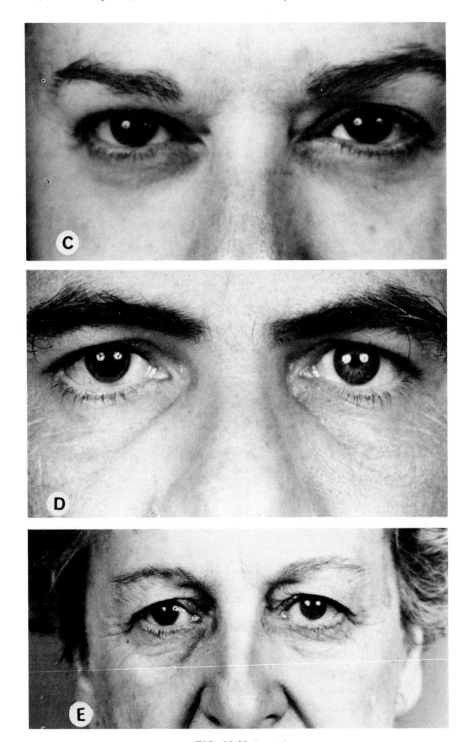

FIG. 13.13 (cont.).

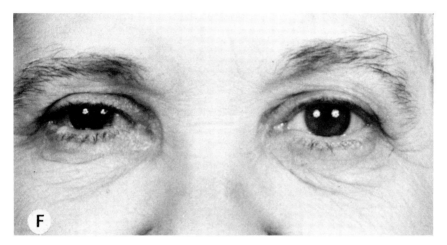

FIG. 13.13 (cont.).

stimulating immunization prior to resection. The resection then may remove the bulk of the tumor mass, possibly allowing the immune surveillance system to destroy any systemic seeding.

Histologic evaluation revealed that all but 1 of the 16 tumors were totally resected with clean margins (Fig. 13.10).

The tumors demonstrated variable degrees of necrosis, some quite extensive (Fig. 13.14). We think this necrosis is due to preoperative diminution of blood supply by photocoagulation and cryotherapy.

Although the eye wall resection procedure is still being refined, we believe that if the criteria and techniques established are strictly adhered to, the results can be most gratifying.

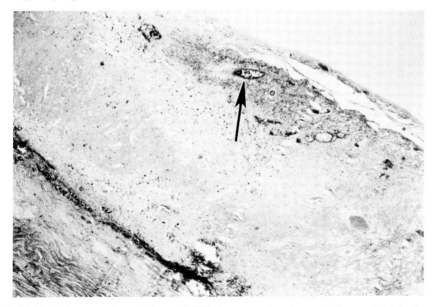

FIG. 13.14. High-power view of Figure 13.10E, demonstrating almost total necrosis of the tumor except for an area surrounding a tumor vessel (arrow). H&E, ×180.

REFERENCES

1. Peyman GA, Dodich NA: Full-thickness eye wall resection: an experimental approach for treatment of choroidal melanoma: I. Dacron graft. Invest Ophthalmol 11:115, 1972
2. Peyman GA, May DR, Ericson ES, Goldberg MF: Full-thickness eye wall resection: an experimental approach for treatment of choroidal melanoma: II. Homo- and heterograft. Invest Ophthalmol 11:668, 1972
3. Peyman GA, Ericson ES, Axelrod AJ, May DR: Full-thickness eye wall resection in primates: an experimental approach for treatment for choroidal melanoma. Arch Ophthalmol 89:410, 1973
4. Peyman GA, Nelsen PT, Axelrod AJ, Graham RO, Daily MJ: Full-thickness eye wall resection: evaluation of preoperative photocoagulation. Invest Ophthalmol 12:262, 1973
5. Peyman GA, Axelrod AJ, Graham RO: Full-thickness eye wall resection: an experimental approach for treatment of choroidal melanoma: evaluation of cryotherapy, diathermy, and photocoagulation. Arch Ophthalmol 91:219, 1974
6. Peyman GA, Diamond JG, Axelrod AJ: Sclero-chorio-retinal (S-C-R) resection in humans. Ann Ophthalmol 6:1347, 1974
7. Peyman GA, Apple DJ: Local excision of choroidal malignant melanoma: full-thickness eye wall resection. Arch Ophthalmol 92:216, 1974
8. Peyman GA, Koziol JM: Limitation of eye wall resection. Can J Ophthalmol 9:328, 1974
9. Peyman GA, Axelrod AJ, Ericson ES, May DR, Goldberg MF: Full-thickness eye wall resection in various species. Mod Probl Ophthalmol 12:556, 1974
10. Peyman GA, Sanders DR: Advances in Uveal Surgery, Vitreous Surgery and the Treatment of Endophthalmitis. New York, Appleton, 1975

Gholam A. Peyman
Donald R. Sanders

14 Treatment of Mass Lesions of the Iris and Ciliary Body: Iridectomy and Iridocyclectomy

TREATMENT OF MASS LESIONS OF THE IRIS

Many benign nonneoplastic as well as neoplastic lesions cannot always be clinically differentiated from malignant melanomas.[1] Fortunately, iris lesions are easily accessible surgically and removal of any form of iris mass for histopathologic diagnosis is usually not difficult. For more than half a century, the accepted form of treatment for mass lesions of the iris has been iridectomy.[2] Several factors govern the choice of therapy.

The vast majority of iris tumors grow slowly. Therefore, before surgical excision is done, the growth rate should be documented. This observation is most ideally accomplished by examining serial photographs. Pigmentary changes in an iris tumor may occur for a number of reasons and should not be considered evidence of definite growth. Distortion of the iris or pupil and incomplete dilatation of the pupil are signs of invasion involving the iris stroma or dilator muscle and are definite signs of growth.

Theoretically, lesions of any size can be excised by iridectomy, provided the lesion is confined to the iris. Practically, however, a mass lesion expands symmetrically, and any lesion larger than two clock hours probably involves angle structures or ciliary body and requires a more radical means of therapy. Ciliary body melanomas that invade the iris typically show a graver prognosis than a primary iris melanoma. Therefore, the differentiation of site of origin of the mass is of extreme importance in determining clinical management and choice of surgical techniques.

Certainly, if iridectomy is to be a successful therapeutic measure, the lesion to be excised must be confined to the iris. Careful examination must demonstrate that the lesion does not involve the cornea, angle structures, or ciliary body. If any of these structures is involved, a more radical surgical approach must be employed.

A lesion that originates closer to the root of the iris may require earlier surgical intervention than will a similar lesion near the pupillary border, as the former may threaten to involve angle structures or the ciliary body, necessitating an iridocyclectomy if it is allowed to grow. A lesion near the pupillary area may grow under observation for a longer time without involvement of adjacent structures.

In the case of malignant melanoma of the iris, heterochromia may indicate that the tumor is diffuse. Similarly, tumor seeding, which may be difficult to distinguish from iris freckles, indicates that the tumor is more widespread. An increase in the intraocular pressure of the affected eye implies that angle structures may be involved, and this suspicion should be verified by gonioscopy. In all such cases, simple iridectomy is insufficient; a more radical surgical approach is necessary.

Technique of Iridectomy

When evaluation of the above factors indicates that the iris lesion is relatively localized, sector iridectomy is the treatment of choice. The purpose of sector iridectomy is to excise completely the possible malignant mass lesion while avoiding contamination and possible tumor seeding of the rest of the eye.

As with a routine cataract extraction, a limbus-based conjunctival flap is made over the area occupied by the tumor. A corneoscleral groove is then made well posteriorly. A clear corneal incision may also be made, but shelving of the incision should be avoided in order to expose the most peripheral part of the iris. The anterior chamber is entered with a knife away from the tumor mass and extended with a corneoscleral scissors. The section should be large enough so that when the cornea is retracted the tumor mass and pupillary border of the iris are well exposed. While an assistant retracts the cornea, the surgeon cuts the iris radially on both sides of the tumor to the iris root with scissors (Fig. 14.1A). The section of iris with the tumor mass is then torn or cut from its insertion (Fig. 14.1B).

To maintain the anatomic conformation of the biopsy specimen after iridectomy, the specimen is pinned flat on a tongue blade, piece of filter paper, or cardboard.[3] It can be fixed by immersion in 10 percent buffered formaldehyde or other fixatives while still attached to the blade or paper.

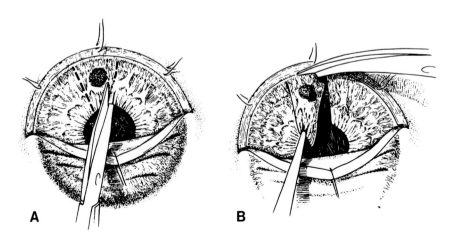

A

B

FIG. 14.1 A. Corneal incision and exposure of the iris tumor prior to iridectomy. B. Resection of iris tumor with scissors.

Prognosis

Rones and Zimmerman[1] reported 3 deaths from metastases in 125 clinically diagnosed cases of malignant melanoma observed for 15 years or more after iridectomy. Of these 125 cases, 87 were benign-appearing nevi, spindle A melanomas, or leiomyomas considered incapable of metastases. Reese and Cleasby[4] reported only 4 deaths in 140 patients followed up for 20 years or more after iridectomy. Ashton and Wybar[5] reported no death from metastasis in 105 histologically proved malignant melanomas. Because of the relatively good prognosis of circumscribed malignant melanoma of the iris, enucleation is almost never justified.

TREATMENT OF MASS LESIONS OF THE CILIARY BODY

Iridocyclectomy is the best acceptable procedure permitting the surgeon to excise a suspicious ciliary body lesion without sacrificing the entire eye, but again there are many factors governing the choice of therapy. The option for observing a lesion of the ciliary body will be determined primarily by the status of the lesion at the time it first appears. By the time a mass lesion causes symptoms, such as retinal detachment, cataract, glaucoma, or visible extension anteriorly, it is probably close to the maximum resectable size, and there will be little time for observation. Activity of the lesion may be inferred from the production of symptoms. However, when a small lesion is discovered incidentally during routine examination, the lesion may, in most circumstances, safely be observed for signs of growth.

Müller et al[6] have stated that a lesion occupying 2½ clock hours is the largest that can safely be excised. Certainly, excision of a larger tumor would involve the removal of more than an entire quadrant of iris–ciliary body. Intraoperative and postoperative complications may be increased with such extensive surgery.

A careful examination is made to reveal the extent of choroidal, corneal, scleral, or angle involvement. An appropriate technique of iridocyclectomy is selected to encompass the entire tumor.

Thorough systemic and ocular examination should reveal no evidence of tumor seeding or metastasis. The presence of seeding or metastasis is a contraindication to iridocyclectomy.

Technique of Iridocyclectomy

Iridocyclectomy was first described by Zirm[7] in 1911, and since then, removals of iris–ciliary body tumors have been reported by many investigators.[2, 5, 8–32] Basically, four techniques and their variations have been used.

"T" INCISION OF STALLARD. A conjunctival flap is prepared to expose bare sclera in the area of the tumor, and a Flieringa ring is sutured to the eye through episcleral tissue. A T-shaped limbal–scleral incision is then made, using a knife and corneoscleral scissors (Fig. 14.2A). Closing sutures may be preplaced. The cornea and the scleral flaps are then reflected, revealing the involved iris and ciliary body (Fig. 14.2B). The ciliary body surrounding the lesion is treated with penetrating diathermy. The pupillary border is grasped, and the iris is cut radically to its base as

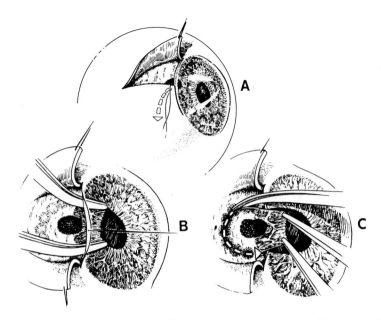

FIG. 14.2 A. T-shaped limbal incision of Stallard. B. Exposure of iris and ciliary body. The pupillary border of the iris is grasped. C. The iris and diathermized ciliary body surrounding the tumor are cut and excised. (Adapted from Stallard: Br J Ophthalmol 45:797, 1961)

described for the iridectomy procedure. The involved portion of ciliary body is then excised with scissors (Fig. 14.2C).[19, 22]

CURVED SCLERAL–LIMBAL INCISION OF FLIERINGA. A conjunctival flap is prepared, and a ring is sutured to the globe. With a knife blade, a half-thickness incision of the limbus and sclera is made along the line shown in Figure 14.3A. Two sutures are placed through the lips of the scleral incision, and the sclera is incised between the sutures to the choroid. As soon as the choroid appears, the remaining incision is completed with blunt-tipped scissors. The scleral–limbal flap is then reflected while the ciliary body is easily dissected free from the sclera with a blunt spatula (Fig. 14.3B).[20] The excision of the iris and ciliary body is performed as shown in Figure 14.2B and 14.2C.

CURVED SCLERAL–LIMBAL INCISION WITH TREPHINE OF MÜLLER ET AL. This procedure[6] is identical to the technique of Flieringa above, except that before the scleral–limbal flap is made, a full-thickness button of cornea and sclera overlying the tumor is trephined (Fig. 14.4A). The button is depressed, and a button of donor sclera is sutured in place (Fig. 14.4B). The scleral–limbal flap is then completed, and the tumor and adjacent portions of iris, ciliary body, cornea, and sclera are removed en bloc in a manner similar to that shown in Figures 14.2B, 14.2C and 14.3B.[6] This procedure has the obvious advantage in that there is less likelihood of disturbing the tumor mass while preparing the scleral flap.

IRIDOCYCLECTOMY OF PEYMAN. Five weeks prior to surgery cryocoagulation is performed at the area of the pars plana and retina in a semi-circular pattern around the tumor to prevent retinal detachment after surgery.[33] At surgery, a 360° limbal peritomy is performed. After localization of the tumor by transillumination and

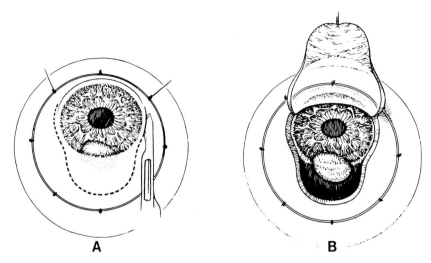

FIG. 14.3 A. Curved scleral–limbal incision of Flieringa. **B.** The scleral–corneal flap is reflected back, exposing the iris and ciliary body containing the tumor. (Adapted from Flieringa: Trans Ophthalmol Soc UK 81:421, 1961)

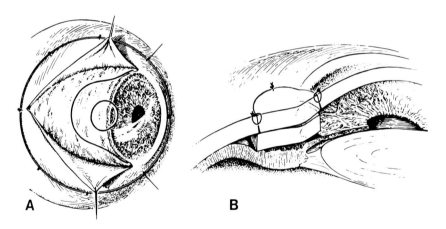

FIG. 14.4 A. Curved scleral–limbal incision of Flieringa combined with the trephine of Müller et al. The circle within the line of incision demonstrates the area to be trephined overlying the ciliary body tumor. **B.** Depression of the trephined corneal–scleral button by a button of donor sclera. (Adapted from Müller et al: Doc Ophthalmol 20:500, 1966)

diathermy marking around the tumor, a cyclectomy basket (Fig. 14.5) is sutured to the sclera close to the limbus. This cyclectomy basket stabilizes the eye and prevents collapse of the eye wall and operative area. Its use may be efficacious with any of the above described techniques. In the past we have performed a full-thickness resection of sclera, choroid, and underlying structures,[33] replacing the removed tissue with a scleral homograft. However, in most instances, we prefer the use of the iridocyclectomy basket with a partial-thickness T-shaped incision of Stallard (Fig. 14.6). This technique has given excellent postoperative results (Fig. 14.7).

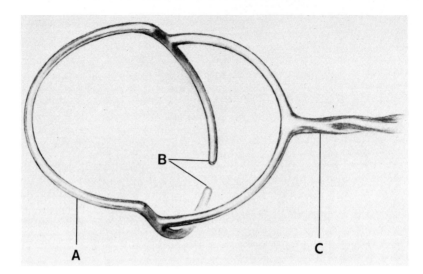

FIG. 14.5. Peyman cyclectomy basket. **A.** Semicircular wire for posterior support. **B.** Arms for limbal support. **C.** Rod for controlled movement of the eye.

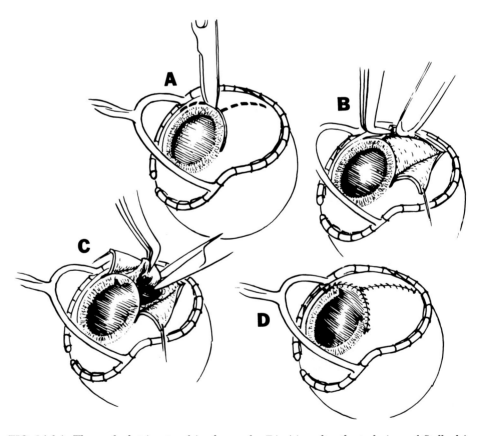

FIG. 14.6 **A.** The eye basket is sutured in place and a T-incision after the technique of Stallard is performed. **B.** A partial-thickness scleral dissection is made with a No. 64 Beaver blade. **C.** Following full-thickness diathermy applications around the tumor, the tumor is resected with curved corneoscleral scissors. **D.** The partial-thickness scleral flaps are sutured with running 9-0 nylon.

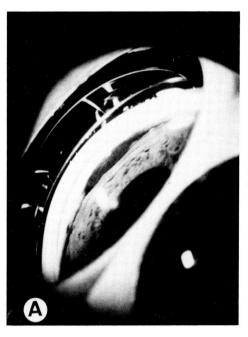

FIG. 14.7. Ciliary body tumor removed by the technique described in Figure 14.6. **A.** Preoperative. **B.** Postoperative. Open arrows indicate edge of lens and long arrow shows one cut edge of iris.

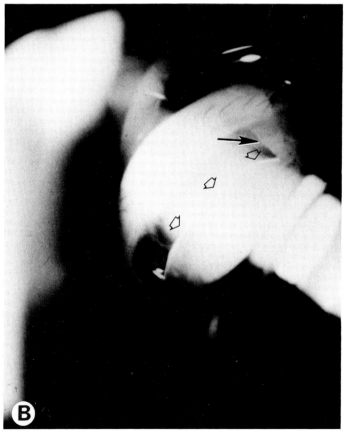

195

Complications of Iridocyclectomy

Many authors have expressed surprise at the small amount of hemorrhage produced by excision of the ciliary body. Nevertheless, hemorrhage (immediate and late) remains a serious complication of this procedure. Encircling the area of ciliary body to be excised with penetrating diathermy may reduce the chances of hemorrhage. Aminocaproic acid (Amicar, 4 g every six hours in an adult) orally may be used to inhibit clot lysis and minimize postoperative bleeding.

Vitreous loss may be unavoidable with large iridocyclectomies, but by using preventive measures, such as osmotic agents, the Flieringa ring, or the cyclectomy basket, one may minimize vitreous loss. If vitreous loss occurs, we perform a vitrectomy with the vitrophage during the procedure.

Cataract and lens dislocation have been reported in as many as 70 percent of patients undergoing iridocyclectomy. They are certainly related to the surgical manipulation and may be unavoidable.

Preoperative prophylactic cryocoagulation or photocoagulation to the retina surrounding the surgical area may help reduce the incidence of postoperative retinal detachment.

REFERENCES

1. Rones B, Zimmerman LE: The prognosis of primary tumors of the iris treated by iridectomy. Arch Ophthalmol 60:193, 1958
2. Raubitschek E: Über Iristumoren. Klin Monatsbl Augenheilkd 52:683, 1914
3. Reese AB: Tumors of the Eye. New York, Hoeber, 1951, p 221
4. Reese AB, Cleasby GW: The treatment of iris melanoma. Am J Ophthalmol 47 (no 5, pt 2):118, 1959
5. Ashton N, Wybar K: Primary tumours of the iris. Ophthalmologica 151:97, 1966
6. Müller HK, Lund OE, Söllner F, Seidel G: Die operative Behandlung von Tumoren des Kammerwinkels und des Ciliarkörpers. Doc Ophthalmol 20:500, 1966
7. Zirm E: Operative Mitteilungen. Arch Augenheilkd 69:233, 1911
8. Mursin AN: Die Trepanation der Hornhaut als Methode operativen Eingriffs auf der Iris. Klin Monatsbl Augenheilkd 85:416, 1930
9. Verhoeff FH: Sarcoma of the iris. Trans Am Ophthalmol Soc 31:270, 1933
10. Vogt A: Soll Man bei wachsendem Irisnaevus und Melanom enukleieren. Klin Monatsbl Augenheilkd 93:108, 1934
11. Haemmerli V: Aussprache-Vogt. Klin Monatsbl Augenheilkd 93:108, 1934
12. Lindner K: Operiertes Ciliarkorpersarkon. Z Augenheilkd 93:97, 1937
13. Franceschetti A: Extirpation d'une tumeur de l'iris et du corps ciliaire par iridectomia transversale. Ophthalmologica 97:1124, 1939
14. Friede R: Über sclero-keratoplastische Eingriffe bei Geschwülsten des Augapfels. Ophthalmologica 126:295, 1953
15. Bangerter A: Maligner Iristumor. Ophthalmologica 127:243, 1954
16. Friede R: Zur Operation maligner Geschwülste des Ciliarkörpers. Ophthalmologica 131:168, 1956
17. Müller HK, Niessen V, Niesel P, Lund DE: Die partielle Resektion des Ciliarkörpers zur Entfernung der Tumoren. Ber Dtsch Ophthalmol Ges 62:80, 1959
18. Stallard HB: Pigmented tumours of the eye. Proc R Soc Med 54:463, 1961
19. Stallard HB: Partial cyclectomy. Br J Ophthalmol 45:797, 1961
20. Flieringa HJ: A method of surgery in the angle of the anterior chamber of the eye. Trans Ophthalmol Soc UK 81:421, 1961

21. Winter FC: Surgical excision of tumors of the ciliary body and iris. Arch Ophthalmol 70:19, 1963
22. Stallard HB: Partial cyclectomy: some further modifications in technique. Br J Ophthalmol 48:1, 1964
23. Diamond S, Borley WE, Miller WW: Partial iridocyclectomy for chamber angle tumors. Am J Ophthalmol 57:88, 1964
24. Borley WE, Miller WW: Iridocyclectomy: a technique for removal of iris melanomas. Am J Ophthalmol 60:829, 1965
25. Korchmáros I: Daten zur operativen Behandlung des Melanoblastoms. In Francois J (ed): Die Tumoren des Auges und seiner Adnexe. Basel, Karger, 1966, p 713
26. Hofmann H: Die Operation von Iris- und Ziliarkörpertumoren. In Francois J (ed): Die Tumoren des Auges und seiner Adnexe. Basel, Karger, 1966, p 622
27. Palm E, Lindner B: Excision of tumours in the iris and the ciliary body. Acta Ophthalmol 46:521, 1968
28. Reese AB, Jones IS, Cooper WC: Surgery for tumors of the iris and ciliary body. Am J Ophthalmol 66:173, 1968
29. Linnic LF: Surgery of tumours of the ciliary body and base of the iris. Br J Ophthalmol 52:289, 1968
30. Müller HK: Die partielle Ausschneidung von Iris und Ciliarkörper. Doc Ophthalmol 26:679, 1969
31. Sears ML: Technique for iridocyclectomy. Am J Ophthalmol 66:42, 1968
32. Vail DT: Iridocyclectomy: a review: gleanings from the literature. Am J Ophthalmol 71:161, 1971
33. Peyman GA, Sanders DR: Advances in Uveal Surgery, Vitreous Surgery, and the Treatment of Endophthalmitis. New York, Appleton, 1975

Robert C. Watzke
Thomas A. Weingeist
John B. Constantine

15 Diagnosis and Management of von Hippel-Lindau Disease

Von Hippel-Lindau disease is a familial condition characterized by angiomatous tumors and cysts of the retina, central nervous system, and viscera. This report describes the important clinical features of the condition, its pathology, and treatment. A pedigree of particular interest demonstrates the protean nature of the disease and the unusual feature of familial disk angiomas.

HISTORY

In 1882 Fuchs[1] described and published drawings of the classical red peripheral retinal tumor with dilated artery and vein. He called the lesion an arteriovenous aneurysm. In 1894, Collins[2] produced the first pathology report (three enucleations in a brother and sister). He found the lesion composed of numerous thin-walled vessels and cystic spaces and termed it a "capillary naevus."

Von Hippel[3] published a description of two patients in 1904 with retinal drawings showing the appearance and progression of new lesions. He had no tissue to examine and, unaware of Collins' work, was unable to explain the disease. Seven years later one of these eyes was enucleated and von Hippel, now acquainted with the report of Collins and, by this time, some others, concluded the tumor was a hemangioblastoma and called the disease "angiomatosis retinae."[4] This patient died four years later, and in 1921 Brandt[5] published the autopsy report revealing that the patient had a cerebellar tumor, a tumor in the base of the brain near the petrous portion of the temporal bone, and one in the cauda equina. There were hypernephromas and multiple cysts in the kidneys and cysts of the pancreas. Epididymal cysts and bladder papillomas were found as well as tumors in several ribs and a vertebra.

In 1926 Lindau's classical paper synthesized the picture.[6] He began with an interest in cerebellar cysts. He found that most of these had mural hemangiomas in them; he collected reports of cerebellar cysts from the literature and added some 16 cases of his own. He noted that many of these patients also had cysts of the pancreas and kidney, renal cell carcinomas (8 of his 16), adrenal and liver

199

adenomas, and epididymal cysts. From the literature he also noted the association of angiomatosis retinae with cerebellar cysts; he searched his own cases for this manifestation and found two instances of it. He then compared the cerebellar tumors with those of the retina and found them to be histologically similar. The picture was complete.

CLINICAL PICTURE

The major manifestations of the disease are found in three different areas: the retina, the central nervous system, and the viscera.

Retinal Manifestations

The retinal picture is well described by von Hippel's term, "angiomatosis retinae." This vascular tumor of the retina classically appears as a localized reddish and/or yellowish mass (up to several disk diameters in size) in the midperiphery of the retina fed by a dilated artery and vein. In many cases more than one tumor is found in a retina (33 percent according to Cordes and Hogan[7]). Bilateral involvement is also frequently seen (30 to 50 percent according to Welch[8]). Eventually the secondary changes dominate the picture. Exudate appears on and around the tumor and often at remote sites. Macular exudates and star figures are frequently seen and may cause the presenting symptom. Localized detachment is a constant feature of all but small tumors. Eventually the exudative detachment enlarges, occupying an entire quadrant or even becoming total. It may appear almost solid, as if the retina lay over coagulated milk.[9] Hemorrhages are also a usual part of the picture. The exudates, hemorrhage, and detachment may actually hide the underlying tumor, rendering the true diagnosis difficult. Often, however, the characteristic dilated artery and vein can be seen entering the involved area, providing the clue to the underlying problem.

In rare instances the angiomas occur in the optic disk, where they may mimic papilledema, neuritis, or another tumor. The diagnostic dilated major vessels are, of course, not there, and, in the absence of a family history or signs of von Hippel-Lindau disease elsewhere, the diagnosis may be elusive. In 1955 Wallner and Moorman[10] found in the literature eight cases of angioma of the disk in which a pathologic examination was done. Six of the eight were diagnosed as von Hippel tumors, the other two as "endotheliomas." There were seven other clinical reports (without pathologic confirmation), five diagnosed as von Hippel tumors. By 1966, Darr et al[11] found 14 reported cases of von Hippel tumors at the disk, 10 confirmed microscopically. Their patient had bilateral disk tumors (the first such case reported), which were misdiagnosed as chronic papilledema by many experienced observers. Most of the angiomas of the nervehead confirmed pathologically were enucleated because of suspected malignancy.[11-15]

Retinal angiomatosis tends to become symptomatic in the third decade. However, the tumors have been discovered in young children (including a premature infant and a fetus) and up to the sixth decade.[16] It is quite common, now that smaller lesions are being found in affected families, to discover lesions during the teenage years.[17] With the advent of better diagnostic techniques and improved modes of treatment, the importance of discovering these angiomas at the earliest possible stage has become recognized.

Joe and Spencer[18] in 1964 called attention to these small lesions when they reported a case in which the subject, with a strong family history of von Hippel-Lindau disease, died of a cerebellar tumor. At autopsy, a 0.5-mm retinal angioma was found, unassociated with dilated vessels or secondary changes. This sign had been unnoticed clinically. In 1968, Jesberg et al[16] demonstrated incipient lesions clinically and pathologically. They emphasized that the lesions were usually found in the equatorial or preequatorial regions in the zone of capillaries between the large vascular trunks. There were no apparent dilated vessels. The lesions were ". . . similar in size and general configuration to diabetic micro-aneurysms and to the round vascular dilatations seen following venous branch occlusion." Welch[8] adds that an early lesion may resemble a small arteriovenous anastomosis. The recognition that small, even microscopic early lesions occur in this disease is not really new. Reports and drawings appeared in 1913,[19] and, indeed, Lindau referred to these early lesions in his original paper.[6]

The recognition of these very small, incipient lesions has become of paramount importance in the modern management of the disease, since they can be easily treated with every expectation of a complete cure. Fluorescein angiography may be of some assistance in confirming the diagnosis if a small nodule can be shown to be highly vascularized or to form a link between artery and vein. Most of the tumors that can be demonstrated will show leakage of the dye. Instances have been recorded in which a small angioma, undiscovered by ophthalmoscopy, has fluoresced during angiography. Only at a later date did the tumor develop enough to become visible without contrast media.[20] On the other hand, Welch[8] discovered an early angioma, without any apparent feeder vessels, which did not fill on fluorescein angiography. Over a period of time the area developed feeder vessels and the tumor filled with fluorescein. Hence, the use of contrast angiography may or may not hasten the discovery of the incipient lesion. It appears that nonfluorescence of a small nodule does not rule out its being an angioma. Nor does it seem likely from experience so far that intravenous fluorescein can reveal a great many angiomas otherwise invisible on indirect ophthalmoscopy, although a systematic study on some large kindreds with von Hippel's disease is needed to investigate this possibility further.

Central Nervous System Manifestations

About 25 percent of patients with angiomatosis retinae eventually develop central nervous system disease.[21] The most common and most important manifestation is the cerebellar hemangioma or hemangioblastoma (as Lindau preferred to call it). This tumor accounts for 2 percent of all brain tumors[22] and 7 to 10 percent of all tumors of the posterior fossa.[23] In 10 percent of cases they are multiple.[24] They usually present symptoms in the mid 30s. Silver and Hennigar[20] reported two age peaks for cerebellar hemangiomas, one from 20 to 40 years of age, and the second from 50 to 60.

While the cerebellum is the usual location of symptomatic central nervous system angiomas, other locations, almost always below the tentorium, have been reported in a significant number of instances. By far the most common of these angiomas are the spinal cord hemangiomas. Otenasek and Silver[22] reported six cases in one family with von Hippel-Lindau disease. In many instances apparently the cord angiomas are not symptomatic. When they are, they often produce symptoms of syringomyelia or spastic paraplegia.

Of less frequency are the angiomas described in the region of the fourth ventricle, medulla, and cerebellar midline which may cause hydrocephalus or syringobulbia. Hemangiomas in von Hippel-Lindau disease have very rarely been described in the cerebrum, and some of these cases have been disputed.

Visceral Manifestations

The systemic and visceral involvement has received less attention than the retinal and central nervous system problems. It was, however, well recognized and amply described by Lindau in his original paper and has been reported many times since.[6] It is far less commonly symptomatic than the retinal and central nervous system lesions, but numerous instances have accumulated in the literature in which it has caused significant symptoms and has aided in the diagnosis of the disease. Table 15.1 summarizes the various organ systems involved. It has been suggested that visceral involvement is found more frequently in cases with spinal cord angiomas.[21] Certainly, visceral cysts and tumefactions are extremely frequent in von Hippel-Lindau disease. Lindau himself was especially impressed with the occurrence of multiple cysts of the pancreas which are never symptomatic. He felt that the finding of a multicystic pancreas in an adult was pathognomonic of his disease.[25]

Epididymal cysts and occasionally adenomas, even carcinomas, are commonly encountered. MacRae and Newbigin described a large kindred in which all male members with retinal angiomatosis also had epididymal cysts.[24]

Clinically, the two most important associated visceral lesions are hypernephromas and pheochromocytomas. Both of these tumors have been the cause of morbidity and mortality in a significant number of cases. Renal lesions (cysts and hypernephromas) have been found in about two-thirds of autopsies.[26] Christoferson et al reported 11 cases of von Hippel-Lindau disease.[27] Eight had renal lesions: six of them had hypernephromas, one an adenoma, and one a hemangioma. Four patients had polycystic kidneys. Numerous other papers have reported hypernephromas, sometimes occurring bilaterally. They are malignant and may metastasize. Melmon and Rosen[26] recommend that renal angiography be done on every patient with confirmed von Hippel-Lindau disease since the urinalysis may be normal and the renal carcinomas may be asymptomatic until metastasis; they may even go unsuspected after intravenous pyelograms (IVP). After initial normal angiograms, a yearly IVP is recommended as the tumor may not show up until late middle age.

The incidence of pheochromocytoma in this syndrome is becoming more and more impressive. Welch[8] had 14 patients with von Hippel-Lindau disease; 5 of them had pheochromocytomas. Goldberg and Duke[28] have found them to occur bilaterally and multifocally. Hagler and Reese reported a family with pheochromocytoma and von Hippel-Lindau disease.[29]

Table 15.1

Pathologic Lesions Described in von Hippel-Lindau Disease

Structure	Lesion
Cerebellum	Hemangioblastoma
	Ependymoma
Medulla oblongata	Hemangioblastoma
Spinal cord	Hemangioblastoma
	Syringomyelia
Retina	Hemangioblastoma
Kidney	Cyst
	Renal cell carcinoma (hypernephroma)
	Fibroma of medulla
	Capillary angioma
	Adenoma
	Hemangioblastoma
Pancreas	Cyst
	Papillary cystadenoma
	Hemangioblastoma
Epididymis	Cyst
	Tumor (hypernephroid)
	Adenoma
Liver	Cyst
	Adenoma
	Angioma
Spleen	Angioma
Lung	Cyst
	Adenoma
	Hyperplasia
Adrenal cortex	Adenoma
	Hyperplasia
Adrenal medulla and sympathetic chain	Cyst
	Pheochromocytoma
	Paraganglioma
Cerebral cortex	Hemangioblastoma
Meninges	Meningioma
Bones	Cysts
	Anomalies of diploic vessels
	?Hemangioma
Bladder	Hemangioblastoma
Skin and mucosa	Nevus (pigmented or vascular)
	Café au lait spots
Omentum	Cyst
Mesocolon	Cyst

It is clear then that nonretinal and nervous system problems are not only of diagnostic but also of clinical importance in von Hippel-Lindau disease. A complete medical work-up is indicated on all patients with angiomatosis and probably on all the family members. Hagler[29] suggested that pharmacologic or biochemical testing for pheochromocytoma should be done even where clinical hypertension is not present since 5 percent of patients with the tumor are normotensive most or all of the time.

The heredofamilial nature of this disease is well established. It is carried as a simple dominant gene with a variable penetrance. Silent tumors and cysts have been found in the central nervous system, in the retina, and especially in the abdomen in clinically "unaffected" members of von Hippel-Lindau families.

Hence, only after an autopsy can an individual be said to be uninvolved. A single study, however complete, of a family at a given point in time tends to understate the number of affected members since some may manifest the disease later in life, or only on the necropsy table. Many pedigrees, in spite of this diagnostic limitation, clearly indicate the dominant genetic pattern with a rather high degree of penetrance.

The same difficulty hinders attempts to estimate the percentage of cases of angiomatosis that show a familial occurrence. The figure "20 percent," which originated with Lindau, is often quoted. Better diagnostic methods and a more aggressive approach today would probably yield a higher familial occurrence.

PATHOLOGY

Two extremes of the pathologic process are seen in histologic studies. In some enucleated globes the damage is likely to be so extensive that any recognizable trace of the original process is obliterated. Complete, organized, and fibrosed hemorrhagic detachments are seen with secondary inflammatory and glaucomatous changes in the anterior segment. At the other extreme, eyes obtained at autopsy may reveal an early lesion that appears only as a tiny red nodule without any appreciable increase in retinal thickness, dilated vessels, hemorrhage, or exudate.

Microscopically, the mature tumor is intraretinal, tending to involve the entire thickness of the retina and to obliterate the normal histologic structure. There are several prominent features of the tumor. First, there is a proliferation of capillaries and small blood vessels in addition to areas of proliferating vascular endothelium without well-formed channels. Second, large numbers of round, lipid-laden "foam" cells are seen. Third, an impressive proliferation of glial cells and fibrosis is usually seen; this finding often comprises the dominant feature of the process.

Other features often seen are cholesterol crystals and other hemorrhagic debris, calcification and bone formation, and pigment proliferation (although the lattermost characteristic is not a prominent feature of untreated tumors). Strands of capillaries and new vessels commonly extend into the vitreous from the tumor surface. There may be old or recent vitreous hemorrhage. Detached retina with subretinal exudate and/or hemorrhage is an almost constant feature. In the area of the macula, if it is still intact, exudates, edema, and cyst formation may be seen, and microaneurysms have been described.[28]

Much of the appearance, activity, destructiveness, and apparent growth of these tumors Reese has ascribed to a spontaneous sclerosing process.[30] The pathologic vessels and vascular spaces undoubtedly contain areas of low or stagnant blood flow, which makes them prone to thrombosis. This feature probably accounts for the foam cells, hemorrhage, and glial reaction. Thrombotic episodes may explain the instances of rapid change in appearance or size or associated complications that may characterize these tumors.

This process is probably a good explanation for much of the behavior of the retinal (and central nervous system) hemangiomas in the more mature stages, but it sheds little light on the very early lesions. Goldberg and Duke in 1968 studied both eyes of a patient who had central nervous system, retinal, and visceral manifestations of von Hippel-Lindau disease and who died of a subarachnoid hemorrhage.[28] They prepared a flat mount of the retinal vasculature with trypsin digestion. Clinically, this retina had contained a very small peripheral lesion that was seen by only one observer on one occasion. No obvious large vessels were seen leading to it. Histologic study of the flat preparation of this lesion revealed a contorted, irregular mass containing many endothelial cells, which stained intensely with PAS. Leading out to the mass from the posterior pole was a relatively large artery, maintaining its caliber all the way to the tumor. Near the terminus of this hyperplastic-appearing artery, but apparently unconnected to the tumor itself, were a number of discrete nodular proliferations of endothelial cells within the wall of the vessel. A large vein returned to the posterior pole.

This case demonstrates clearly that the earliest abnormalities in this disease are vascular. The small nodules of endothelial hyperplasia in the arteriolar wall are intriguing. Whether they represent a primary malformation or endothelial cells from which the vascular tumor originates, or are secondary to abnormal vascular hemodynamics is not established. However, since they were not found elsewhere in the retina except contiguous to the angiomatous mass and probable arteriovenous shunt, it seems unlikely that they represent preexisting lesions from which the angiomas arise. Goldberg and Duke contend that the presence of a hyperplastic artery and these nodules in the case of such a small early tumor suggests that the disease process from the beginning is an abnormality of the entire vascular unit (artery, vein, and capillary).[28]

Jesburg et al[16] also studied the retina with trypsin digestion and demonstrated a solitary small nodule appearing quite similar to that described above. The nodule was a collection of proliferating endothelial and mural cells causing an irregular thickening of a branch venule in the periphery of the retina. There were two vessels of capillary size extending from it. However, in this case there was no hypertrophied vessel leading to or from the nodule, the surrounding retinal vasculature being quite normal. This finding suggested that the tumors arose from a previously normal retinal vascular channel and not from a congenital rest of undifferentiated cells. In addition, the implication is that the hypertrophy of the vessels leading to and from these nodules was a secondary phenomenon.

Notable in both of these cases was the fact that the early nodules lay essentially in the capillary area with communication to both the arterial and venous systems. This finding, of course, has been long recognized as a feature of the disease. In the past some early lesions have been observed that consisted only of one or a group of small vessels without any tumefaction forming a direct connection between artery and vein. One such early case was presented in the classic set of drawings published by Ditroi and reprinted in Welch's paper.[8] The first drawing showed an early lesion composed of a small fan of vessels making an arteriovenous communication. The second picture, at a later examination, showed the network to have transformed into a tumor nodule.

Other observers also reported instances in which the original lesion appeared to be a simple arteriovenous shunt.[31] It is often observed, for example, that the color of the efferent vein from these tumors is similar to that of the artery (suggesting "arterialized" blood). Fluorescein angiography has demonstrated that the flow through this shunt may be so extensive that it effects the surrounding retinal circulation, causing, in effect, a "steal" syndrome.[32] This may be the best explanation for the maculopathy and papilledema so commonly seen in angiomatosis retinae even when the tumors are quite distant from the posterior pole.

REPORT OF A KINDRED
WITH CLINICOPATHOLOGIC CORRELATION

The family described here demonstrates the protean nature of this disease and the presence of disk angiomas in several generations (Fig. 15.1).

Patient III-1

A 19-year-old man was first examined December 30, 1955, because of failing vision in the left eye. Vision was 6/30 in the left eye and 6/4.5 in the right eye. The left eye showed a large sclerosed angioma in the superior temporal quadrant with a large feeding artery and draining vein. The right fundus revealed a vascular malformation at the superior nasal margin of the disk with a surrounding localized flat retinal detachment and circinate exudate (Fig. 15.2). Results of complete neurologic work-up, including cerebrospinal fluid analysis, was within normal limits; IVP was normal. Radiation therapy was administered to the posterior segment of the left eye, but hemorrhagic glaucoma developed in that eye and an enucleation was performed in 1967. Histologic examination revealed a retinal hemangioma with extensive secondary exudative detachment and scarring. Examination of the right eye in November 1971 revealed slight enlargement of the serous detachment nasal to the disk with some fibrotic alteration in the original disk neovascularization. The disk had become more elevated with some new vascular tissue on the superior temporal margin (Fig. 15.3). The patient is still being followed up.

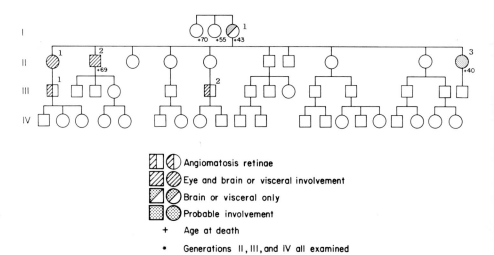

FIG. 15.1. Pedigree of family with von Hippel-Lindau disease.

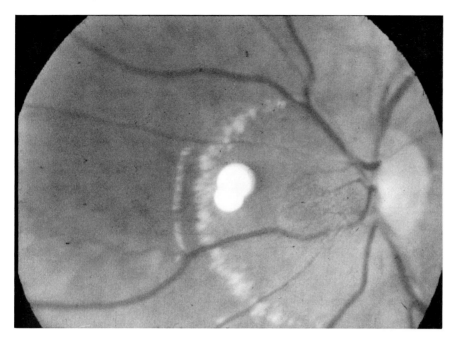

FIG. 15.2. Disk angioma with serous detachment and exudate in a 19-year-old man with von Hippel-Lindau disease. Vision was 20/20. Patient III-1 in the kindred study.

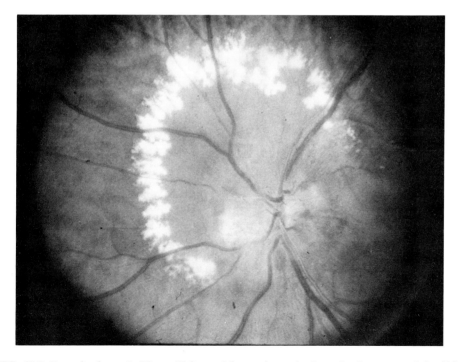

FIG. 15.3. Same fundus as in Figure 15.2 seen 15 years later. Angioma involves more of the disk and serous detachment has enlarged slightly. Vision was 20/20.

Patient II-2

A 66-year-old man, the maternal uncle of the previous patient, was seen on February 17, 1971, because of difficulty in walking. The patient gave a history of a brief period of unconsciousness 16 years before, which had been attributed to a spontaneous brain hemorrhage. Ocular examination at this time revealed 20/20 vision in each eye and bilaterally blurred disk margins, which were felt to be due to chronic papilledema. An area of neovascularization was noted on the superior temporal margin of the right disk. Neurologic examination revealed signs of a posterior fossa tumor. An occipital craniotomy and cervical laminectomy was performed, revealing an extensive arteriovenous malformation on the posterior aspect of the spinal cord. Decompression was performed to the level of T-1. Following the operation the patient did well, with complete clearing of his papilledema and no progression of his ataxia.

In November 1971 the fundus examination revealed regression of the papilledema and a small disk angioma at the temporal aspect of the margin of the right disk (Fig. 15.4). Fluorescein angiography showed filling and leakage from this lesion during the late arteriovenous phase (Fig. 15.5). Subsequent examination in 1972 revealed no other retinal lesions or changes in the vessels adjacent to the disk. In May 1974 the patient died of bronchopneumonia at home.

The most significant findings at autopsy were in the spinal cord, stomach, and eyes. A large vascular neoplasm located adjacent to the right lateral spinal cord extended through the lower cervical and upper thoracic regions. There was hemosiderosis and necrosis of the spinal cord in that area. On cut sections this mass consisted of vascular channels of variable size, the largest of which was filled with laminated thrombus as well as numerous small cystic spaces. There was marked left lateral compression of the substance of the spinal cord and distortion of the normal gray and white matter.

A polypoid lesion attached to the serosal surface of the stomach was found, on microscopic examination, to be a capillary hemangioma. No cysts were found in either the kidneys or pancreas, as might be expected in von Hippel-Lindau disease.

Examination of the right eye was unremarkable except for the presence of an angiomatous lesion extending from the optic nervehead, which consisted of many small endothelium-lined vessels. These thin-walled channels were similar in structure and size to capillaries (Fig. 15.6). No lipid deposits or foam cells were observed with special stains. No other vascular lesions were observed grossly or microscopically. The left globe was within normal limits except for the presence of dilated retinal vessels and evidence of chronic papilledema.

Patient II-1

This 68-year-old woman, the mother of patient III-1, was first seen in October 1971 because of chronic ataxia, generalized weakness, lethargy, and decreased vision in the right eye. Ocular examination revealed an edematous right disk due to an angioma surrounded by a localized retinal detachment. The left fundus was normal. The patient underwent an occipital craniotomy on November 9, 1971, and a large cyst of the left cerebellar hemisphere was found. It was drained and excised, and a small hemangioma was found in the cyst wall. Since surgery the patient's general condition has markedly improved and the disk angioma has not changed.

A complete family survey was undertaken of over 40 members of the kindred from three generations. Because of this screening the following patient was found.

Patient III-2

This patient was a 34-year-old man, the first cousin of patient III-1. He had a typical retinal angioma in the superior temporal quadrant of the left eye. This angioma was 3 disk diameters in size, with a very large feeding artery and draining

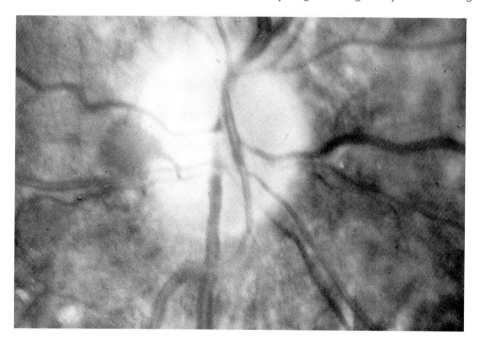

FIG. 15.4. Disk angioma in the 66-year-old maternal uncle (patient II-2) of patient III-1.

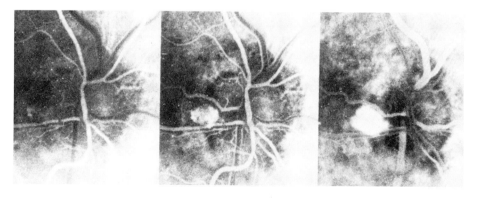

FIG. 15.5. Fluorescein angiography of this angioma shows typical early filling and late leakage of the dye.

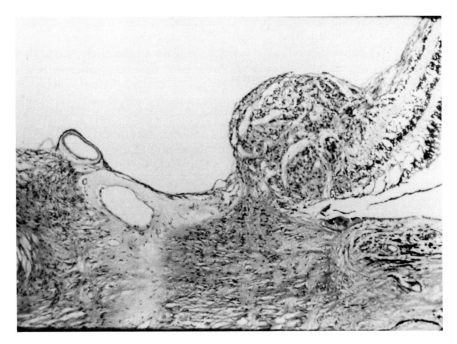

FIG. 15.6. Histologic section of this angioma reveals a tumor composed of endothelial cells lining vascular channels. H&E, ×300.

vein. The tumor regressed satisfactorily after combined cryotherapy and photocoagulation. Because of neurologic symptoms, in 1974 a frontal lobe tumor was resected that proved to be a meningioma and *not* an angioma.

Patient I-1

This patient died at the age of 43 because of a "brain hemorrhage."

Patient II-3

This patient has had severe hypertension since age 17 and also had a history of loss of consciousness due to a brain hemorrhage. Adequate fundus examination was never performed. A phentolamine test for pheochromocytoma was "probably negative," and an assay of urinary catacholamine levels was normal. Stenosis of the right renal artery was found and was corrected by a venous bypass. The patient died in an automobile accident two months after the surgery, and no autopsy was performed.

TREATMENT OF VON HIPPEL-LINDAU DISEASE

Family Management

Management of a family with von Hippel-Lindau disease presents three problems: survey and recognition of early ocular angiomas and their treatment, management of systemic manifestations, and genetic counseling.

Obviously, all blood relatives of patients found to have retinal angiomas must have a complete ocular examination. In children this examination should be performed as soon as possible without resorting to general anesthesia, usually at age four or five. We do not feel it necessary to examine infants under anesthesia since most early lesions are small and there appears to be little danger of significant growth prior to the age when examination is practical. In adults no patient should be considered too old for such a survey.

The examination should be performed with indirect ophthalmoscopy. With repeated effort enough cooperation can be achieved to perform an adequate examination even in four- or five-year-old patients. The most important point in fundus examination of these individuals is to realize that we are looking for a lesion that is the size of a diabetic microaneurysm. Any unusual arteriovenous malformation, irregularity, kinking, or anastomosis should be studied under as high a magnification as is possible (Fig. 15.7). After an indirect ophthalmoscopic survey the particular lesions in young children can be studied with a direct ophthalmoscope, and in older individuals as soon as possible by slit-lamp biomicroscopy.

Since it is now well substantiated that angiomas can appear in areas that have clinically appeared normal, we generally advise that patients be examined every six months during the first two or three years of observation and once yearly thereafter.

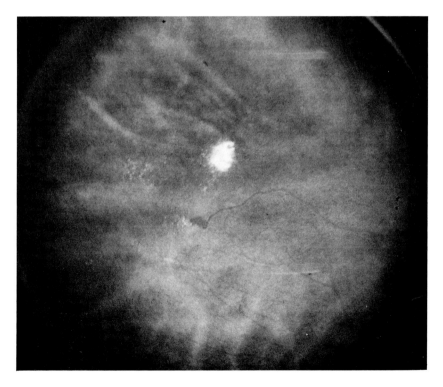

FIG. 15.7. A typical early angioma in a 26-year-old man. The lesion is slightly larger than a microaneurysm with the afferent arteriole and efferent venule already present. Nearby is a white exudate.

The frequency of examination depends somewhat on the age of the patient. In adults past the age of 30, yearly examination is usually sufficient.

We believe that all angiomas should be treated as soon as they are seen. For logistic and scheduling reasons, however, particularly when one is dealing with a large family, treatment may safely be postponed for several months to schedule treatment of many children at one time. In our experience, the growth of small lesions has been fairly slow and this approach has not caused complications.

We have not found routine fluorescein angiography helpful as a survey mechanism to find small, clinically unrecognized angiomas. It is of value in some patients to confirm the presence of suspected angiomas.

Every patient from a kinship of von Hippel-Lindau disease should be informed in a general way of the cerebral and visceral manifestations. Young adults should have a neurologic examination and a general physical examination. These consultants will determine the type and extent of work-up according to their own philosophy and experience. Our own neurologic consultants feel that invasive procedures should not be performed on these patients unless neurologic signs and symptoms have occurred. Our urologic consultants feel that young adults should have a good urologic examination including yearly IVPs. The ophthalmologist should inform all consultants of his concern for the presence of cerebellar and spinal cord tumors, kidney cysts, hypernephromas, and pheochromocytomas.

Patients should be told of the protean and extensive organ system involvement of this condition and the dominant nature of its inheritance. In the past most of the patients we have seen have not been told of its genetic dominance, and while it may not be appropriate for the counseling physician to advise family planning unless asked, patients should be given enough information to make a rational and well-informed decision.

Treatment

Treatment of retinal angiomas consists of either photocoagulation or cryosurgery or a combination of the two. We no longer use diathermy or radiation therapy.

Experimental cryosurgery has demonstrated that low temperature causes choroidal exudation, choroidal vascular alteration, vascular stasis in the choriocapillaris, and platelet agglutination. Thrombosis of the vessels, particularly in the choriocapillaris, follows.[33] There is also necrosis of retinal capillaries with pigment deposition and hypercellularity, particularly around retinal venules. By six weeks retinal vessels of capillary size are completely hyalinized and destroyed, and there is considerable loss of mural and endothelial cells.[34] These changes are intensified by a triple freeze–thaw technique.[33] Such heavy and repetitive cryosurgery also seems to stimulate a hyaline metaplasia of the pigment epithelium with formation of new collagen tissue[35] (Fig. 15.8).

Cryotherapy is convenient when treating peripheral lesions and tumors in eyes with opaque media. It is particularly advantageous in eyes with a rather thick and large tumor mass, for the entire depth of the tumor in which all the cellular components are reached by freezing. This penetrance is not possible with photo-

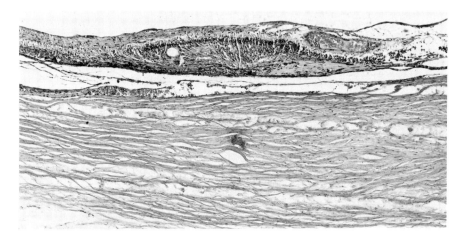

FIG. 15.8. Retinal angioma in a 14-year-old boy treated with three sessions of triple-freeze cryotherapy eight months previously. No endothelial cells or vascular channels are present. A hyalinized pigment epithelial scar replaces the outer retina. Arteriole and venule are patent. H&E, ×100. (From Watzke: Arch Ophthalmol 92:399, 1974)

coagulation. Cryotherapy is particularly efficacious in angiomas surrounded by an exudative retinal detachment that has lifted the angioma above the surface of the surrounding fundus. Finally, cryotherapy is safe in angiomas that are large and thin-walled. Such tumors may be shrunken down and surrounded by a fibrotic reaction much more safely than with photocoagulation. In our experience severe secondary exudative detachments following treatment are less common with cryotherapy than with photocoagulation.

There are several disadvantages of cryotherapy. It invariably produces a rather large scar, which is undesirable when treating very tiny and flat angiomas. Cryotherapy must be repeated at least three times with an interval of six weeks to three months between treatments, for the full effect of these treatments is delayed for that period. Finally, even with a completely fibrotic alteration in a retinal angioma, the feeding artery and veins do not appear to be narrowed. Consequently, these lesions must be followed up for a long time before we can know the ultimate and permanent results of cryotherapy for retinal angiomatosis.

The advantages of photocoagulation are also numerous. By altering the size of the photocoagulation beam one may treat only the angioma and reduce the scarring of surrounding retina to a minimum. Photocoagulation is extremely effective for small to medium-size flat tumors that do not have a surrounding secondary detachment. It is more convenient to treat angiomas located in the posterior pole with photocoagulation, and treatment of feeder arteries and draining veins can also be accomplished at the time of treatment.

The disadvantages of photocoagulation, in addition to the usual technical problems of treating eyes with opaque media and peripherally located tumors, are the exudative reaction commonly following extensive photocoagulation treatment and the difficulty in treating more than superficial cells in thick multicellular tumors.

In our experience it is also very difficult to completely obliterate and scar large retinal angiomas with surrounding retinal detachments.

Photocoagulation also involves the choice between xenon and argon modalities. Clinically there is little difference between the two except for the technical problems of using a contact lens and slit-beam delivery system with the argon modality. Both require retrobulbar anesthesia in all except the tiniest and flattest angiomas since only the most phlegmatic patients can tolerate the intensity and duration necessary to obliterate these lesions. In using the argon laser one must avoid small 50- and 100-μ spot sizes with short-duration burns when treating rather large angiomas since it is possible to cause a vitreous hemorrhage with such small and intense burns. The spot size should be fitted to the size of the tumor and purposely made rather large and of long duration to avoid perforation of an angioma wall and consequent hemorrhage.

EARLY RETINAL ANGIOMAS. Retinal angiomas that are flat and smaller than ¼ disk diameter in size with no surrounding retinal detachment should be treated as soon as possible with photocoagulation unless the tumors are so peripheral that this procedure is not possible. The tumors are treated directly; then the feeding artery and then the draining vein are photocoagulated. Cryotherapy is not used because the resulting scar is too large for such small tumors. Treatment of these tumors is very satisfactory, usually requiring only one session. Local anesthesia is used if possible.

MODERATELY ADVANCED TUMORS WITHOUT RETINAL DETACHMENT. Retinal angiomas of ¼ to 1 disk diameter in size without a surrounding retinal detachment may be treated with either cryotherapy or photocoagulation, depending on the location of the tumor and the opaqueness of the media. If cryotherapy is elected a cryosurgical unit is selected that freezes to at least −60C. The tumor is indented precisely with the probe tip and the tissue is frozen until the maximum whiteness develops throughout the tumor; during freezing, the fundus is monitored with the indirect ophthalmoscope. Some angiomas turn completely white and others retain a faint, reddish flush in the center. The mass is allowed to thaw and is then refrozen twice more. We do not advise treatment of the feeding artery and vein with cryotherapy since they are usually not affected significantly and quite a bit of retina is scarred in the process.

Photocoagulation can also be used for these tumors, particularly in the posterior pole. The treatment is the same as for small tumors. Of course, an exudative reaction is usually produced, which seems to subside, invariably, without complications.

If cryotherapy is used, these tumors are followed up and retreated when the fibrotic reaction appears to be maximum, usually after about six weeks to three months. Cryotherapy may and should be repeated until the tumor appears to be satisfactorily regressed. Even though the feeding artery and vein have not regressed, we usually do not treat these with photocoagulation and have not found it necessary to do so as yet.

MORE ADVANCED TUMORS WITH OR WITHOUT RETINAL DETACHMENT. Surrounding exudative detachment rarely occurs with angiomas smaller than about 1 disk diameter. Tumors this large or larger are best treated with a combination of cryotherapy and photocoagulation. These angiomas are first treated with cryotherapy, as previously described, for a total of three treatments approximately six

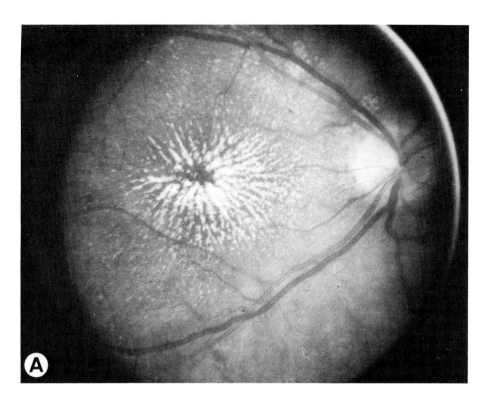

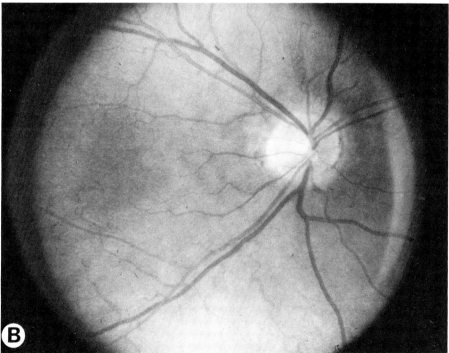

FIG. 15.9 **A.** Macular star and edema in an 18-year-old woman with a disk-size angioma in the retinal periphery. Vision was 20/100. **B.** Nine years after treatment of the angioma the central fundus was normal. Vision was 20/20.

weeks to two months apart. Such treatment shrinks the tumor remarkably and produces an intense fibrotic reaction within it. It then is usually possible to treat the inner surface of the angioma with photocoagulation and finally to treat the feeding artery and vein. Unfortunately many of the large tumors never completely lose their surrounding retinal detachment and continue to have a certain vascular flush in them.

Fluorescein angiography may be used to monitor the effectiveness of therapy since incompletely scarred tumors continue to leak fluorescein. It may be impossible, however, to completely scar large tumors, and these eyes may simply have to be followed up periodically. Such tumors are always a menace, and we have patients in whom progressive traction retinal detachments and chorioretinal scarring have progressed after a latent period of several years.

Patients with macular exudates and decreased central vision due to a peripheral angioma may recover remarkably if the peripheral tumor can be completely scarred. However, this success is *only* possible in small tumors (Fig. 15.9).

In some patients who have very large retinal detachments with large active multiple tumors, drainage of the detachment, cryotherapy, and even diathermy in the operating room may be attempted. The prognosis for these patients is very poor, however.

REFERENCES

1. Fuchs E: Aneurysma arterio-venosum retinae. Arch Augenheilkd Weisb 11:440, 1882
2. Collins ET: Intra-ocular growths: I. Two cases, brother and sister, with peculiar vascular new growth, probably primarily retinal, affecting both eyes. Trans Ophthalmol Soc UK 14:141, 1894
3. Von Hippel E: Über eine sehr seltene Erkrankung der Netzhaut. Albrecht von Graefes Arch Ophthalmol 59:83, 1904
4. von Hippel E: Die anatomische Grundlage der von mir beschriebenen "sehr seltenen Erkrankung der Netzhaut." Albrecht von Graefes Arch Ophthalmol 79:350, 1911
5. Brandt R: Zur Frage der Angiomatosis retinae. Albrecht von Graefes Arch Ophthalmol 106:127, 1921
6. Lindau A: Studien über Kleinhirncysten: Bau, Pathogenese und Beziehungen zur Angiomatosis retinae. Acta Pathol Microbiol Scand (Suppl) I:1, 1926
7. Cordes FC, Hogan MJ: Angiomatosis retinae (Hippel's disease): Report of a case in which roentgen therapy was used in an early stage. Arch Ophthalmol 23:253, 1940
8. Welch RB: Von Hippel-Lindau disease: the recognition and treatment of early angiomatosis retinae and the use of cryosurgery as an adjunct to therapy. Trans Am Ophthalmol Soc 68:367, 1970
9. Cordes FC, Dickson OC: Angiomatosis retinae (von Hippel's disease): results following irradiation of three eyes. Am J Ophthalmol 26:454, 1943
10. Wallner EF, Moorman LT: Hemangioma of the optic disk. Arch Ophthalmol 53:115, 1955
11. Darr JL, Hughes RP Jr, McNair JN: Bilateral peripapillary retinal hemangiomas. Arch Ophthalmol 75:77, 1966
12. Souders BF: Justapapillary hemangioendothelioma of the retina. Arch Ophthalmol 41:178, 1949
13. Cross AG: Angioma of the retina. Br J Ophthalmol 27:372, 1943
14. Carr TA, Stallard HB: A case of angio-gliomatosis retinae with pathological report. Br J Ophthalmol 17:525, 1933

15. Manschot WA: Juxtapapillary retinal angiomatosis. Arch Ophthalmol 80:775, 1968
16. Jesberg DO, Spencer WH, Hoyt WF: Incipient lesions of von Hippel-Lindau disease. Arch Ophthalmol 80:632, 1968
17. Blodi FC, Watzke RC: The treatment of von Hippel-Lindau disease. In XXI Concilium Ophthalmologicum, Mexico, 1970. Amsterdam, Excerpta Medica, 1971, p 880
18. Joe S, Spencer WH: Von Hippel-Lindau disease. Arch Ophthalmol 71:508, 1964
19. Seidel E: Über ein Angiom der Netzhaut. Ber Versamml Ophthalmol Ges 38:335, 1913
20. Silver ML, Hennigar G: Cerebellar hemangioma (hemangioblastoma): a clinico-pathological review of 40 cases. J Neurosurg 9:484, 1952
21. Rho YM: Von Hippel-Lindau disease: a report of 5 cases. Can Med Assoc J 101:135, 1969
22. Otenasek FJ, Silver ML: Spinal hemangioma (hemangioblastoma) in Lindau's disease. J Neurosurg 18:295, 1961
23. Hoff JT, Ray BS: Cerebral hemangioblastoma occurring in a patient with von Hippel-Lindau disease. J Neurosurg 28:365, 1968
24. MacRae HM, Newbigin B: Von Hippel-Lindau disease: a family history. Can J Ophthalmol 3:28, 1968
25. Lindau A: Capillary angiomatosis of the central nervous system. Acta Genet Statist Med 7:338, 1957
26. Melmon KL, Rosen SW: Lindau's disease: review of the literature and study of a large kindred. Am J Med 36:595, 1964
27. Christoferson LA, Gustafson MB, Petersen AG: Von Hippel-Lindau disease. JAMA 178:280, 1961
28. Goldberg MF, Duke JR: Von Hippel-Lindau disease: histopathologic findings in a treated and an untreated eye. Am J Ophthalmol 66:693, 1968
29. Hagler WS in Reese AB: Tumors of the Eye. New York, Harper & Row, 1963
30. Reese AB: Tumors of the Eye. New York, Harper & Row, 1963
31. Ballantyne AJ, Michaelson IC: Textbook of the Fundus of the Eye, 2nd ed. Baltimore, Williams & Wilkins, 1970
32. Norton EWD, in discussion, Goldberg MF, Duke JR: Von Hippel-Lindau disease. Trans Am Ophthalmol Soc 66:243, 1968
33. Amoils SP, Honey DP: Early cryosurgical chorioretinal microcirculatory changes. Arch Ophthalmol 82:220, 1969
34. Wood LW, Watzke RC: Effects of cryopexy upon the retinal vasculature. Arch Ophthalmol 81:254, 1969
35. Watzke RC: Cryotherapy for retinal angiomatosis: a clinicopathologic report. Arch Ophthalmol 92:399, 1974

Morton F. Goldberg

16 Clinicopathologic Correlation of von Hippel Angiomas after Xenon Arc and Argon Laser Photocoagulation

Treatment of von Hippel retinal angiomas is often successful when the size of the hamartoma is not excessive and when one or more of several destructive modalities (radiation, electrocautery, diathermy, xenon arc photocoagulation, argon laser photocoagulation, and cryocoagulation) is correctly applied.[1-4] Of the available energy sources, the xenon arc, argon laser, and cryocoagulator are most useful clinically. Although the goal of therapy is total destruction of all angiomas with preservation of an attached, functioning retina, this goal may not always be successfully achieved. Palliative diminution in size of an angioma, with reduction in its propensity for further growth, transudation, and hemorrhage, may be all that can be accomplished. Ophthalmoscopy and fluorescein angioscopy or angiography are important in clinical decision making when the therapist must determine whether or not retreatment of an angioma is indicated because of persistent perfusion of an angioma. Even angiography, however, may occasionally be misleading, because nonperfusion does not necessarily mean nonviability of one of these hamartomatous malformations.

In this report von Hippel angiomas are described that were treated by either xenon arc or argon laser photocoagulation and that were clinically improved and thought to be eradicated on the basis of ophthalmoscopic and angiographic evidence. After the deaths of the patients from complications of cerebellar hemangioblastomas, histopathologic studies showed viable angiomatous tissue in some areas of photocoagulation. In other areas, smaller angiomas were completely destroyed.

XENON ARC PHOTOCOAGULATION

Case Report: A 49-year-old black man had a 2- to 3-disk diameter von Hippel angioma inferonasally near the equator of his right eye.[1] Vision was 20/20. The tumor had a whitish appearance and was covered with small blood vessels;

This study was supported in part by Research to Prevent Blindness, Inc., the Robbins Fund, and by the Illinois Society for the Prevention of Blindness.

it had bled locally into the vitreous, and was supplied by typically enlarged feeder and drainer blood vessels (Fig. 16.1).

Two photocoagulation sessions were carried out. Initially, an attempt was made to reduce the perfusion of the tumor by coagulating the borders of the feeding and draining major vessels (Fig. 16.2). Several brief coagulations along the edges of these vessels were accomplished with the W. German Zeiss xenon arc photocoagulator set at normal intensity number 2, the 3° field diaphragm, and the iris diaphragm completely open. Fifteen months later, the angioma appeared unchanged by ophthalmoscopy. Fluorescein studies were not performed. Dense pigment accumulations were seen about the major supply vessels. Repeat photocoagulation was performed, with the creation of 12 moderately intense burns directly on the body of the angioma itself and at its border. The photocoagulator was set at normal intensity number 2, the 4.5° field diaphragm, and a completely open iris diaphragm. A typical self-limited serous retinal detachment occurred about the tumor, but there was no hemorrhage.

Twenty-four months after the initial photocoagulation and nine months after the second photocoagulation, he died from a large intraventricular cerebral hemorrhage.[1] The gross pathologic specimen of the right eye showed a 1 × 2 × 2-mm white nodule where the angioma had been treated (Fig. 16.3). Pigmented scars were noted about the major supply vessels, which remained patent.

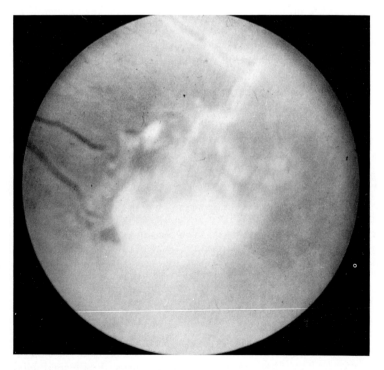

FIG. 16.1. Prior to treatment, von Hippel angioma measures 2 to 3 disk diameters. Note white coloration (From Goldberg and Duke: Am J Ophthalmol 66:693, 1968).

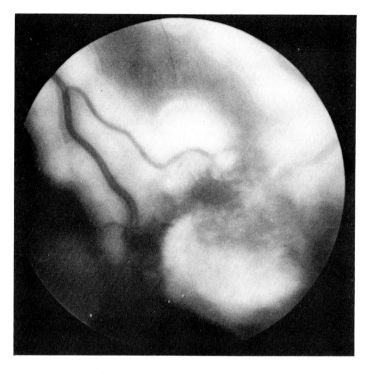

FIG. 16.2. Fresh xenon arc photocoagulation burns about major supply vessels of von Hippel angioma (From Goldberg and Duke: Am J Ophthalmol 66:693, 1968).

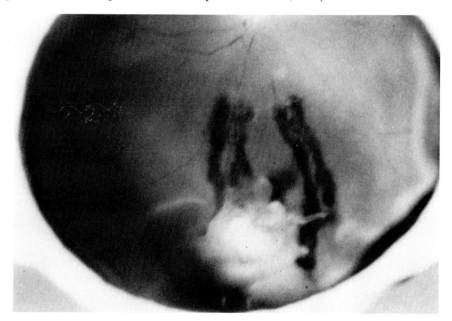

FIG. 16.3. Two years after Figure 16.2, autopsy specimen shows pigmented scars at sites of previous photocoagulation (From Goldberg and Duke: Am J Ophthalmol 66:693, 1968).

Serial sections through the coagulated angioma were obtained. Centrally, there was no normal retinal tissue present, but many endothelial cells with vascular channels of various sizes were found in irregular angiomatous masses. At the periphery of the tumor, there was extensive glial cell proliferation and circumscribed nests of proliferating endothelial cells (Fig. 16.4). At the vitreoretinal interface, neovascular channels grew out of the retina into the vitreous (Figs. 16.4, 16.5). Adjacent to the angioma, bleeding from the sensory retina into the space between it and the retinal pigment epithelium caused localized retinal detachment (Fig. 16.6).

ARGON LASER PHOTOCOAGULATION

Case Report: A 47-year-old white man had four von Hippel angiomas in the right eye near the equator.[2] Vision was 20/50. Angioma 1 at 9:45 o'clock was the largest, measuring 1 disk diameter. It had well-defined supply vessels, but they were not excessively dilated or tortuous (Fig. 16.7). The angioma leaked fluorescein.[2] Angiomas 2 and 3 at 9 o'clock were 0.1 to 0.2 disk diameter in size, and only one of them leaked fluorescein. There were no obvious major supply vessels. Angioma 4 at 6 o'clock was 0.6 to 0.8 disk diameter in size, and had supply vessels that were not excessively enlarged or tortuous.[2, 3]

Two photocoagulation sessions were carried out. Initially, angiomas 2, 3, and 4 were focally and directly coagulated (Fig. 16.7). Angioma 1 was initially treated only by coagulation of its feeding arteriole (Fig. 16.7). The Coherent Radiation argon laser was set at 50 to 200 μ, 150 to 450 mW, and 0.1 to 0.5

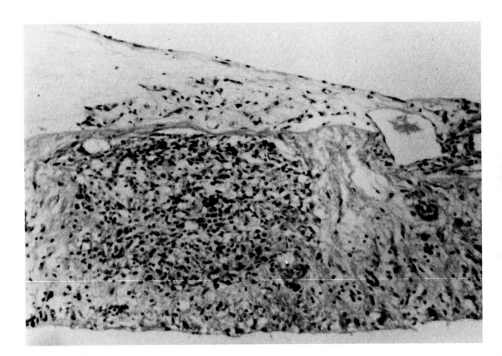

FIG. 16.4. Despite prior photocoagulation of angioma, nests of viable and proliferating hamartomatous cells persist. In addition, neovascular tissue is seen at vitreoretinal interface. H&E, ×51.

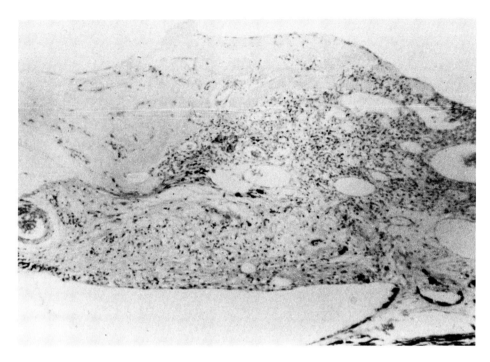

FIG. 16.5. Neovascular tissue extending from retina into vitreous is seen on internal surface of photocoagulated angioma. H&E, ×60.

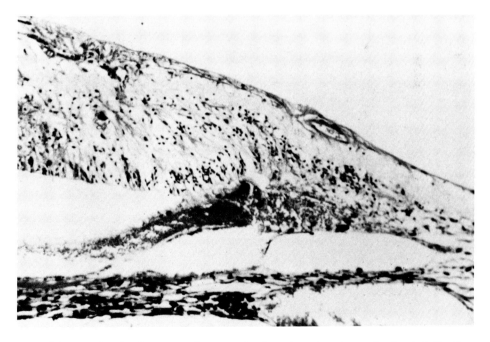

FIG. 16.6. Immediately adjacent to photocoagulated angioma is a focus of subretinal bleeding. H&E, ×40 (From Goldberg and Duke: Am J Ophthalmol 66:693, 1968).

second. The three small angiomas appeared obliterated, and subsequent photocoagulation was not performed upon them. The feeding arteriole of angioma 1 was interrupted, and none of the angiomas leaked fluorescein immediately after the initial treatment session.[2] Two months later, angiography showed that the feeding arteriole of angioma 1 had regained perfusion. Accordingly, this arteriole was recoagulated, and the angioma itself was coagulated directly (Fig. 16.8). The laser was set at 200 μ, 200 mW, and 0.5 second. A day later, angiography showed nonperfusion of all angiomas (Fig. 16.9), except for two tiny spots in angioma 1 that appeared to fill in retrograde direction. A month later, a 2-disk diameter spontaneous hemorrhage occurred transiently over angioma 1 (Fig. 16.10). Eleven months thereafter, all angiomas appeared scarred and eradicated (Fig. 16.11), and none had fluorescein perfusion or leakage.

Eighteen months after the first treatment and 16 months after the second treatment, the patient died of cerebellar hemangioblastoma. Light and electron microscopy was performed on all angiomas.[3]

Gross inspection of the specimen showed no obvious tumor nodules, and the feeder arteriole to angioma 1 appeared occluded (Fig. 16.12). Histologic examination confirmed total occlusion of this vessel (Fig. 16.13). Angioma 1 was largely intact, however, and showed many viable, actively proliferating spindle-shaped cells (Fig. 16.14). Numerous cells containing large amounts of lipid (Fig. 16.15) were also present. A fibrous membrane covered the internal surface of this angioma (Fig. 16.14) and obscured it from clinical

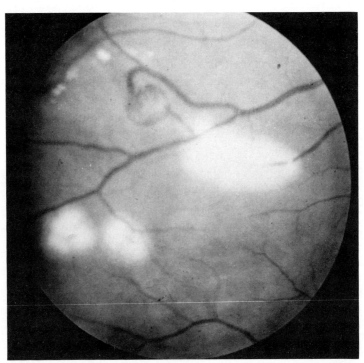

FIG. 16.7. Fresh argon laser photocoagulation of feeding arteriole to angioma 1 is seen in upper part of photograph. Angiomas 2 and 3 have been directly treated by argon laser (lower left) (From Goldberg and Koenig: Arch Ophthalmol 92:121, 1974).

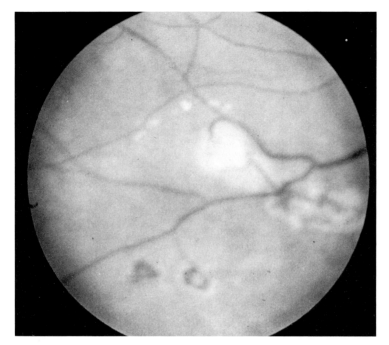

FIG. 16.8. Two months after Figure 16.7 the feeding arteriole to angioma 1 had reopened. This photograph shows the fresh appearance of repeat argon laser photocoagulation of this arteriole and direct focal photocoagulation of angioma 1 itself. Angiomas 2 and 3 appear scarred and obliterated (From Goldberg and Koenig: Arch Ophthalmol 92:121, 1974).

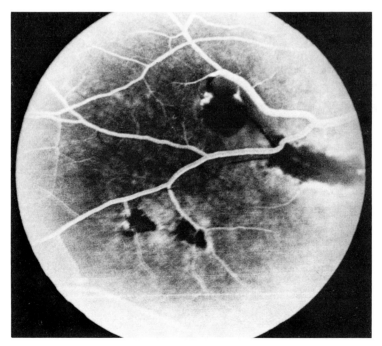

FIG. 16.9. One day after Figure 16.8 fluorescein angiography confirms repeat closure of feeding arteriole. What little perfusion there is in angioma 1 appears to have occurred in retrograde direction. Angiomas 2 and 3 are nonperfused (From Goldberg and Koenig: Arch Ophthalmol 92:121, 1974).

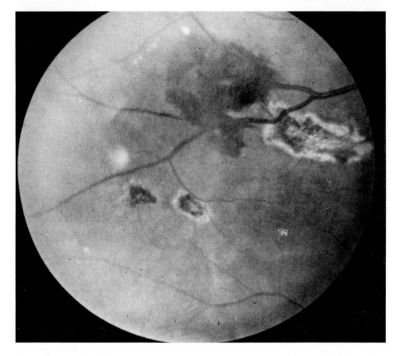

FIG. 16.10. One month after Figures 16.8 and 16.9 a small spontaneous hemorrhage occurred over angioma 1 (From Goldberg and Koenig: Arch Ophthalmol 92:121, 1974).

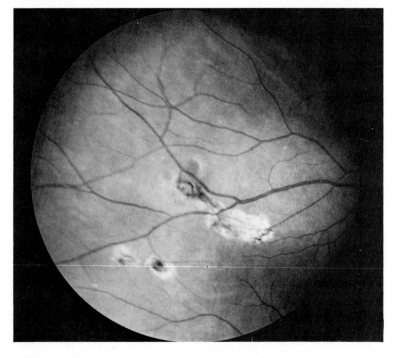

FIG. 16.11. Eleven months after Figure 16.10 all angiomas appear eradicated.

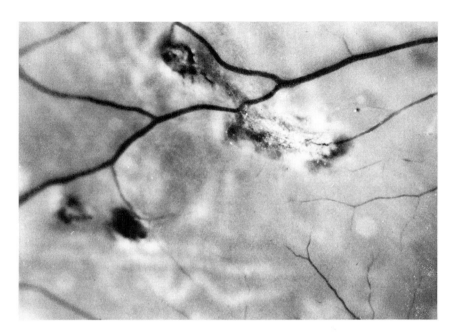

FIG. 16.12. Gross autopsy specimen 18 months after first treatment and 16 months after second treatment. All angiomas appear eradicated, and the feeding arteriole to angioma 1 appears obliterated (From Apple et al: Arch Ophthalmol 92:126, 1974).

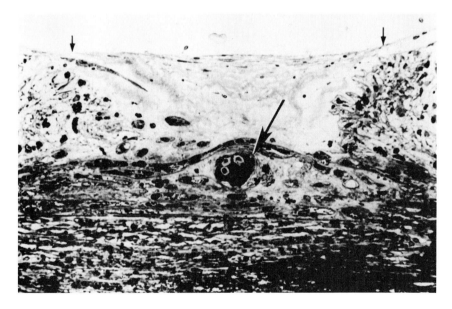

FIG. 16.13. Histologic examination confirms occlusion of major feeding arteriole (large arrow) to angioma 1. Two small arrows demonstrate dense scar after argon laser photocoagulation. Mallory blue, ×110 (From Apple et al: Arch Ophthalmol 92:126, 1974).

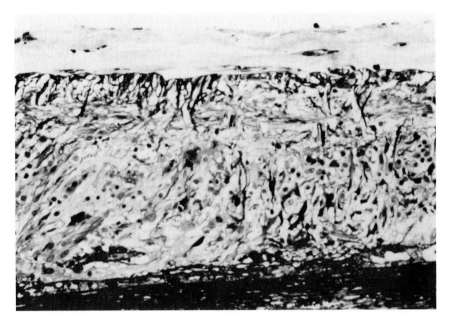

FIG. 16.14. Angioma 1 after argon laser photocoagulation. Note fibrous membrane along internal margin of tumor. The tumor contains many viable spindle-shaped cells. Mallory blue, ×100 (From Apple et al: Arch Ophthalmol 92:126, 1974).

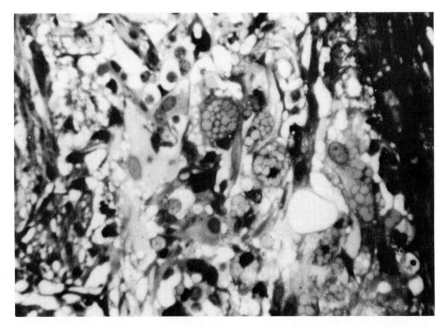

FIG. 16.15. Higher magnification of viable cells remaining after argon laser photocoagulation of angioma 1. Note numerous lipid clusters within several macrophages. Mallory blue, ×250 (From Apple et al: Arch Ophthalmol 92:126, 1974).

detection. Angiomas 2 (Fig. 16.16) and 3 (Fig. 16.17) were completely replaced by nonhamartomatous fibroglial membranes and dispersed pigment. There was no microscopic evidence of viable tumor. Angioma 4, which also appeared clinically obliterated (Figs. 16.18–16.20), was largely eradicated and replaced with dense fibrous tissue and intermingled, migrating pigment epithelial cells (Fig. 16.21). At one edge of this lesion, clusters of viable spindle-shaped hamartomatous cells persisted (Fig. 16.22).

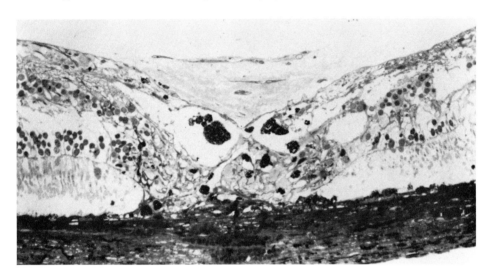

FIG. 16.16. Angioma 2 has been completely replaced by laser-induced scar tissue and migrated pigment. Mallory blue, ×110.

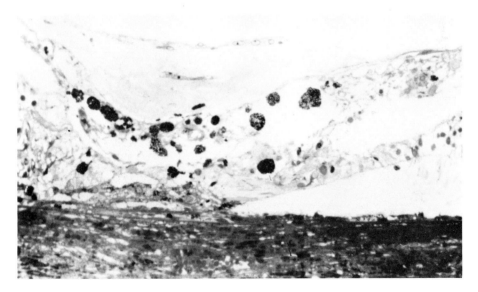

FIG. 16.17. Angioma 3 has been completely eradicated. In its place are scar tissue and numerous pigment-filled macrophages. Mallory blue, ×100.

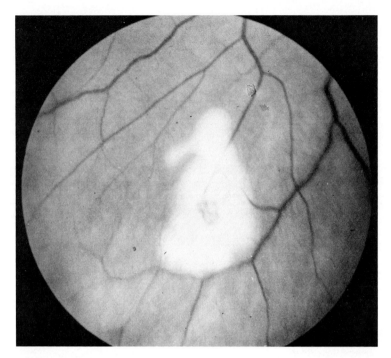

FIG. 16.18. Appearance of angioma 4 immediately after argon laser photocoagulation.

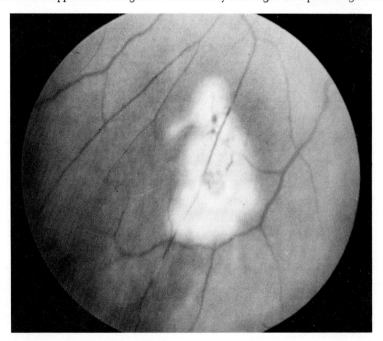

FIG. 16.19. One day after Figure 16.18 a few tiny hemorrhages are seen within fresh photocoagulation scar.

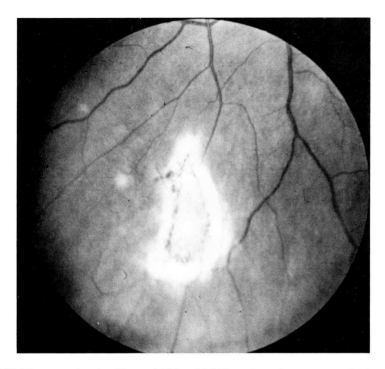

FIG. 16.20. Three months after Figures 16.18 and 16.19 angioma 4 appears completely eradicated (cf. Fig. 16.22).

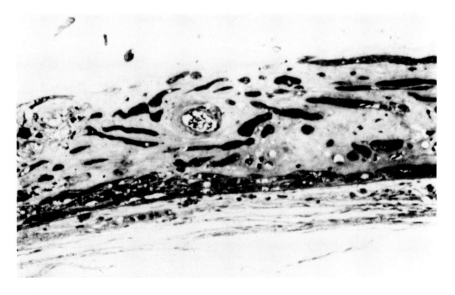

FIG. 16.21. Eighteen months after Figures 16.18 and 16.19 histopathologic appearance of angioma 4 shows dense scar tissue with many melanin-containing cells. Mallory blue, ×110 (From Apple et al: Arch Ophthalmol 92:126, 1974).

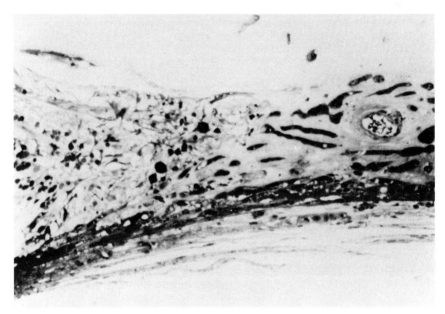

FIG. 16.22. Adjacent to area pictured in Figure 16.21 are clusters of viable hamartomatous cells (to left of photograph). Mallory blue, ×110.

DISCUSSION

Because of theoretical considerations, it might be supposed that the complementary wavelengths of red angiomas and blue-green argon laser light would enhance the utility of this laser in this clinical setting. However, clinical and histopathologic experience suggests that there is no inherent clinical advantage in using the wavelengths of an argon laser instead of the white light of a xenon arc for such lesions. Both sources of light energy may be incapable of total eradication of larger retinal angiomas of the von Hippel type, as shown in some of the accompanying histopathologic illustrations (Figs. 16.4, 16.14, 16.15, 16.22). A similar inability of the argon laser to eradicate malignant melanomas of the choroid has been documented by clinicopathologic correlation.[5] With both types of tumors photocoagulation (with either xenon arc or argon laser) converts pigmented tissue initially to white or whitish gray. The net effect is to reflect much of the incident light beam once a narrow superficial layer (0.2 to 0.75 mm thick) of tumor tissue has been coagulated.[5] If prior bleeding or tumor growth has caused the deposition of a white fibroglial mantle on the internal surface of a retinal angioma, a similar reflection of photocoagulating light is likely, and this effect may partially explain the subtotal effect in our xenon-treated case. Retinal angiomas and many choroidal malignant melanomas contain large and numerous vascular channels, sometimes with a very rapid flow of blood. The obvious heat sink created by these blood vessels may dissipate sufficient light-induced heat energy such that the clinically desired coagulating effect is minimized.

Xenon arc photocoagulation may actually be preferred to argon laser photocoagulation for eradication of von Hippel angiomas because of larger beam diameters, more prolonged burn durations, and inclusion of more wavelengths of light. On the other hand, there is little reason to believe that the argon laser cannot cause lesions similar to those of the xenon arc when it is used with retrobulbar anesthesia and instrument settings that simulate those of the xenon arc (beam diameter greater than 200 μ, burn duration greater than 0.5 second, etc.).[6]

A definite advantage held by commercially available argon laser photocoagulators over older xenon arc photocoagulators is their biomicroscopic delivery systems with highly magnified, stereoscopic, and brightly illuminated views of the lesions to be coagulated. With the advent of a similar, though somewhat less convenient, delivery system for xenon arc photocoagulators,[7] much of the advantage of the argon laser systems has been obviated. With biomicroscopic control over burn placement, either an argon laser or xenon arc can be used for precise placement of coagulating burns. It is rarely, if ever, necessary to occlude feeder arterioles of von Hippel angiomas with the obligatory infarction of dependent retina and corresponding loss of retinal function. Even the argon laser can be aimed directly at retinal angiomas, with little probability of immediate hemorrhage (assuming that beam diameters of 200 μ or more are employed). Preservation of visual field is thus optimized. Focal treatment of this sort is liable to be followed by self-limited serous detachments of the retina.

When angiomas are large (2 or more disk diameters), multiple focal treatments at intervals of weeks to months are likely to be necessary. Some of the treatment, particularly in very large angiomas, can be carried out to advantage with either cryotherapy or diathermy, because neither argon nor xenon photocoagulators seemed capable by themselves of eradicating the largest (many disk diameters) of these tumors. In some cases, even the combination of a variety of energy sources repetitively applied may be unsuccessful, and retinal detachment, vitreous hemorrhage, subretinal hemorrhage, or macular transudation may irreversibly destroy normal retinal function.

Fluorescein angioscopy or angiography is a valuable adjunct in the clinical management of von Hippel angiomas, particularly when perfusion of such a tumor can be demonstrated. Repeat treatment is clearly indicated in such a circumstance. The absence of fluorescein perfusion is not as helpful in determining management, because very small angiomas, even prior to treatment, may show no fluorescein,[2] and because, once treated, viable angiomas may also show no fluorescence on occasion.[2,3] There are several explanations for such a false-negative contrast study using intravascular fluorescein. As shown in Figures 16.14–16.17, photocoagulation can induce fibroglial scarring on the internal surface of the burned area. This tissue can obstruct visualization of more externally located fluorescence. Freshly coagulated tissue is also usually opaque to underlying fluorescence. The presence of melanin from migrated retinal pigment epithelial cells (Fig. 16.21) and the presence of a layer of blood may also interfere with visualization of a fluorescing tumor mass, due to quenching of its fluorescence. Thus, viable tumors may persist despite absence of visible fluorescence.

CONCLUSIONS

Argon lasers can be effective in directly coagulating small (< 0.8 disk diameter) von Hippel angiomas. Larger angiomas may require additional or different sources of energy, such as xenon arc photocoagulation, diathermy, or cryocoagulation. The wavelength of argon laser photocoagulators does not appear to have inherent clinical advantages for the treatment of von Hippel angiomas, but biomicroscopic delivery systems for either argon lasers or xenon arcs appear useful in preserving the visual field. Direct photocoagulation of the angioma (rather than prior occlusion of its major supply vessels) appears warranted and not excessively dangerous with either source of light energy. Fluorescein angiography is valuable when persistent perfusion of a tumor documents incomplete prior treatment. In this situation, retreatment is indicated. Absence of visible perfusion, however, can occur in the presence of viable tumor and is thus not as useful a clinical sign.

ACKNOWLEDGMENT

Histopathologic studies were performed in collaboration with David Apple, M.D., James R. Duke, M.D., and George Wyhinny, M.D.

REFERENCES

1. Goldberg MF, Duke JR: von Hippel-Lindau disease: histopathologic findings in a treated and an untreated eye. Am J Ophthalmol 66:693, 1968
2. Goldberg MF, Koenig S: Argon laser treatment of von Hippel-Lindau retinal angiomas: I. Clinical and angiographic findings. Arch Ophthalmol 92:121, 1974
3. Apple DJ, Goldberg MF, Wyhinny GJ: Argon laser treatment of von Hippel-Lindau retinal angiomas: II. Histopathology of treated lesions. Arch Ophthalmol 92:126, 1974
4. Watzke RC: Cryotherapy for retinal angiomatosis: a clinicopathologic report. Doc Ophthalmol 34:405, 1973
5. Apple DJ, Goldberg MF, Wyhinny GJ, et al: Argon laser photocoagulation of choroidal malignant melanoma: tissue effects after a single treatment. Arch Ophthalmol 90:97, 1973
6. Goldbaum MH, Goldberg MF, Nagpal K, et al: Quantitative photocoagulation and the treatment of proliferative sickle retinopathy. In L'Esperance F (ed): Current Diagnosis and Management of Chorioretinal Disease. St. Louis, Mosby, 1976
7. Peyman GA, Wyhinny GJ, Goldberg MF: Optical radiation and Zeiss short-pulsed xenon photocoagulators: I. Clinical considerations of articulation with the Fankhauser slit-lamp delivery system. Arch Ophthalmol 92:341, 1974

David J. Apple
Nancy A. Hamming
David K. Gieser

17 Differential Diagnosis of Leukocoria

Three major diagnostic considerations come to mind when evaluating a white (or pink-white or yellow-white) pupillary reflex in a child: retinoblastoma (Fig. 17.1), cataract, and the so-called pseudogliomas.[1] The diagnosis of a congenital cataract is usually relatively easy with adequate history and clinical examination and in general does not pose a diagnostic problem in the differential diagnosis of retinoblastoma. The numerous conditions characterized as pseudoglioma include a wide range of diseases affecting the lens, vitreous, and retina–choroid, and at times they are extremely difficult to differentiate from retinoblastoma.[2,3] The clinician must be aware of these diseases if he is to evaluate a child for retinoblastoma correctly. A retrolental white mass should always evoke an awareness of this malignant neoplasm, which is, of course, the most serious cause of a white pupil in children, both with respect to vision and to life. This chapter describes the numerous retrolental and fundus disorders that may mimic this important tumor and therefore must be considered in a differential diagnosis in order to insure appropriate management of the patient.

Early investigators, going back to the era of Virchow in the mid-nineteenth century, considered retinoblastoma to be a glial tumor or glioma. Treacher Collins, in a clinicopathologic study, first applied the term "pseudoglioma" to a variety of disorders that often caused a white pupil, thereby mimicking the appearance of a retinoblastoma.[4] Although we now know that a retinoblastoma is not strictly a glial tumor, but more typically shows differentiation toward neuronal elements,[5,6] the term pseudoglioma has persisted as representing the various conditions causing the white retinal mass that may mimic a retinoblastoma. The term "pseudoretinoblastoma" would be more accurate, but the older term is firmly entrenched in the literature and will be very difficult to dislodge from clinical usage.

There are numerous classifications of pseudoglioma, most of them grouped according to a very rough approximation of incidence.[1,2,7–11] A sufficiently large and statistically significant series that would allow an accurate determination of the true incidence of the various conditions is difficult to obtain. One of the better

This study was supported in part by a fellowship from the Alexander von Humboldt Foundation, Schillerstr. 12 D-5300 Bonn-Bad Godesberg, West Germany.

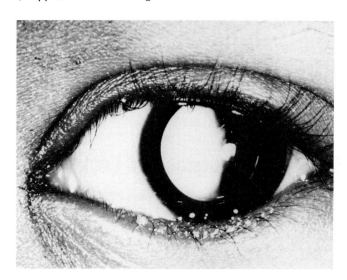

FIG. 17.1. Retinoblastoma. The retrolental white mass (leukocoria, white pupil, amaurotic cat's eye, or pseudoglioma) is a common presenting sign of the disease.

classifications to date is that of Howard and Ellsworth[2] (Table 17.1), in which the diseases are listed in order of approximate frequency. They studied 500 consecutive patients referred to their clinic for possible retinoblastoma. Of these 500 patients, most of whom had unilateral or bilateral leukocoria, other (nonretinoblastoma) diagnoses were made in 265 cases (53 percent). Naumann[10] and Naumann and Lommatzsch[11] grouped the conditions causing a pseudoglioma according to unilateral or bilateral occurrence (Table 17.2). Table 17.3 lists the differential diagnosis of pseudoglioma in terms of the etiologic factors, pathogenesis, and structural characteristics of each disease. Such a grouping provides a perspective as to the nature of the basic tissue changes occurring in each disease and offers insight as to the rationale for the basic laboratory and clinical procedures necessary to evaluate each patient.

As is clear from Table 17.3, the differential diagnosis of a white pupil or leukocoria (not including primary opacities of the lens, but only retrolental lesions) in an infant or child includes disturbances of different tissues by different pathologic processes. These possibilities include defects in embryogenesis, vascular anomalies, lipid exudations, oxygen toxicity, infectious conditions, genetic aberrations, and neoplasms. Clinical diagnosis is greatly improved by proper genetic history, history of previous oxygen therapy, careful clinical examination under general anesthesia, fluorescein angiography, ultrasonography, and electroretinography. The determination of lactic acid dehydrogenase (LDH) levels on aspirated aqueous fluid can assist in differentiating retinoblastoma from other retrolental lesions.[12] (See Chapter 19 for a detailed discussion.)

In the older reports dealing with pseudoglioma, the most common diagnosis demonstrated pathologically was metastatic endophthalmitis with vitreous abscess. With the exception of larval granulomatosis, such conditions are rarely encountered. Even today we sometimes encounter cases in which pathologic examination of an enucleated globe may not always allow distinction between the various types

Table 17.1

265 Patients with Suspected Retinoblastoma
in whom Other Diagnoses Were Made*

Diagnosis	No. of Cases	Percent of Total
Persistent hyperplastic primary vitreous	51	19.0
Retrolental fibroplasia	36	13.5
Posterior cataract	36	13.5
Coloboma of choroid or optic disk	30	11.5
Uveitis	27	10.0
Larval granulomatosis	18	6.5
Congenital retinal fold	13	5.0
Coats' disease	10	4.0
Organizing vitreous hemorrhage	9	3.5
Retinal dysplasia	7	2.5
Tumor other than retinoblastoma	4	1.5
White-with-pressure sign	3	1.0
Juvenile xanthogranuloma	3	1.0
Retinoschisis	3	1.0
Tapetoretinal degeneration	2	1.0
Endophthalmitis	2	1.0
Persistent tunica vasculosa lentis and pupillary membrane	2	1.0
Miscellaneous	9	3.5
Anteriorly dislocated lens with secondary glaucoma	1	
Congenital corneal opacity	1	
Incontinentia pigmenti (Bloch-Sulzberger syndrome) with total funnel-shaped retinal detachment	1	
Cyst in remnant of hyaloid artery	1	
Anomalous optic disks	1	
Hematoma under retinal pigment epithelium	1	
High myopia with advanced chorioretinal degeneration	1	
Medullation of nerve fiber layer	1	
Traumatic choroiditis	1	
Total	265	100.0

* *From Howard and Ellsworth: Am J Ophthalmol 60:610, 1965.*

Table 17.2

Clinical Classification of Pseudoglioma
According to Unilaterality and Bilaterality*

Unilateral	Bilateral
Trauma or hemorrhage	Retrolental fibroplasia
Persistent hyperplastic primary vitreous	Trisomy 13
Coats' syndrome	von Hippel-Lindau angiomatosis
Toxocariasis (larval endophthalmitis)	Norrie's disease
Medulloepithelioma	Incontinentia pigmenti
	X-linked retinoschisis

* *Adapted from Naumann and Lommatzsch: In Opitz H and Schmid F (eds): Handbuch der Kinderheilkunde: Tumoren in Kindesalter, vol 8, pt 2, 1972. Courtesy of Springer Verlag.*

Table 17.3

Leukocoria: Classification According to Pathogenesis or Structural Characteristics

Persistence and hyperplasia of embryonic ocular vasculature
  Persistent hyperplastic primary vitreous (PHPV)
  Posterior PHPV, epipapillary and peripapillary lesions, and congenital falciform fold

Retinal vascular anomalies with lipid exudation
  Coats' syndrome
  Leber's military aneurysms
  von Hippel-Lindau angiomatosis

Toxic retinopathy
  Retinopathy of prematurity (retrolental fibroplasia)

Inflammatory conditions
  Toxocariasis (nematode endophthalmitis)
  Uveitis, pars planitis
  Metastatic endophthalmitis

Conditions exhibiting abnormal retinal embryogenesis and/or retinal dysplasia as prominent
    features
  Norrie's disease
  Trisomy 13 syndrome
  Fundus colobomas
  Incontinentia pigmenti (Bloch-Sulzberger syndrome)
  X-linked retinoschisis

Prenatal and infantile trauma, organizing vitreous hemorrhage, and massive retinal gliosis

Neoplastic and proliferative lesions
  Medulloepithelioma
  Miscellaneous proliferative lesions, hamartomas, and choristomas of the fundus

of the intraocular diseases that lead to opacification of the media. In particular, in cases where the history and clinical findings are lacking, it is often impossible to determine the correct diagnosis in end-stage, phthisical eyes in which advanced fibrosis, tissue degeneration, and bone formation may obscure all traces of the primary process.

The diseases described in this chapter are grouped according to the classification in Table 17.3. Because PHPV is one of the more important and frequent conditions mimicking a retinoblastoma,[2] we will describe it in detail.

PERSISTENCE AND HYPERPLASIA OF EMBRYONIC INTRAOCULAR VASCULATURE

PHPV is the most serious lesion induced by abnormal development of the embryonic intraocular vasculature. The basic lesion is a persistence of various portions of the primary vitreous with hyperplasia of the associated embryonic connective tissue. In untreated cases the condition is often characterized by progression toward secondary complications such as rupture of the lens capsule and cataract formation, resorption of lens cortex,[13, 14] intraocular hemorrhage, secondary glaucoma, traction and retinal folds with occasional associated detachment, and eventual phthisis bulbi.

Components of Primary Vitreous

To understand the development and anatomy of the vitreous and the embryonic intraocular vasculature, it is useful to review the early phases of ocular embryogenesis.[3, 15-18] The embryonic fissure of the optic cup (see below, Fig. 17.25, page 269) creates a notch or temporary defect that allows ingrowth of vascular elements into the eye. These transient vessels, which are necessary for growth and development of the eye, include the hyaloid artery trunk and its tributaries, which eventually form the central retinal artery and its branches (Fig. 17.2).

The hyaloid vascular system, combined with a scaffolding of delicate fibrillar strands, forms the primary vitreous (Fig. 17.2), which fills the entire vitreous space for the first three months of life. Thereafter the avascular secondary or adult vitreous forms and proceeds to occupy an increasingly greater proportion of the vitreous space (Fig. 17.3). The tertiary vitreous or zonules of Zinn also begin to form about the fourth month of gestation. Eventually the primary vitreous is confined to a small area (Cloquet's canal) extending from the disk to the back of the lens.

The embryonic intraocular vascular system may be divided into two main components (Table 17.4): an anterior system in the region of the iris and a

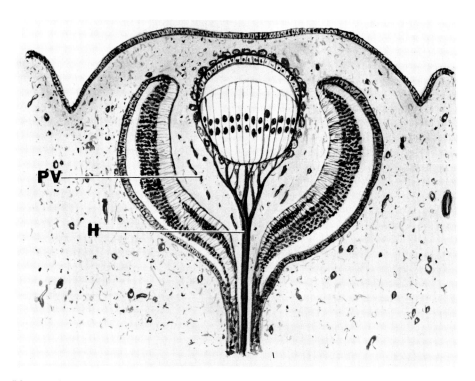

FIG. 17.2. Embryonic eye during first trimester. The hyaloid artery (H) enters the globe through the embryonic fissure. Its anterior tributaries form the vascular tunic of the lens and the vascular component of the primary vitreous (PV). (From Apple: In Peyman and Sanders (eds): Advances in Uveal Surgery, Vitreous Surgery and the Treatment of Endophthalmitis, 1975. Courtesy of Appleton-Century-Crofts.)

Table 17.4

Components of the Embryonic Ocular Vasculature

Anterior aspect (anterolental)
    Pupillary membrane (anterior tunica vasculosa lentis and minor iris circle), iris stroma
    Capsulopupillary vessels (lateral tunica vasculosa lentis)

Posterior aspect (retrolental, or primary vitreous)
    Posterior tunica vasculosa lentis and vasa hyaloidea propria
    Main hyaloid trunk and its surrounding sheath
    Bergmeister's papilla

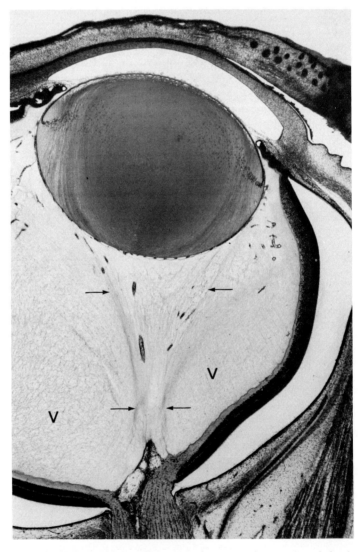

FIG. 17.3. Six-month-old human fetus. The arrows demarcate the margins of the funnel-shaped, retrolental remnants of the primary vitreous (Cloquet's canal), which is replaced by the avascular secondary (adult) vitreous (V). H&E, ×2.5. (Courtesy of Prof. G.O.H. Naumann)

posterior (retrolental) component within the vitreous.[3, 15–20] This division is useful for descriptive purposes, but it is somewhat artificial since all the components of the embryonic vascular system are intricately interrelated, both structurally via rich anastomoses, and functionally in development and regression.

The pupillary membrane is formed by small, blind buds from the annular vessel that grow centrally to vascularize the mesoderm anterior to the lens. These vessels form the anterior vascular tunic of the lens. This central portion is destined to disappear during fetal life. The peripheral pupillary membrane, which is thick and cellular, persists throughout life as the collarette.

The posterior tunica vasculosa lentis is formed by the terminal branches of the main trunk of the hyaloid artery.[17, 21] The hyaloid artery[22–24] branches from the dorsal ophthalmic artery during the third week of life and enters the interior of the optic cup by passing through the embryonic fissure. It grows anteriorly from the optic nervehead toward the lens (Fig. 17.4), where its terminal branches envelop the posterior surface of the lens and extend around the equator of the lens as the

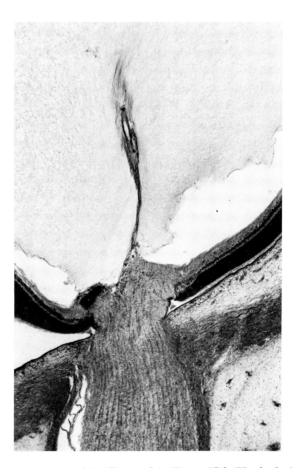

FIG. 17.4. Deeper section in the globe illustrated in Figure 17.3. The hyaloid artery enters the vitreous from the optic nervehead (Bergmeister's papilla) and passes out of the plane of the section. H&E, ×4. (Courtesy of Prof. G.O.H. Naumann)

lateral tunica vasculosa lentis or capsulopupillary vessels (Fig. 17.2, Table 17.4). This route provides an anastomosis with the anterior tunica vasculosa lentis and a drainage system via the annular vessel and, later in gestation, the ciliary vessels. The intravitreal branches located outside the confines of the posterior tunica vasculosa lentis are termed the vasa hyaloidea propria.

The hyaloid vascular system begins to show signs of regression even before some of its components have reached their height of development. The retrolental tunica vasculosa lentis reaches the height of development at three months. By the end of gestation it is typically almost entirely atrophied, except for the termination of the hyaloid artery, which may form a clinically insignificant opacity on the posterior lens surface, the so-called Mittendorf dot.[25, 26]

The glial sheath of Bergmeister (Fig. 17.5) envelops the hyaloid artery. It begins to atrophy about the seventh month of gestation, even before the main vessel itself atrophies. The extent of this atrophy below the surface of the disk may be partially responsible for the depth of the physiologic cup. If the atrophy of the sheath is less complete, a tuft of glial tissue may be seen throughout life as persistent Bergmeister's papilla.

Persistent Hyperplastic Primary Vitreous

CLINICOPATHOLOGIC CORRELATION. Howard and Ellsworth[2] determined that PHPV was the most frequent of the conditions causing a white pupillary reflex, accounting for 51 of the 265 diagnoses in their series. For many years PHPV was described by several different terms, such as persistence and thickening of the posterior fibrovascular sheath of the lens, persistent tunica vasculosa lentis, persistent thickened hyaloid artery with secondary changes, persistent hyaloid canal and artery, congenital membrane behind the lens, pseudophakia fibrosa, and retrolental

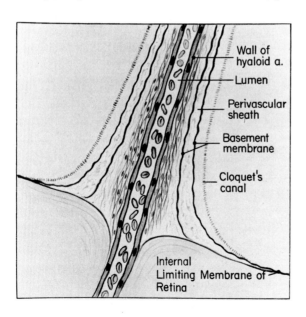

Wall of
hyaloid a.

Lumen

Perivascular
sheath

Basement
membrane

Cloquet's
canal

Internal
Limiting Membrane of
Retina

FIG. 17.5. Schematic drawing of optic nervehead showing emergence of hyaloid artery and sheath of Bergmeister's papilla.

fibroplasia. The last term is, of course, now reserved for the blinding condition due to extended, high-concentration oxygen therapy in premature infants.

In 1955 Reese[27] suggested "persistent hyperplastic primary vitreous" as a more appropriate term, thus emphasizing that the entity involved not only the tunica vasculosa lentis, but all components of the primary vitreous including the main hyaloid trunk. It should be emphasized that this entity in its full-blown form does not merely represent a simple persistence of the embryonic vessels, but may also be characterized by extensive proliferation of the involved tissues, including the fibrillar framework on which it is situated.

The clinical appearance of PHPV may be quite varied, depending on the amount and character of the hyperplasia of the embryonic vitreous components and the extent and nature of the secondary complications. The Mittendorf dot[25, 26] is very common, but because it is so innocuous, it does not warrant classification as PHPV.

In the great majority of cases of PHPV, the abnormality is unilateral in a fully developed, full-term, otherwise normal infant, and there is no apparent predisposition to sex or race (Table 17.5). Most cases are isolated and sporadic with no apparent hereditary influence. The presence of the lesion is usually discovered by either the physician or the parents immediately after birth or within a few weeks. Leukocoria is the most common presenting sign (Fig. 17.6). In rare instances the presenting sign may be a nystagmus or squint due to maldevelopment of visual function. The affected eye is usually microphthalmic (Fig. 17.7), which is one of the important features differentiating PHPV from retinoblastoma. The leukocoria is initially due to the opacity induced by a funnel-shaped mass of fibrovascular tissue occupying the retrolental space and the site of Cloquet's canal (Figs. 17.8, 17.9). The stem of the funnel often contains remnants of the hyaloid artery (Fig. 17.9). The retrolental mass may vary in size from a small localized plaque just nasal of center to a complete covering of the posterior surface of the lens. Sometimes the tissue may extend as far peripherally as the ciliary processes, ora serrata, and vitreous base, or anteriorly along the equator of the lens. The mass is usually gray-

Table 17.5

Features Differentiating PHPV from Retinoblastoma

PHPV	Retinoblastoma
Unilateral	Unilateral, but often (20 to 40 percent) bilateral
No (or very rare) hereditary disposition	May be transmitted as autosomal dominant
Relative microphthalmia	Usually normal-size eye
Elongated ciliary processes	Ciliary processes not elongated
Retrolental mass early	Retrolental mass usually later when entire globe is filled with tumor
Relatively early cataract	Cataract is rare or occurs in later phases
Relative microphakia often present	Normal lens size
Hyaloid remnants present (seen when media is sufficiently clear)	Hyaloid remnants not characteristic
No calcification seen on x-ray except in very late stages where phthisis bulbi occurs	Calcification of necrotic tumor foci is common
Normal LDH levels in aqueous	Increased levels of aqueous LDH

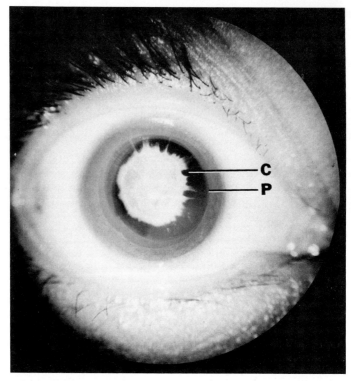

FIG. 17.6. PHPV with elongated ciliary processes (C) dragged into the pupillary space, pupillary border (P). From Goldbaum: In Peyman and Sanders (eds): Advances in Uveal Surgery, Vitreous Surgery, and the Treatment of Endophthalmitis, 1975. Courtesy of Appleton-Century-Crofts)

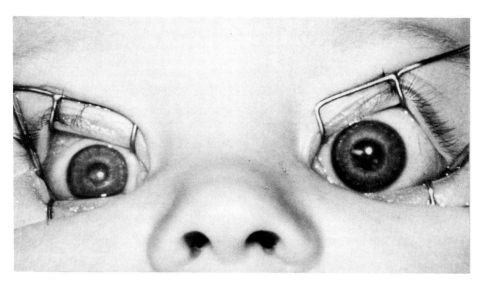

FIG. 17.7. PHPV and microphthalmia in the right eye, associated with a faint retropupillary white reflex. (Courtesy Prof. G.O.H. Naumann)

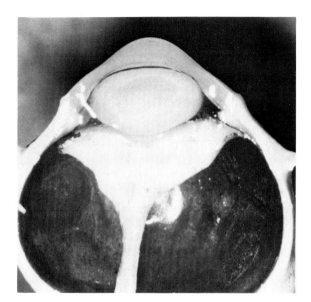

FIG. 17.8. Globe enucleated for a retrolental white mass suspected to be retinoblastoma. The dense white fibrovascular mass behind the lens suggests persistence of the tunica vasculosa lentis (PHPV). The persistent hyaloid artery should be located by serial sectioning to confirm this diagnosis. Note the total retinal detachment due to traction from the mass. (From Apple and Rabb: Clinicopathologic Correlation of Ocular Disease, 1974. Courtesy of CV Mosby)

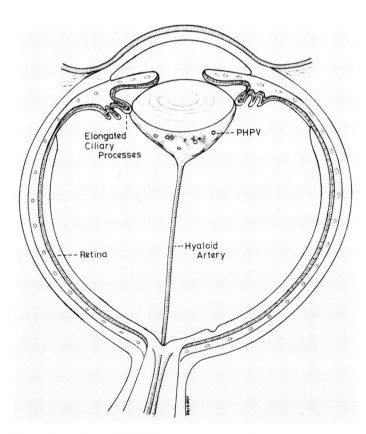

FIG. 17.9. Schematic drawing of PHPV showing retrolental fibrovascular mass, elongated ciliary processes, and persistent hyaloid artery.

white or pink, and the anterior aspect of the retrolental mass is usually concave, following the shape of the posterior lens surface. Identification of the hyaloid artery is extremely useful in confirming the diagnosis and differentiating this lesion from other causes of a funnel-shaped retrolental mass. The hyaloid artery may be patent or occluded. Usually the artery is represented by vascular remnants extending from the mass for various distances into the vitreous. If the hyaloid artery reaches the optic disk, the original interconnection of the artery with the central retinal vessels may be maintained.

The tissue is usually richly vascular, and repeated hemorrhages within the retrolental mass, the vitreous, and the perilenticular area are common, occurring most frequently in the first few months of life. It is not surprising that hemorrhage is a fairly common complication since the proliferating vessels that occur in the fibrovascular membrane are essentially new vessels that might be considered analogous to the neovascular tissue seen in the numerous proliferative retinopathies. Such vessels are characteristically very delicate and friable. Furthermore, the traction of the contracting fibrovascular membrane on the retina and ciliary body may induce rupture of normal vessels in these structures. With mydriasis, elongated, stretched ciliary processes may extend centrally within the pupillary aperture (Figs. 17.6, 17.9). This finding in conjunction with microphthalmia constitutes one of the better clinical indications differentiating this lesion from retinoblastoma and the other causes of leukocoria.

Because the retrolental mass is composed primarily of tissue of mesenchymal origin, it is not surprising that other mesodermally derived heteroplastic tissues may form as the aberrant proliferative process continues. An interesting form of metaplasia occasionally occurs in which adipose tissue is derived from the mass.[28] Fat may be observed in the plaque, the vitreous body, and even the lens after capsular rupture (so-called pseudophakia lipomatosa). Rarely, in cases of massive infiltration, the fat cells may almost completely replace the vitreous body or the lens substance.

Several iris abnormalities may be clinically apparent. The pupil usually dilates poorly, and with advanced, long-term cases ectropion uveae occurs. Although not a common feature, remnants of the fetal pupillary membrane may simultaneously persist. Rarely, a large vessel derived from the tunica vasculosa lentis extends anteriorly around the equator of the lens through the pupil, anastomosing with iris stromal vasculature. As might be expected with persistence of such remnants, colobomas of the iris and lens may be seen. The diameter of the lens is usually small, often even smaller than one would expect when compared to the degree of microphthalmia present. In fact, with mydriasis, the equator of the lens occasionally may be seen within the pupillary margin.

Characteristically, the lens is clear at first, but with time it becomes cataractous, usually due to rupture of the posterior capsule. The fibrovascular tissue eventually invades the lens cortex, creating cortical fiber degeneration, liquefaction, and cataract formation. This occurrence is often accompanied by swelling of the lens, which in turn may lead to secondary closed-angle pupillary block glaucoma. Sometimes the lens border becomes slightly luxated or displaced anteriorly through the dilated pupil due to swelling of the lens and traction created by the fibrovascular tissues. In long-standing, severe cases the lens cortex may slowly resorb, leaving only remnants of calcified cortex or a wrinkled capsule adjacent to the fibrovascular mass—so-called pseudophakia fibrosa or membranous cataract (Fig. 17.10).

When the fundus can be seen through the retrolental mass, the retina appears normal in early stages. In more advanced cases signs of old and recent intravitreal hemorrhage in various stages of organization may be seen. As the fibrovascular mass contracts, the retina is drawn peripherally by traction onto the pars plana or ciliary processes. This effect typically induces numerous folds in the retinal periphery. However, severe retinal detachment is relatively unusual.

Secondary closed-angle pupillary block glaucoma is a major cause of a blind painful eye that requires enucleation. The glaucoma is usually caused by either swelling of the lens or anterior displacement of the lens–iris diaphragm. Rarely, the lens may be so anteriorly displaced that it comes into opposition with the posterior surface of the cornea. This effect disrupts the integrity of the corneal endothelium, leading to corneal edema, opacification, and pannus formation. When severe secondary glaucoma ensues, one observes an apparently paradoxical situation in which an originally microphthalmic eye eventually becomes grossly enlarged or buphthalmic.

CLINICAL COURSE AND TREATMENT. Following diagnosis of PHPV, the immediacy and type of treatment chosen by the physician are critical due to the constantly changing and complication-ridden course of this syndrome. PHPV is progressive and dynamic in nature. Reese[27] firmly asserts that untreated cases will eventually progress to phthisis bulbi. This rather tragic clinical course applies only

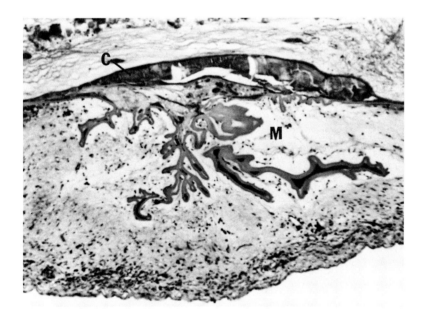

FIG. 17.10. PHPV. Retrolental fibrovascular mass (M) contains numerous wrinkled, coiled fragments of lens capsule. Remaining lens cortex (C) is shown. There is also invasion anterior to the lens by the fibrous membrane (above). This profile was formerly termed pseudophakia fibrosa. H&E, ×200.

to severe, full-blown cases and contrasts markedly with the static nature of simple persistence without hyperplasia of a hyaloid artery or pupillary membrane remnants.

Most eyes with full-blown PHPV do not survive to adult life. Quite often such eyes are enucleated for fear of a retinoblastoma. A case of PHPV in a 71-year-old man[13] represents the most spectacular exception to the rule that affected eyes usually undergo early enucleation. The unrelenting, often rapid progression of secondary complications frequently forces enucleation. These sequelae include unrelenting absolute glaucoma, repeated massive hemorrhages, retinal detachment and atrophy, and phthisis bulbi.

Because the natural course of PHPV is ill fated, early intervention is extremely important. Present concepts of surgery are based on the fact that hemorrhage may occur relatively early in life; it appears that "conservative, watchful waiting" only results in eventual progression, necessitating a more radical surgical procedure or even enucleation in the future.

Reese[27] emphasizes that the objectives of surgical intervention are to preserve the globe, to salvage useful vision, and to attempt to relieve existing complications. Although details regarding surgical techniques are beyond the scope of this chapter, the reader should be aware of the most important discussions of surgical treatment of PHPV, including the reports of Reese,[27] Acers and Coston,[29] Gass,[30] van Selm,[31] and Smith and Maumenee.[32]

The recent paper by Smith and Maumenee[32] summarizes the results of previous authors and incorporates information gained by previous investigators into a series of useful recommendations for surgical management. All authors agree that early intervention is necessary to preserve the globe. Indications for surgical intervention include shallowing of the anterior chamber (by a clear or cataractous lens), which almost inevitably leads to secondary glaucoma if untreated. The presence of progressive traction on the ciliary processes is also an indication for surgical interruption because in such cases hemorrhage and glaucoma are likely to occur. Any other evidence of progression of the disease, such as development of a cataract in a previously clear lens, is also suggested as an indication for treatment.

Smith and Maumenee[32] emphasize that contraindications to surgical treatment include the inability to rule out retinoblastoma on clinical or laboratory grounds, long-standing intractable glaucoma or hemorrhage, and severe microphthalmia. In the last two circumstances, the eyes inevitably require enucleation.

If surgery is decided on, the surgeon must evaluate visual function, such as direct and consensual pupillary reactions, response to light, and electroretinogram, to determine whether visual function would be possible even after removal of the membrane. Although Gass[30] has observed hypoplasia of the macula by clinical examination in some eyes with PHPV, this finding is not yet widely accepted or proved, and it is yet to be determined whether this phenomenon is a consistent component of this syndrome. Histopathologic studies have not confirmed the presence of an anatomically observable macular hypoplasia.[32]

The basic surgical approach of Smith and Maumenee[32] is twofold: the aspiration of all lens material and the creation of a clear pupillary space by excision of part of the retrolental membrane. The aspiration is completed first. The decision to proceed immediately with discission of the PHPV membrane then depends on the nature of the membrane itself. If the membrane is relatively avascular, the surgeon can proceed immediately to excise the membrane. If the membrane contains engorged vessels, there is a danger of hemorrhage if treatment is undertaken immediately. In the latter instance treatment is delayed and a second operation is performed at a later date, at which time the degree of vascular engorgement is usually decreased and there is less danger of hemorrhage. The membrane may be excised using Vannas or other fine scissors, by iridocapsulomembranectomy utilizing the Holth punch, or by simple discission. One can also use a pars plana approach to complete removal of PHPV with one of the recently developed vitrectomy instruments.[33]

The final visual acuity is generally poor; an acuity greater than 20/200 is rarely achieved. Nevertheless, most globes are salvaged, enucleation is not necessary, and cosmetically acceptable results are achieved, thus justifying the use of these techniques. Because there is a possibility of some visual return in at least a small percentage of cases, such early intervention does indeed seem warranted. Complications of surgery are rare, and the return of useful vision would require appropriate use of contact lenses and consideration of amblyopia therapy.

Posterior PHPV, Epipapillary and Peripapillary Lesions, and Congenital Falciform Fold

An understanding of the pathogenesis of various abnormalities that may occur in the posterior segment of the eye requires an awareness that the primary vitreous is of a dual nature.[34, 35] All of the intravitreal embryonic vessels are derived from embryonic mesoderm. The second component of the primary vitreous is fibrillar, possibly derived from the inner layer of the optic cup. The second component of the primary vitreous consists of (1) the delicate fibrils that form the supporting scaffolding between the intravitreal vascular network and (2) the fibroglial sheath of Bergmeister's papilla, including the surrounding sheath of the hyaloid artery as it passes into the vitreous (Figs. 17.5, 17.11). Interspersed among vessels, sheath, and fibrils is a ground substance composed of hyaluronic acid.

The appearance of each posterior polar anomaly is determined by the degree of retention of one or more of these components. Variations in the fundus pattern can only be explained when one recalls that different components may persist and proliferate in any case.

Lesions based on the persistence of the mesodermal or vascular component of the hyaloid trunk at the posterior pole are well recognized.[36-44] Marked variations occur, ranging from a very short stump of persistent hyaloid trunk arising from the disk (Fig. 17.12) to a longer trunk, which may be relatively straight or tortuous, extending up to the posterior aspect of the lens. The persistent vascular strand may be patent or occluded.

The pathogenesis of so-called vascular loops or corkscrew vessels arising from the optic disk (Fig. 17.12) is unclear. Some investigators feel that such loops are totally unrelated to the persistence of any component of the hyaloid system (reviewed by Bisland[38]). However, when one considers that the retinal and hyaloid vessels arise from a common embryologic vascular bulb in the optic nerve, such a

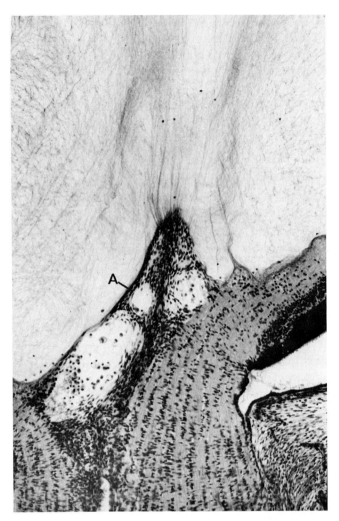

FIG. 17.11. Human fetal globe at six months of gestation. The glial sheath of Bergmeister protrudes anteriorly from the optic nervehead. Note also the myriad delicate fibrils that course anteriorly from the retinal surface. Portion of residual lumen of the hyaloid artery trunk (A) is indicated. H&E, ×250. (Courtesy of Prof. G.O.H. Naumann)

neglect of the hyaloid artery in the pathogenesis of vascular loops appears arbitrary and is actually a matter of semantics. It is likely that the vascular loop consists of the proximal trunk of the hyaloid system, which gives rise to an aberrant persisting branch within the vitreous. Normally such branches in the vitreous regress or are only seen within the optic nerve and retina during formation of the major retinal vessels. Such aberrant formation and persistence of a channel associated with the main hyaloid trunk would conceivably result, after atrophy of the anterior aspect of the hyaloid artery, in the presence of a vascular loop.

The term "persistent Bergmeister's papilla" is loosely used to describe a

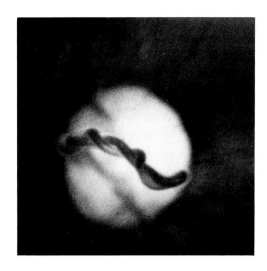

FIG. 17.12. Vascular loop arising at the disk, probably a form of persistence of the posterior aspect of the hyaloid trunk.

variety of conditions. Recalling that Bergmeister's papilla is a structure with two components, the central vascular core surrounded by the fibroglial sheath (Figs. 17.5, 17.11), one could theoretically expect persistence of either component. Therefore, a persistent Bergmeister's papilla might represent a simple vascular remnant usually associated with fibroglial tissue or the fibroglial component alone. The vascular remnant may be either patent or occluded.

The persistence of at least a minimal component of Bergmeister's papilla is such a common phenomenon that it is actually an anatomic variant. Some other authors consider that the extent of resorption of the epipapillary tissue may be partially responsible for determination of the depth of the physiologic optic cup— ie, the greater the resorption, the deeper the cup.

The retention of elements of the glial sheath of Bergmeister is usually clinically manifest by the formation of epipapillary or peripapillary, delicate, white to gray membranes or glial cysts. Such membranes rarely present visual difficulties, but they are important in relation to the differential diagnosis of lesions on and around the optic nerve, particularly small retinoblastomas. Medullated retinal nerve fibers represent a relatively common developmental condition that must be differentiated from persistent elements of Bergmeister's papilla. Normally, myelination is completed shortly after birth and extends only up to the posterior aspect of the lamina cribrosa. When myelination extends into the nerve fiber layer, the photoreceptive area of the retina is obscured from light by the opaque myelinated fibers, resulting in a visual field defect.

Epipapillary membranes based on the persistence of primary vitreous must also be differentiated from drusen of the optic nervehead, hamartomatous growths (such as astrocytomas occurring in tuberous sclerosis), and, most important, small retinoblastomas in the region of the optic disk. An inflammatory lesion can be another significant cause of a white epipapillary or peripapillary membrane.

The fibrils of the primary vitreous insert into the sensory retina not only in the region of the optic disk, but also in the midperiphery and periphery of the fundus.

Therefore, retention and proliferation of these elements may lead to occasional thickening of the nerve fiber layer and formation of small inner retinal or preretinal fibroglial tufts.[34, 40, 42] Pruett and Schepens[40] classified this effect as posterior hyperplastic primary vitreous. Traction exerted by shrinkage of fibroglial remnants at the vitreoretinal interface may produce retinal folds anywhere in the fundus. One can thereby explain the attachment of abnormal vitreous fibrils to any portion of the retina as anterior as the ora serrata. Indeed, the traction produced by such abnormal vitreoretinal development may create giant retinal tears and may be occasionally associated with lens colobomas. Pruett and Schepens[40] also postulated that some congenital remnants of the primary vitreous may be operative in the causation of rhegmatogenous retinal detachment. Furthermore, preretinal proliferation of these membranes may explain the presence of preretinal, intravitreal, or epipapillary cysts which form a distinct clinical entity.[36, 37, 44]

Pruett and Schepens[40] believe that congenital falciform fold is a form of posterior hyperplastic primary vitreous. This condition[40, 41, 45–50] is a rare cause of leukocoria or pseudoglioma. It is clinically recognizable as an elongated folding or tenting-up of retinal tissue, usually, coursing from the optic nervehead toward the retinal periphery or ciliary region. It is sometimes inherited in an autosomal recessive manner. It is often bilateral (4 of 13 cases in Howard's and Ellsworth's series[2]) and usually affects the lower temporal quadrant. Falciform folds are sometimes associated with abnormal persistence of the hyaloid artery, and the artery may actually be located along the apex of the ridge of retina. Most authors postulate that traction exerted by the persistent components of the primary vitreous induces traction on the inner aspect of the retina, thereby creating a tenting-up of the retina. The disease is usually progressive and eventual massive retinal detachment and phthisis bulbi generally occur.

Howard and Ellsworth[2] have noted that there is a striking similarity between congenital retinal fold and grade 3 cicatricial retrolental fibroplasia; some observers have considered them the same entity. However, Howard and Ellsworth emphasize that there is reason to classify them separately. Retrolental fibroplasia nearly always occurs in infants of low birth weight who have been maintained in an incubator for a time. Such a history is not obtained in patients with congenital retinal folds. Microscopic examination of histologic sections provides another reason for segregating these two entities. The retina in congenital retinal fold is disposed in dysplastic rosettes, indicating an early disturbance in embryogenesis, whereas in retrolental fibroplasia, it is characterized by vascular proliferation leading to secondary gliosis and secondary degenerative changes.

RETINAL VASCULAR ANOMALIES WITH LIPID EXUDATION

Coats' syndrome, Leber's miliary aneurysms, and von Hippel-Lindau angiomatosis are retinal vascular diseases, which, despite differences in pathogenesis and variations in clinical appearance, are often characterized by the outpouring of lipid exudates. Indeed, it is not simply the presence of the vascular anomaly of the former two diseases or the hemangioblastoma of von Hippel disease that is responsible for the marked visual loss associated with these diseases. The more important factor is the exudation that leads to retinal detachment, secondary glaucoma, hemorrhage, and eventually phthisis bulbi. Because the lipid exudation can be massive and each disease may mimic a retinoblastoma, these three conditions are described together.

Coats' Syndrome

In 1908, when George Coats first described the syndrome that bears his name, he divided it into three groups.[51] Groups 1 and 2 showed massive retinal exudation and lipid deposition, but differed in the clinical appearance of their vessels. Group 1 vessels appeared normal ophthalmoscopically; group 2 vessels exhibited clinically evident changes such as telangiectasia (Figs. 17.13, 17.14), aneurysms, vascular sheathing, and neovascularization. Coats' group 3 is now recognized as von Hippel-Lindau angiomatosis.

The classic Coats' syndrome[51-54] consists of a nonfamilial, unilateral affection primarily occurring in infants or juveniles in the absence of other systemic findings. Males are more commonly affected. The diagnosis is usually made at a slightly

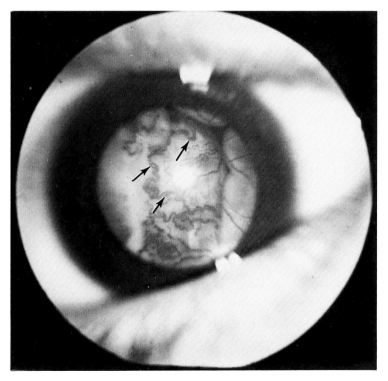

FIG. 17.13. Fundus photograph of a retrolental mass in a young boy. Two features were noted clinically that led to the correct clinical diagnosis of Coats' syndrome: (1) marked retinal vascular telangiectasia (arrows) and (2) a yellow discoloration of the mass, due to massive lipid exudation. (From Apple and Rabb: Clinicopathologic Correlation of Ocular Disease, 1974. Courtesy of CV Mosby)

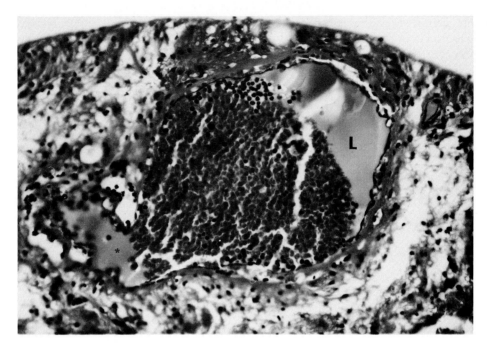

FIG. 17.14. Coats' syndrome. Photomicrograph of retina with vitreoretinal interface and internal limiting membrane above. Note the markedly enlarged, telangiectatic vessel containing serum and coagulated erythrocytes. The enlarged vessel is continuous with a nonenlarged channel at lower left (asterisk). L indicates vessel lumen. PAS, ×400.

later age than for retinoblastoma, this syndrome manifesting toward the end of the first decade. Characteristically, subretinal and intraretinal deposition of cholesterol-containing lipid exudates are clinically and pathologically evident (Figs. 17.15, 17.16). The clinical differentiation from retinoblastoma is facilitated by recognition of the characteristic retinal telangiectasia seen in Coats' syndrome (Figs. 17.13, 17.14).[52] Although vascular engorgement may occur in retinoblastoma, the severe vascular changes outlined in Table 17.6 are much more characteristic of Coats' syndrome.

Table 17.6

Primary Histopathologic Hallmarks of Coats' Syndrome

Vascular changes
    Coats' type 1: no vascular changes apparent ophthalmoscopically
    Coats' type 2
        Irregular vessel caliber, including telangiectasia, aneurysms
        Hyalination, sheathing
        Arteriovenous anastomoses
        Neovascularization

Lipid exudation
        Intraretinal and subretinal deposits of lipid (cholesterol clefts)
        Hemorrhage and gliosis, deposition of hemosiderin-laden and lipoidal macrophages
    Intraretinal PAS-positive deposits

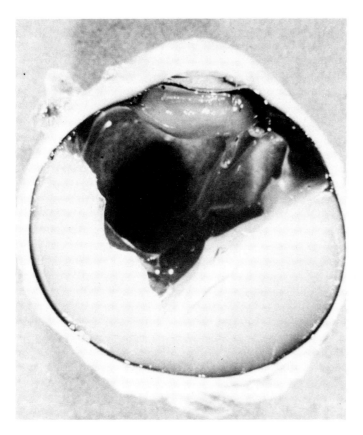

FIG. 17.15. Coats' syndrome, gross photograph. There is massive retinal detachment with a yellow-white, milky, turbid subretinal fluid.

Additionally, in many cases the exudative retrolental mass assumes a yellow color due to the large component of lipid within the lesion and a yellow-green bullous retinal detachment is very characteristic of this disease. This feature contrasts with the usual chalk white or pink-white appearance of retinoblastoma, which is often calcified. The yellow, glistening, crystalline deposits of cholesterol within the exudates in Coats' syndrome should not be confused with the chalk white calcium deposits seen in necrotic retinoblastomas. The progression to retinal hemorrhage, retinal detachment, secondary glaucoma, and phthisis bulbi, which typically occurs in untreated cases (Fig. 17.17), is primarily due to the outpouring of these massive intraretinal and subretinal exudates, the organization of blood breakdown products and lipid deposits, and the subsequent secondary gliosis. Photocoagulation is one of the few modalities of treatment available and may be successful in early cases in achieving resorption of the exudates.

The three major histopathologic hallmarks that together are pathognomonic of Coats' syndrome are listed in Table 17.6. The vascular changes probably represent the primary etiologic factor. There is a deficiency due to loss of functional endothelial cell tight junctions in the blood–retinal barrier. Blood fluids and lipids

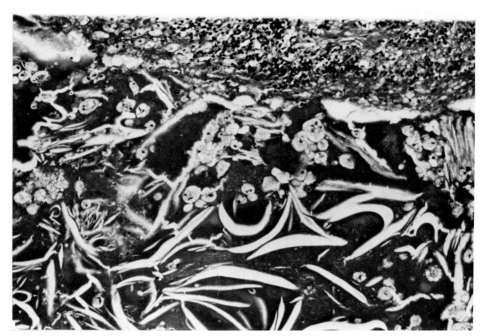

FIG. 17.16. Coats' syndrome. The retina (above) overlies a subretinal exudate composed of protein, lipid, cholesterol clefts (narrow slits), and hemosiderin- and lipid-laden macrophages. The macrophages are round, poorly staining cells with small nuclei. The small granules seen in many of the macrophages are hemosiderin deposits derived from blood. PAS, ×280.

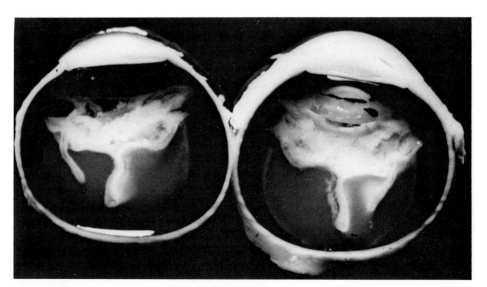

FIG. 17.17. Gross photograph of a globe enucleated for Coats' syndrome showing end-stage changes, including total retinal detachment. (Courtesy of Prof. G.O.H. Naumann)

bridge this gap and are deposited within the vessel wall (plasmatic vasculosis) and perivascular interstitial tissues.[53, 54] The nature of the intraretinal, PAS-positive deposits is unclear, but these probably are also foci of blood fluids deposited in the retina following passage from the blood. They are very useful for diagnosis and, if present in large amounts, are highly characteristic of the syndrome.

Similar clinical and pathologic findings may be seen unilaterally in eyes of adults without systemic disease.[54] In such cases the complex of lesions is similar to that seen in the juvenile form, but a unifying etiology between the adult and the juvenile forms has not been demonstrated. Such adult cases are, of course, usually not in question with regard to the differential diagnosis of retinoblastoma because of the age distinction.

Leber's Miliary Aneurysms

There is continuing controversy as to the relationship between Leber's miliary aneurysms and Coats' syndrome.[55, 56] Some authors consider them to be variations of the same disease with similar etiology and pathogenesis; others consider them totally separate entities. Leber's multiple miliary aneurysms with retinal degeneration most commonly occur in young to middle-age individuals. Therefore, these patients are generally somewhat older than those with typical juvenile Coats' syndrome, and the lipid deposition is seldom as severe. The most distinguishing feature of this disease is a saccular or bulbous dilatation of retinal arterial channels (Fig. 17.18). These aneurysms should be distinguished from the much smaller capillary microaneurysms characteristic of diabetes mellitus. The saccular or bulbous arterial aneurysmal dilatation seen in this syndrome is often focal, involving discrete foci on the involved vessel. Therefore, although there is considerable overlap between the two conditions, this characteristic differs slightly from the more diffuse telangiectasia sometimes associated with the classic Coats' syndrome. The aneurysmal dilatations of the retinal vessels show perfusion by fluorescein angiography but do not leak and do not represent new vessels. Plasma fluids and lipids leak into the retina, apparently from associated arteriovenous shunts and damaged capillaries and veins rather than from the larger dilated arterial channels.

Many of the aneurysmal lesions spontaneously regress, and visual impairment is often minimal if the fovea is uninvolved. Visual impairment is largely related to tissue destruction by the lipid exudates. The most satisfactory treatment of threatening lesions is photocoagulation. Destruction of leaking channels within and adjacent to the exudative ring leads to resorption of the exudates.

Von Hippel-Lindau Angiomatosis

Von Hippel-Lindau angiomatosis (angiomatosis retinae) is generally categorized with the phakomatoses, that is, a group of diseases characterized by formation of lesions affecting the skin, eyes, central nervous system, and the viscera.[3, 57] The other three major phakomatoses are tuberous sclerosis, neurofibromatosis, and the Sturge-Weber syndrome. Differentiation of angiomatosis retinae from retinoblastoma is usually not difficult because the typical feeder vessels and retinal an-

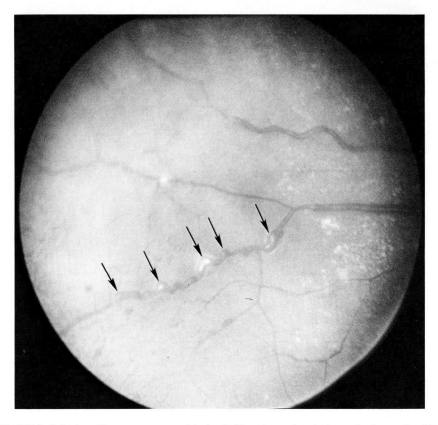

FIG. 17.18. Leber's miliary aneurysms, with focal dilatations of retinal vessels (arrows). (From Apple and Rabb: Clinicopathologic Correlation of Ocular Disease, 1974. Courtesy of CV Mosby)

giomas present a pathognomonic fundus picture (Fig. 17.19). Furthermore, the patient usually reveals symptoms at a later age, and the symptoms and findings created by the cerebellar angioma serve to differentiate this lesion from retinoblastoma. Occasionally, however, when massive intraretinal and subretinal lipid outpouring is a prominent feature (Fig. 17.20), this condition can clinically resemble retinoblastoma or Coats' syndrome.

Angiomatosis retinae, like retinoblastoma, is transmitted as an autosomal dominant trait with incomplete penetrance. The characteristic fundus lesion consists of a feeder arteriole and draining venule that enters into and exits from a well-circumscribed yellow to white or red retinal tumor (Fig. 17.19). The retinal lesions are frequently multiple in each eye and are often bilateral. The disease affects both sexes. The onset of symptoms generally occurs during the teens or early twenties. Although clinical symptoms and signs are rarely evident at birth, intraretinal microvascular abnormalities that are not clinically evident are present very early in life.[58] These lesions probably evolve into the clinically evident, progressive vascular anomalies apparent in later life.

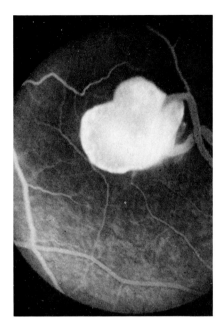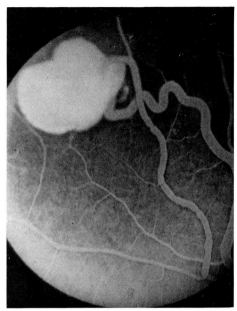

FIG. 17.19. Typical fluorescein angiographic pattern of a von Hippel intraretinal hemangioblastoma with associated feeder arteriole and draining venules.

The angiomatous tumor itself may be capable of forming lipid. However, extensive exudation of lipid usually occurs in areas remote from the primary angioma, particularly in the macular region (Fig. 17.20). When lipid exudation is profuse, the fundus picture of angiomatosis retinae is even more similar to that of Coats' syndrome than to retinoblastoma. Indeed, in his original description, Coats classified what we now designate as von Hippel-Lindau disease as group 3 of the syndrome that bears his name.

Several features differentiate the two diseases. Coats' syndrome is usually unilateral; von Hippel retinal angiomatosis is often bilateral. Coats' syndrome is usually diagnosed at a much earlier age than von Hippel-Lindau disease. The clinical appearance of the diffuse retinal vascular telangiectasia seen in Coats' syndrome differs markedly from the clinical picture of the vascular anomalies seen in retinal angiomatosis. However, the clinical appearance of the intraretinal and subretinal exudates can be identical.

The retinal hemangioblastoma can be obliterated by diathermy, photocoagulation,[59] or cryotherapy. Destruction of the tumor is highly desirable because untreated lesions almost invariably lead to complications that may cause blindness. If the tumor is not destroyed, the subsequent subretinal and preretinal hemorrhage and outpouring of lipid will lead to retinal detachment, secondary glaucoma, and ultimately phthisis bulbi. The diagnosis and treatment of von Hippel-Lindau disease are discussed in further detail in Chapters 15 and 16.

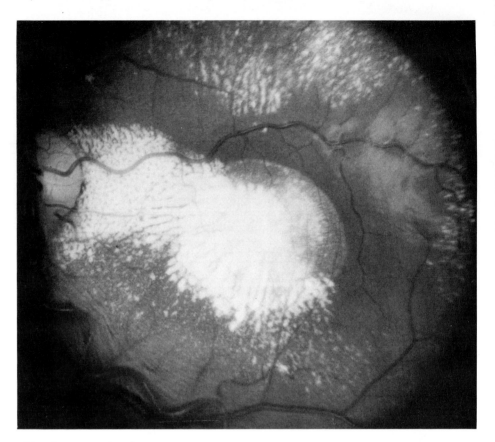

FIG. 17.20. Von Hippel-Lindau disease. This fundus photograph reveals the deposition of lipid exudates within the papillomacular region. The main tumor and the associated feeder arteriole and draining venule are out of the photograph. Only a portion of the draining venule is shown (lower left). It is characteristic of this disease that lipid may be formed both within the main tumor and, as is illustrated in this case, in areas (usually in the macular region) removed from the primary hemangioblastoma. Such lipid deposits are similar to those seen in Coats' syndrome and Leber's miliary aneurysms. Lipid exudation, neovascularization of the retina and anterior segment, retinal detachment, secondary glaucoma, and eventual phthisis bulbi are frequent complications of untreated cases. (From Apple and Rabb: Clinicopathologic Correlation of Ocular Disease, 1974. Courtesy of CV Mosby)

TOXIC RETINOPATHY
(RETINOPATHY OF PREMATURITY)

Terry, in 1942, first described the clinicopathologic characteristics of toxic retinopathy and coined the term "retrolental fibroplasia."[60] He described the condition as a "fibroplastic overgrowth of persistent vascular tissue behind each crystalline lens." At that time and in subsequent years the role of oxygen administration in the pathogenesis of this disease was unknown. The tendency toward widespread administration of oxygen to premature infants in the 1940s and early 1950s led to a dramatic increase in blindness due to this disease. The mechanism of oxygen toxicity was elucidated in the 1950s by several investigators (reviewed by several authors[2, 61–67]), and the tendency toward aggressive oxygen therapy was correspondingly reduced.

The observations made by Terry generally dealt with cases in advanced stages of the disease in which a hypervascular retrolental band or mass was the primary feature (Fig. 17.21). Actually, retrolental fibroplasia is primarily a proliferative vascular disease in which neovascular buds penetrate the inner membrane of the retina, invade the vitreous, and subsequently undergo exuberant proliferation and fibrous metaplasia (Fig. 17.22). These fibrovascular bands in the vitreous then induce traction on the retina, and there is retinal detachment in which the retina is sequestered into a position behind the lens. It is this retrolental involvement seen in the later stages that produces the leukocoria and that is responsible for the term "retrolental fibroplasia." In the milder clinical form, in which this intravitreal proliferation is minimal, only a small peripheral mass is seen.

The fully developed or mature vasculature of the retina of a full-term infant is relatively insensitive to oxygen damage. However, the incompletely vascularized retina of the premature infant is susceptible to toxic damage induced by high levels of oxygen inhalation. It is important to recall that the most peripheral areas of the sensory retina are incompletely vascularized prior to birth. During normal embryogenesis, the vascular buds emanate from the disk and reach the nasal ora serrata at eight months of gestation. The temporal ora serrata is not fully vascularized until several weeks after birth. Maturation of the vascular tree of the temporal sensory retina is presumably delayed because of the greater distance from the optic disk to the temporal aspect of the eye. This phenomenon is largely responsible for the greater incidence of damage on the temporal aspect of the globe seen in this condition. Because the temporal retina is not fully vascularized until several weeks after birth, this disease may occasionally be seen in full-term infants.

When oxygen is administered to the premature infant, the still developing angioblastic tissue of the retinal periphery is stimulated toward an initial primary stage of vasoconstriction and vasoobliteration. During this stage oxygen administration induces actual damage or necrosis of the capillary endothelium and partial obliteration of the retinal vascular tree. Following removal of oxygen, a secondary stage ensues, with vasodilation and a marked proliferation of the remaining vascular channels. This effect leads to exuberant neovascularization and formation of glomeruloid buds and tufts of vessels (Fig. 17.22). These elements proliferate and eventually invade the vitreous in a fashion analogous to that observed in other neovascular conditions, such as diabetic retinopathy or sickle cell retinopathy. The secondary proliferative response following oxygen removal is best explained as an overreaction by the tissue in response to the relative hypoxia and ischemia.

The final evolutionary stage is the terminal or cicatricial stage.[63] Howard and Ellsworth[2] emphasized that there is a specific form of the cicatricial stage of this disease (grade 3) that is particularly noteworthy because of its resemblance to congenital falciform retinal fold. In this form, a "dragged disk" is observed where there is traction on the retina, producing a sharply demarcated, elevated retinal septum that arches forward into the vitreous body; it usually reaches temporally from the disk to the extreme periphery of the fundus. The latter stages are also

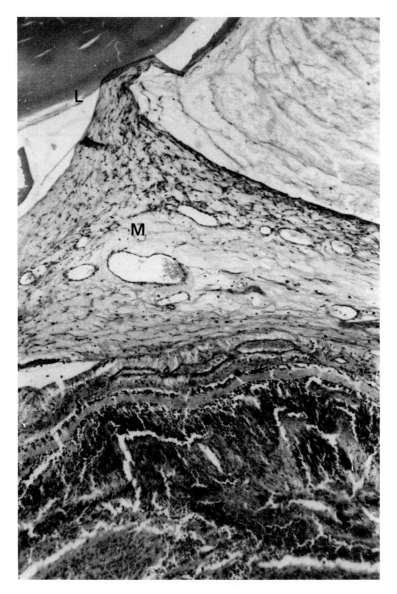

FIG. 17.21. Retrolental fibroplasia. This photomicrograph demonstrates the retrolental fibrovascular mass (M) that has formed secondary to neovascular proliferation from immature peripheral retinal vessels. The edge of the lens is seen superiorly (L). The sensory retina (below) has been pulled into the retrolental membrane, forming a funnel-shaped detachment. Note the new-formed vessels within the mass. PAS, ×25.

characterized by glaucoma, hemorrhage, scarring and fibrosis, and eventual phthisis bulbi. Although phthisis bulbi is a common sequela, the changes are not necessarily progressive and the disease may become quiescent at any stage.

Several features differentiate retrolental fibroplasia from retinoblastoma and other causes of leukocoria. The relationship of the disease to premature birth and

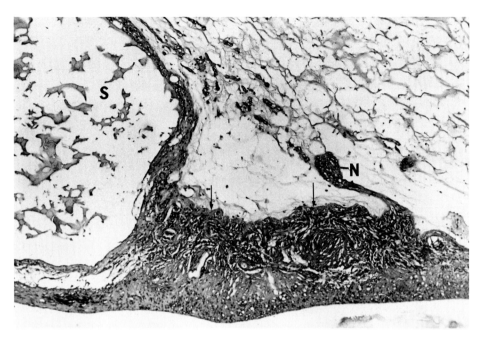

FIG. 17.22. Retrolental fibroplasia. The markedly degenerate peripheral retina (below) shows a large schisis cavity (S). Neovascular buds (N) form the basis for the pathogenesis of the retrolental fibrovascular membrane. There is marked condensation of vitreous fibrils (above, right). Arrows indicate internal limiting membrane of the retina. PAS, ×100.

oxygen therapy is obvious. The formation of the retrolental membrane is usually not present immediately at birth, but develops subsequently. The condition is often bilateral, and the eyes are normal in size at birth, although they may show growth retardation and relative microphthalmia later. In later stages, the dragged disk may resemble congenital falciform fold, but is usually easily differentiated from retinoblastoma. As in PHPV, elongated, centrally displaced ciliary processes may be seen clinically. This finding is due to contracture and shrinkage of the retrolental mass, which causes elongation of the ciliary processes. Such vitreous traction is usually not a major component in retinoblastoma.

Clinical management of the premature infant requires judgment with regard to the use of oxygen to preserve life and potential blindness due to oxygen toxicity. Current emphasis is on the use of a titration of oxygen at which systemic complications due to hypoxia and ocular complications due to hyperoxia might be avoided.

INFLAMMATORY CONDITIONS

Toxocariasis (Nematode Endophthalmitis)

In 1952, Beaver and coauthors[68] described a syndrome of childhood secondary to *Toxocara* invasion and coined the term "visceral larva migrans." Typically affecting children in the first decade of life, the *Toxocara* ova, usually *T. canis*, but occasionally *T. catis*, are ingested and hatch in the small intestine[69] (Fig. 17.23). There is usually a history of the child being exposed to the family pet, more commonly a puppy rather than an adult dog.[69] The larvae are distributed to the peripheral organs, particularly the liver, lungs, brain, and eyes, via the arterial circulation; there they are deposited and consumed or encapsulated by an eosinophilic granulomatous response.[70] The life cycle is never completed in humans and ends at this point.

Intraocular toxocariasis was first described by Wilder in 1950.[71] She found larvae in histologic sections of over half of a selected series of pseudoglioma cases. Ocular toxocariasis may create a picture of leukocoria closely resembling retinoblastoma (Fig. 17.24). The infection usually takes one of three forms: (1) a retrolental, intravitreal lesion forming a vitreous abscess and endophthalmitis[71-75]; (2) an isolated posterior polar lesion, often confined to the macula[73, 76]; or (3) well-localized peripheral retinal or ciliary body inflammatory masses.[69, 77] Although these three primary sites of infestation are recognized, Wilkinson and Welsh[70] believe that the initial site of the larva is determined solely by chance. It is an interesting but puzzling fact that patients with the systemic form, eg, hepatic infestations, rarely contract the ocular lesion, and vice versa. As in most parasitic diseases, eosinophilia of the peripheral blood often occurs. However, the eosinophil count

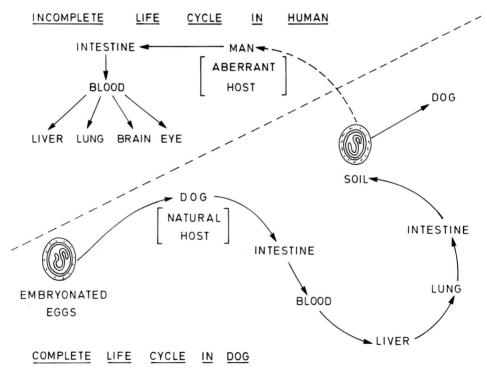

FIG. 17.23. Life cycle of *T. canis* in dog (natural host) and man (unnatural host). (From Zinkham: Johns Hopkins Med J 123:41, 1968[69])

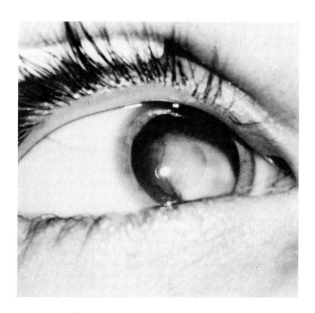

FIG. 17.24. Toxocariasis. This white intravitreal mass from a young boy required enucleation to rule out a retinoblastoma. Microscopic examination revealed a vitreous abscess and endophthalmitis, also containing numerous eosinophils. (From Apple and Rabb: Clinicopathologic Correlation of Ocular Disease, 1974. Courtesy of CV Mosby)

is more consistently elevated in cases of systemic visceral larva migrans than in cases localized to the eye.

It is usually quite difficult to demonstrate the organisms in histopathologic sections of enucleated globes without the benefit of extensive serial sectioning. Indeed, there is no inflammatory reaction until the organism dies. However, because the cellular infiltrative pattern is quite distinct, a tissue diagnosis can be made confidently, even without localization of the actual organism. The infected intraocular tissues typically show a central focus of necrosis, usually surrounding the worm, accompanied by abundant eosinophils. The eosinophil, characterized by eosinophilic-staining cytoplasm and bilobed nucleus, is usually associated with an accompanying infiltration rich in neutrophils and plasma cells, as well as epithelioid cells and other nonspecific chronic inflammatory elements. Generally, one can safely conclude that this combination of eosinophils and plasma cells within a retinal or vitreous abscess in a child with leukocoria is sufficient for a presumptive diagnosis of nematode endophthalmitis. In very late stages of the disease, there is extensive fibrosis and organization of the involved tissues and a decrease in cellularity of the lesion. Even in these cases, however, there are usually residual cellular infiltrates differentiating this condition from the other conditions causing a white pupil.

When a vitreous abscess and severe endophthalmitis occur, differentiation from retinoblastoma is often difficult by simple clinical examination. In such cases, the aqueous humor LDH assay described by Swartz et al[12] may prove exceedingly useful. (See also Chapter 19.)

The localized posterior polar form of *Toxocara* granuloma shows little or no active inflammation, is nonprogressive, and should not be confused with retinoblastoma.

Wilkinson and Welsh[70] emphasized the relatively high incidence of a peripherally (anteriorly) situated center of inflammation. In four of ten of their enucleated cases, the lesion was within the peripheral retina or ciliary body. Because this form is often associated with retinal folds, it is more likely to be confused with grade 3 cicatricial retrolental fibroplasia or congenital falciform fold.

Peripheral toxocariasis may also be confused with pars planitis.[78] Indeed, the syndrome of pars planitis has occasionally been described secondary to proved toxocariasis, toxoplasmosis, chorioretinitis, cytomegalic inclusion retinitis, or other forms of posterior and peripheral focal endophthalmitis. Howard and Ellsworth[2] observed pars planitis in 4 of 265 cases of pseudoglioma. The caked yellow exudate in the lower half of the retina and the large, fluffy exudates within the vitreous may closely resemble retinoblastoma.

Metastatic Endophthalmitis

Prior to the era of antibiotic therapy, metastatic endophthalomitis was a significant cause of pseudoretinoblastoma. Today this condition is quite rare and is usually differentiated from retinoblastoma by recognition of the concurrent disease.

CONDITIONS EXHIBITING ABNORMAL RETINAL EMBRYOGENESIS AND/OR RETINAL DYSPLASIA AS PROMINENT FEATURES

Retinal Dysplasia

A dysplasia signifies a failure of normal development of a tissue during embryonic life. The tissue never achieves maturity. Furthermore, the noxious influence (such as a chromosome abnormality) responsible for growth retardation usually causes a deviation in the growth pattern so that the final appearance of the tissue not only reveals a retardation of growth with retention of the embryonic configuration but also shows a distinctly abnormal structure. Embryonic tissues are relatively pluripotential in their capacity to develop along several lines, and dysplastic growth often reflects this state in that bizarre tissue differentiation sometimes occurs.

Retinal dysplasia[79, 80] is best considered a lesion with specific morphologic characteristics rather than a disease or syndrome in itself. It may occur in otherwise normal individuals as an isolated, unilateral lesion, or it may be observed as a component of several syndromes with intraocular involvement.[3, 81] Such syndromes include Norrie's disease and trisomy 13 syndrome.

The primary feature of retinal dysplasia that renders histopathologic diagnosis relatively easy is the formation of rosettes. A rosette, which may be monolayered, bilayered, or trilayered, represents an attempt to form embryonic retinal tissue, primarily rods and cones. The nuclei lining the rosette are analogous to the nuclear layers of the retina. The benign rosettes of retinal dysplasia, which show no anaplasia, can be clearly distinguished from the malignant Flexner-Wintersteiner rosettes formed in retinoblastoma. The latter rosettes possess the same propensity toward formation of rods and cones but, unlike dysplastic rosettes, they exhibit neoplastic differentiation with malignant behavior. In addition to the formation of rosettes, retinal dysplasia occasionally involves an attempt by the faulty neuro-epithelium to form tubules and cords of simple cuboidal epithelium resembling that of embryonic ciliary body or retina.

Norrie's Disease

Norrie's disease[48, 82–86] is a rare syndrome with an X-linked recessive inheritance pattern characterized by bilateral congenital amaurosis and varying degrees of hearing impairment and mental retardation. Ophthalmoscopically, the usual clinical presentation is that of a white, often hemorrhagic retrolental mass noted during the first few months of life. This retrolental opacity categorizes this syndrome as a pseudoglioma.

Affected eyes have rarely had histopathologic examination, but the evidence available to date suggests that the basic mechanism of pathogenesis is a defect in the development of the embryonic retina. The changes are primarily neuroecto-dermal in origin. There is not only an arrest (hypoplasia) in the development of the inner layer of the optic cup (the sensory retina), there is also an aberrant growth of some segments of the retina, leading to the retinal dysplasia. Retinal dysplasia is evidenced by the formation of rosettes and cords of proliferating embryonic cuboidal epithelium resembling primitive optic cup epithelium forming within the retrolental mass.

The primary defect in optic cup differentiation offers a pathogenetic explanation as to the origin of the myriad findings of this disease. In addition to the neuro-glial proliferation from the retina into the vitreous, there are extensive secondary changes that are largely responsible for the formation of the large preretinal mass that sometimes mimics a retinoblastoma. These effects include secondary retinal detachment and intraretinal and preretinal hemorrhage. The organization of blood breakdown products with the formation of granulation tissue creates a large fibrous mass that may comprise the bulk of the retrolental mass. It is not entirely clear from histopathologic studies whether the intravitreal capillary buds formed in affected globes are derived in greater proportion from pure neovascularization or whether a certain percentage of these vascular elements are derived from PHPV.[86]

Trisomy 13 Syndrome

Trisomy 13 (Patau's syndrome, Bartholin's syndrome, Reese-Blodi-Straatsma syndrome) is the chromosomal aberration that is most closely associated with severe intraocular abnormalities. The specific clinical findings characteristic of the disease, the diagnostic pattern seen by karyotypic analysis, and the fact that almost all affected infants die in the first few months of life clearly differentiate this syndrome from retinoblastoma. Therefore, although leukocoria is a prominent feature of trisomy 13, the general aspects of the disease differ enough from retinoblastoma such that it is not an important factor in the differential diagnosis and a detailed review here is unnecessary. The ocular findings are listed in Table 17.7. Detailed

Table 17.7

Ocular Findings in Trisomy 13*

Microphthalmia; sometimes apparent (clinical) anophthalmia

Colobomas (usually of ciliary body and iris, less commonly of the optic nerve); colobomas seen in almost 100 percent of affected eyes

PHPV; communication of extraocular connective tissue of mesodermal origin with intraocular hyaloid system and tunica vasculosa lentis via ciliary body coloboma; sometimes pigmented

Intraocular cartilage formed in mesoderm within the ciliary body coloboma; ingrowth of uveal melanocytes into globe through the coloboma

Retinal dysplasia, including abnormal, anteriorly dislocated sensory retinal tissue formed over pars plana

Cataracts; primary aphakia (rare)

Rudimentary differentiation of angle structures

Corneal opacities; posterior corneal ulcers (rare)

Optic nerve hypoplasia, atrophy, occasional coloboma of the optic nerve

Cyclopia (rare)

* From Apple and Rabb: Clinicopathologic Correlation of Ocular Disease, 1974. Courtesy of CV Mosby.

clinicopathologic descriptions and a review of the literature of this disease have been published by Apple[87] and Apple and Rabb.[3]

Fundus Colobomas

Howard and Ellsworth[2] noted fundus colobomas in 30 of 265 children with suspected retinoblastoma, ranking this entity fourth (after PHPV, retrolental fibroplasia, and posterior cataract) as a cause of leukocoria (Table 17.1). In most cases, the colobomas are of the "typical" type, based on malclosure of the embryonic intraocular fissure.[3]

The fissure is a transient cleft along the ventral aspect of the cup (Fig. 17.25); in effect, it creates a defect or notch in the inferior wall of the future eyeball. This defect provides an entrance and exit pathway for the transient embryonic blood vessels and creates a temporary slit in the optic stalk through which the retinal nerve fibers pass from the ganglion cell layer of the retina into the brain. Fusion of the lips of the embryonic ocular fissure, of critical importance in the normal development of the eye, leads to closure of the cleft and formation of an intact, complete globe. Defective closure of the embryonic ocular fissure produces the typical coloboma. Because the embryonic fissure normally courses along the inferior nasal aspect of the eye, the typical colobomatous defect occupies the same position. The defect may involve the iris, creating the so-called keyhole pupil, and less commonly involves the ciliary body. The colobomatous defect may involve any portion of the inferior fundus, including the optic nervehead.

The white color imparted to the fundus by a massive coloboma is primarily due to maldevelopment of the involved retina and choroid permitting visualization of the underlying sclera (Fig. 17.26). This phenomenon is responsible for the white reflex in the pupil, but careful fundus examination usually suffices to differentiate the colobomatous defect from retinoblastoma. The affected maldeveloped retina often shows the features of retinal dysplasia.

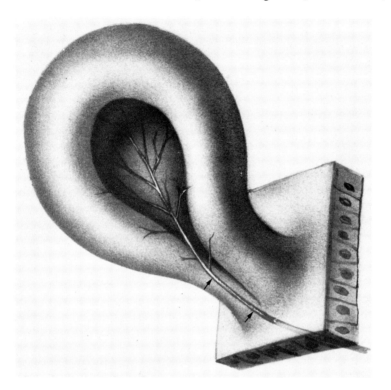

FIG. 17.25. Schematic model of embryonic eye showing the inferonasal embryonic fissure through which the hyaloid artery (arrows) enters the globe. Malclosure of this fissure creates a "typical" coloboma.

Incontinentia Pigmenti (Bloch-Sulzberger Syndrome)

The skin lesions of incontinentia pigmenti (described by Bloch[88] and Sulzberger[89, 90]) are usually present at birth or shortly thereafter. The disease is almost exclusively confined to females (210 of 216 cases collected by Lenz[91]). Many hereditary cases have been noted, and Lenz suggests that the disease is transmitted by a gene on the X chromosome. The skin lesions occur in three stages.[92] In the initial stage, occurring immediately after birth, intraepidermal vesicles are a prominent feature. They occur mainly on the extremities and last several months. The second stage consists of linear, verrucous lesions. In the third stage, the characteristic disseminated pigmented skin lesions become evident. They are located mainly on the sides of the trunk (so-called Blascho's lines)[93] and arise de novo. That is, they arise totally independent of the vesicular and verrucous lesions located primarily on the extremities. The histopathologic appearance of these pigmented lesions is responsible for the term "incontinentia pigmenti." There is loss of melanin from the cells of the basal layer of epithelium, with deposition and accumulation of the pigment in the dermis. Sulzberger[90] assumed that primary damage to the cells of the basal layer causes them to become incapable of holding and metabolizing melanin. The pigmented skin lesions often fade with aging and may be difficult

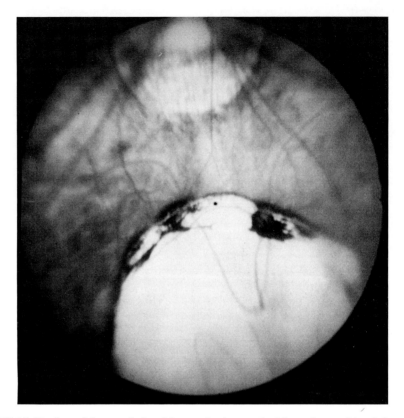

FIG. 17.26. Fundus coloboma of the right eye is characterized by a large white defect infero-nasally, which caused a leukocoria, but which was readily differentiated from retinoblastoma by ophthalmoscopy. This "typical" coloboma is due to faulty closure of the embryonic intraocular fissure. (Courtesy Prof. G.O.H. Naumann)

to observe in later life. Analogous subepithelial melanin deposits have also been described in the conjunctiva.[93] Clinical differentiation of this lesion from retino-blastoma is best attained by localization and biopsy of this skin lesion. In addition to the cutaneous lesions, other ectodermal structures are often affected, including the nails, hair (alopecia), teeth, central nervous system, and eyes. Eosinophilia is sometimes present.

Ocular findings occur in one-quarter to one-third of cases (reviewed by Scott and coauthors,[94] Wollensak,[95] and Best and Rentsch[96]). Relatively unusual findings include myopia, strabismus, nystagmus, microphthalmia, optic atrophy, and blue sclera. More common, and more important in relation to the differential diagnosis of retinoblastoma, is the occurrence of posterior and retrolental changes that create a pseudoglioma (Fig. 17.27). It has been variously described as resembling an exudative or proliferative retinitis, falciform retinal fold, metastatic endophthalmitis, or retrolental fibroplasia. Many of these cases reveal a cataract, which usually arises secondary to the retrolental mass.

It is extremely difficult to relate the pathogenesis of the intraocular changes

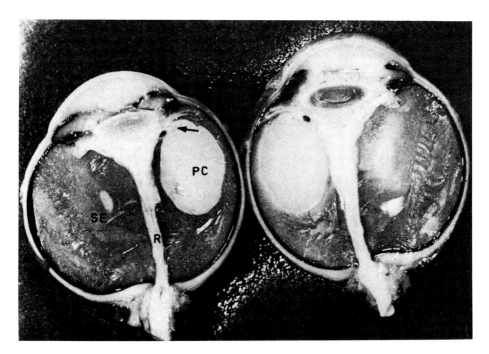

FIG. 17.27. Pseudoglioma in incontinentia pigmenti. Note total funnel-shaped retinal detachment (R) and formation of retinal pseudocysts (PC). The connection of the cyst to the retina is indicated by the arrow. Subretinal exudate (SE) is shown. (From Best and Rentsch: Klin Monatsbl Augenheilkd 164:19, 1974)

that lead to a leukocoria to the pathogenesis of the skin lesions. Three major theories of pathogenesis have been proposed: (1) Intraocular inflammation, eg., exudative chorioretinitis, is one possibility[95-97]; however, many cases have been histologically studied in which an inflammatory response was absent. (2) A form of PHPV has been proposed,[98] although it has been found in only a few instances and more cases must be added before it can be considered a significant cause. (3) Although the etiology of the intraocular changes of incontinentia pigmenti clearly differs from that of retrolental fibroplasia (oxygen toxicity), Findlay,[99] Cole and Cole,[100] and Best and Rentsch[96] point out the striking similarity of the pathologic changes in these two diseases and suggest a similar pathogenesis, ie, the formation of new vessels with subsequent proliferative retinopathy as a response to a hypoxic stimulus (Figs. 17.28, 17.29).

A theory of pathogenesis was recently proposed by Best and Rentsch.[96] They asserted that the primary insult consists of a congenital defect in the development of the retinal vascular system. They reported a case in which the initial fundus findings included what appeared to be a vessel-free zone, ie, an extensive hypoplasia of the peripheral retinal arterial system (analogous to the immature peripheral retinal vessels associated with retinopathy of prematurity). This phenomenon, also observed by other authors and by fluorescein angiography, has also been described as an obliterative endarteritis. The pseudoglioma probably results from the hypoxic

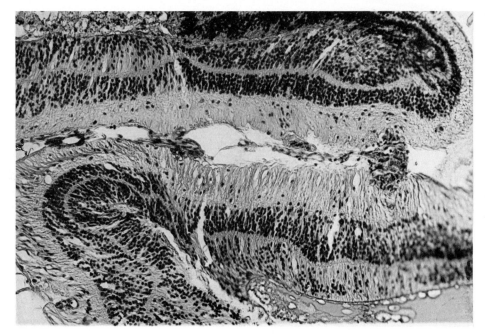

FIG. 17.28. Incontinentia pigmenti. Proliferation of glomeruloid buds of new-formed vascular endothelium between folds of retina. It is probable that the retinal folds and pseudorosettes represented secondary changes due to the proliferative process rather than a primary retinal dysplasia. (From Best and Rentsch: Klin Monatsbl Augenheilkd 164:19, 1974)

stimulus induced by the arterial insufficiency, in a fashion totally analogous to that seen in retrolental fibroplasia when the oxygen is withdrawn and a state of relative hypoxia is induced. As with many neovascular retinopathies (eg, in diabetes and sickle cell disease), the proliferative process may largely be a nonspecific response to oxygen insufficiency. The histopathologic appearance, consisting of proliferation of buds of new-formed vascular endothelium and eventual preretinal neovascularization and proliferative retinopathy is similar in both diseases (Figs. 17.28, 17.29). These changes, incidentally, are similar to those Apple and associates[86] found in Norrie's disease, and the pathogenesis of this disease may also relate to a primary defect in development of the retina and/or retinal vessels.

In a more recent study, Watzke et al[101] also observed vascular anomalies. Of 19 patients with incontinentia pigmenti, 7 had a bizarre retinal anomaly that consisted of a zone of abnormal arteriovenous connections and preretinal fibrotic tissue at the temporal equator, with no perfusion peripheral to it. These authors postulate that the retinal lesion may represent an early stage of the pseudoglioma.

Best and Rentsch found no evidence to support the theories that inflammation or PHPV plays a role in the pathogenesis of incontinentia pigmenti. The formation of retinal rosettes and pigment epithelial plaques in incontinentia pigmenti is probably secondary to the proliferative neovascular process and does not represent a primary retinal dysplasia. The atrophy and elongation of the ciliary processes produced by traction from the proliferative retrolental fibrovascular mass may resemble

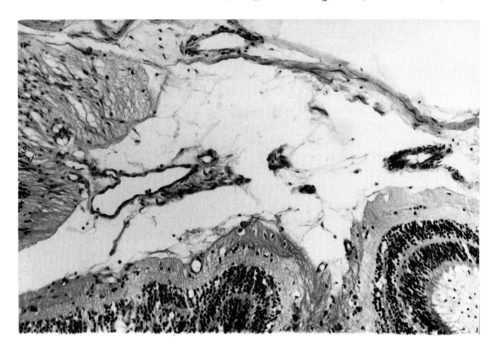

FIG. 17.29. Incontinentia pigmenti. Peripheral retina below with preretinal neovascularization and formation of a fibrovascular membrane. (From Best and Rentsch: Klin Monatsbl Augenheilkd 164:19, 1974)

that seen in PHPV and retrolental fibroplasia. The massive retinal detachment that occurs in full-blown cases can also be easily explained by the preretinal proliferative process.

X-Linked (Juvenile) Retinoschisis

X-linked juvenile retinoschisis (congenital vascular veils in the vitreous) is a condition in which ophthalmologic evidence of the disease is usually present at birth.[102] The clinical appearance is usually readily differentiated from retinoblastoma, but occasional cases have been reported in which leukocoria is a prominent feature. The fovea is almost always involved; therefore, this disease is a potential source of significant visual loss. This loss may occur in either of two ways: either the inner layer of the retinoschisis comes to lie immediately behind the lens, producing the white reflex, or, rarely, a retinal detachment ensues. The expression of the gene is often low, so that the multiple signs characteristic of the disease are seen in only a small percentage of cases.

The presence of foveal retinoschisis, which is typically bilateral and symmetric, is pathognomonic. Ophthalmoscopically, foveal retinoschisis consists of an optically empty zone from which radial, spoke-like folds may emanate. Actual vitreous veils and cysts appear in fewer than 50 percent of cases. The veils representing the inner layer of the retina (Fig. 17.30) may or may not contain vessels; they are translucent and are sometimes perforated with one or more lacunae. A common complication of this disease is hemorrhage into the vitreous from ruptured retinal vessels (usually venules) in the areas of retinoschisis. However, true retinal detachment is rarely a complication. Visual acuity can remain normal for a long period, but there is gradual diminution of vision with increasing age. As with other forms of schisis, a complete and sharply delimited scotoma corresponds to the outlines of the split region. The electroretinographic response is diminished but not extinguished. Chorioretinal atrophy and macular degeneration lead to decreased visual acuity; however, complete blindness is rare.

Histopathologically, the plane of cleavage in the retina is at the level of the nerve fiber layer.[103, 104] The veils that float in the vitreous actually form from the inner stratum of the split retina. This thin membrane extends internally into the vitreous due to traction exerted by the posterior vitreous. Therefore, the inner stratum of the schisis cavity is composed of the internal limiting membrane and

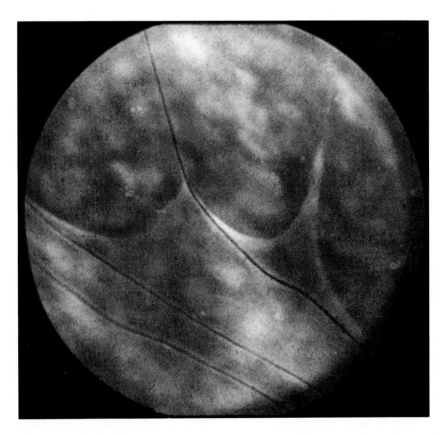

FIG. 17.30. X-linked juvenile retinoschisis. The inner schisis wall is displaced in a vitreal direction, forming so-called vascular veils within the vitreous. The plane of cleavage is at the level of the nerve fiber layer. (From Apple and Rabb: Clinicopathologic Correlation of Ocular Disease, 1974. Courtesy of CV Mosby)

immediately adjacent fragments of retinal neural and glial tissue. This plane of cleavage differs from that observed in simple peripheral cystoid degeneration of the Blessig-Iwanoff type and from that seen in senile retinoschisis. In the latter conditions, the plane of cleavage is in the outer plexiform layer.

PRENATAL AND INFANTILE TRAUMA, ORGANIZING VITREOUS HEMORRHAGE, AND MASSIVE RETINAL GLIOSIS

Kogan and Boniuk[9] have determined that trauma accounted for 50 percent of enucleations from children less than 15 years of age and was the most frequent cause for eye removal in children 3 years of age or older. Therefore, trauma can be considered one of the most important causes of pseudoglioma; it is particularly important in the differential diagnosis when a definite history of trauma is not available, as is the case with most prenatal trauma or with an unreliable history.

Howard and Ellsworth,[2] in their series of 265 patients, observed 9 in whom an organizing vitreous hemorrhage was encountered that mimicked retinoblastoma. As the large vitreous hemorrhage undergoes organization, it may assume a yellow-white color and produce leukocoria. This result can follow either trauma or hemorrhagic disease of the newborn. Indirect ophthalmoscopy can localize the lesion within the vitreous cavity, often in an inferior position, and confusion with retinoblastoma should not occur.

Friedenwald,[105] in 1926, coined the term "massive gliosis of the retina." Such cases are characterized by massive fibroglial proliferation within the retina and vitreous to such an extent that the lesion resembles a neoplasm (Fig. 17.31). Reese[106] reported a similar series of cases in which the eyes were characterized by a protrusion of a gray-white mass from the retina; it primarily occurred in young individuals due to the organization of hemorrhage at birth or trauma after birth. He first emphasized that the picture resembles a retinoblastoma and must be differentiated from it. Moreover, following hemorrhage in either the newborn or infant, there is contracture of fibrous tissue, and more and more retina is pulled into the lesion, giving it the appearance of progressing, thereby leading all the more to the suspicion of a retinoblastoma.

In a review of 38 cases of massive gliosis of the retina at the Armed Forces Institute of Pathology,[107] it was shown that the lesion configuration of massive retinal fibrosis varied from rather obviously reactive proliferations to growths that appeared neoplastic (Fig. 17.31). It was also shown that massive gliosis occurs not only in conjunction with prenatal and infantile trauma and hemorrhage, but also occasionally in relation to congenital malformations, chronic inflammatory processes, and vascular disorders such as Coats' syndrome. It was emphasized that one problem in the differential diagnosis of retinoblastoma from massive retinal gliosis is the fact that both diseases undergo calcification and that x-ray differentiation is of no benefit (Fig. 17.32). However, the calcification seen in massive retinal gliosis usually occurs in later stages and, therefore, in an older age group than does retinoblastoma. Therefore, the two main features assisting in the distinction from

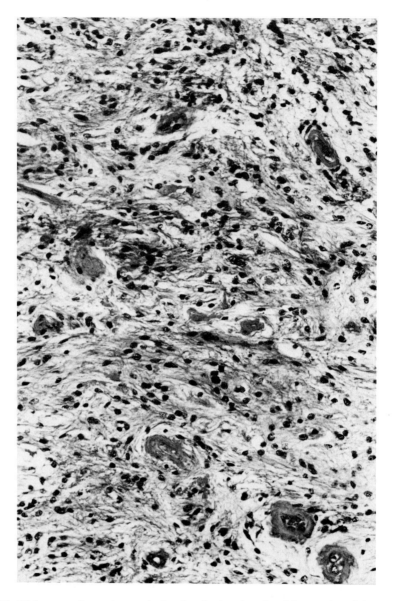

FIG. 17.31. High-power photomicrograph showing the interior of a globe enucleated from a child with massive hemorrhage of the newborn and massive retinal gliosis. The reactive fibrosis is so extensive that it resembles a neoplastic growth (glioma). H&E, ×250.

retinoblastoma are a history of trauma or other antecedent disease and the fact that massive gliosis is more commonly manifest in young adulthood rather than in infancy and childhood, as is retinoblastoma. Occasionally the differentiation of a posttraumatic phthisis bulbi with massive retinal gliosis from a spontaneously regressed retinoblastoma[108] may be clinically difficult.

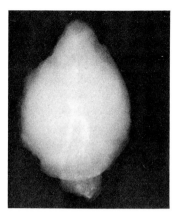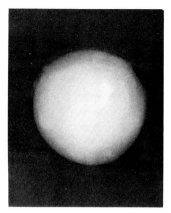

FIG. 17.32. Postenucleation x-ray films of globes filled with a large, calcified retinoblastoma. Globes with massive retinal gliosis may also exhibit calcification, but usually in an older age group than is seen with retinoblastoma. (Courtesy of Prof. G.O.H. Naumann)

NEOPLASTIC AND PROLIFERATIVE LESIONS

Medulloepithelioma

In 1908 Fuchs coined the term "diktyoma" to describe a group of ciliary body tumors occurring in infancy and childhood (cited by Zimmerman[109]). He chose this term because the microscopic arrangement of the tumor cells was such that interlacing rows of cords of epithelial cells created the appearance of a lacework or network (Greek *diktyon*, net). This term is unsatisfactory, and tumors of this type are best classified as neuroepithelial tumors of the ciliary body, medulloepithelioma subtype.

The most satisfactory classification of neuroepithelial tumors of the ciliary body was proposed by Zimmerman[109] (Table 17.8). The tumor appearing in the pediatric age group, formerly called the diktyoma, is designated the medulloepithelioma. (These tumors are described in detail in Chapter 21.) The prefix *medullo* signifies an origin from cells resembling the medullary epithelium that lines the neural tube. This is the same cell line that, following evagination from the brain, forms the primitive bilayered optic cup during normal ocular development.

The medulloepithelioma consists of two cellular components—the epithelial and the stromal (Fig. 17.33). Rows of epithelial cells are arranged in convoluted patterns of various sizes and shapes. Sometimes the cells are arranged in cords or in a circular pattern around a lumen, forming a rosette-like structure or a structure that resembles an embryonic neural tube. Similar to most other epithelial neoplasms, the medulloepithelioma forms a tumor stroma. Occasionally, the stroma is quite extensive and sometimes forms the bulk of the mass. The stromal component consists of loose, delicate fibrils that strongly resemble embryonic mesenchyme or myxoid tissue. This component of the tumor represents an attempt by the growth to form embryonic vitreous.

The teratoid medulloepithelioma (Table 17.8) exhibits epithelial and stromal

Table 17.8

Neuroepithelial Tumors of the Ciliary Body*

Congenital
  Glioneuroma
  Medulloepithelioma
    Benign
    Malignant
  Teratoid medulloepithelioma
    Benign
    Malignant

Acquired
  Pseudoadenomatous hyperplasia
  Adenoma
    Solid
    Papillary
    Pleomorphic
  Adenocarcinoma
    Solid
    Papillary
    Pleomorphic

From Zimmerman LE: Am J Ophthalmol 72:1039, 1971.

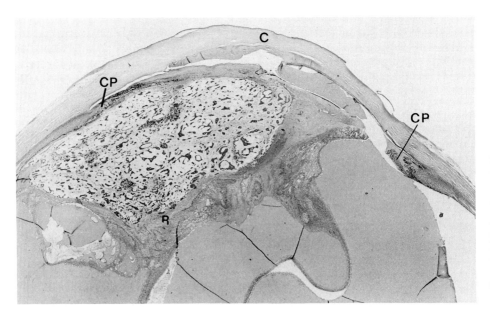

FIG. 17.33. Medulloepithelioma of the ciliary body in a child. The tumor mass (area showing honeycomb pattern) may induce a leukocoria and mimic a retinoblastoma. The tumor is composed of cords of deeply staining epithelium and a loose background stroma. Cornea (C), ciliary processes (CP), and totally detached retina (R) adherent to posterior aspect of tumor are indicated. H&E, ×10. (From Apple and Rabb: Clinicopathologic Correlation of Ocular Disease, 1974. Courtesy of CV Mosby)

growth identical to that of the simple medulloepithelioma. However, a teratoid medulloepithelioma is further distinguished by the presence of one or more heteroplastic elements (abnormally positioned tissues that are not normally present in the globe, or cells that one would not generally expect to form from the optic anlage) in addition to the simple epithelial and stromal components. The most frequently observed heteroplastic element formed by this tumor is hyaline cartilage. This tumor, therefore, shares with trisomy 13 the finding of cartilage within the ciliary body. Cartilage formed within the ciliary body coloboma in trisomy 13 represents an example of a dysplastic growth; the cartilage seen within a teratoid medulloepithelioma is directly formed from the neoplasm. Other heteroplastic elements occasionally seen in a medulloepithelioma are brain tissue and rhabdomyoblastic cells. In rare instances, the rhabdomyoblastic component may predominate, and the microscopic pattern is that of a rhabdomyosarcoma.

Most medulloepitheliomas are relatively benign or are only locally invasive. Even when malignant differentiation occurs, metastasis to distant organs is unusual.

Miscellaneous Proliferative Lesions, Hamartomas, and Choristomas of the Fundus

Solitary fundus lesions may occasionally mimic retinoblastoma. In many instances these lesions occur as a component of the various phakomatoses. As noted previously, the phakomatoses (Greek *phako*, birthmark) comprise a group of diseases characterized by formation of lesions affecting the skin, the eye, the central nervous system, and the viscera. Certain combinations of lesions reappear in families with sufficient consistency to allow categorization of the various symptoms and sign complexes into specific syndromes. The four major phakomatoses are von Hippel-Lindau angiomatosis, tuberous sclerosis, neurofibromatosis (von Recklinghausen's disease), and the Sturge-Weber syndrome.

Although the various neuroglial and angiomatous fundus lesions seen in these syndromes may simulate retinoblastoma, the diagnosis is usually readily confirmed by adequate history, physical examination, and documentation of growth or lack of growth. Font and Ferry[57] and Apple and Rabb[3] provide more detailed descriptions of the phakomatoses.

ACKNOWLEDGMENT

Portions of the manuscript were prepared during a period of sabbatical research in collaboration with Prof. Dr. med. G. O. H. Naumann at the Universitäts Augenklinik, Tübingen, West Germany. Irena Suvaizdis assisted in preparation of the photographs and Rita J. Toohey typed the manuscript.

REFERENCES

1. Sarin LK, Shields JA: Differential diagnosis of leukocoria. In Harley RD (ed): Pediatric Ophthalmology. Philadelphia, Saunders, 1975
2. Howard GM, Ellsworth RM: Differential diagnosis of retinoblastoma. Am J Ophthalmol 60:610, 1965
3. Apple DJ, Rabb MF: Clinicopathologic Correlation of Ocular Disease. St. Louis, Mosby, 1974
4. Collins ET: Pseudoglioma. Lond Ophthalmol Hosp Rep 13:361, 1892
5. Ts'o MOM, Zimmerman LE, Fine BS: The nature of retinoblastoma: I. Photoreceptor differentiation; a clinical and histopathological study. Am J Ophthalmol 69:339, 1970
6. Ts'o MOM, Fine BS, Zimmerman LE: The nature of retinoblastoma: II. Photoreceptor differentiation; an electron microscopic study. Am J Ophthalmol 69:350, 1970
7. Sanders TE: Pseudoglioma. Trans Am Ophthalmol Soc 48:575, 1950
8. Duke J: Pseudoglioma in children. South Med J 51:754, 1958
9. Kogan L, Boniuk M: Causes of enucleation in childhood with special reference to pseudogliomas and unsuspected retinoblastomas. Int Ophthalmol Clin 2:507, 1962
10. Naumann GOH: Intraoculare tumoren beim Kinde. In: Bericht über die 69 Zusammenkunft der Deutschen Ophthalmologischen Gesellschaft in Heidelberg 1968. Munich, Bergman, 1969, p 12
11. Naumann GOH, Lommatzsch P: Tumoren der Augen und Augenhöhle. In Opitz H, Schmid F (eds): Handbuch der Kinderheilkunde: Tumoren in Kindesalter, vol 8, pt 2. Berlin, Springer, 1972, p 350
12. Swartz M, Herbst R, Goldberg MF: Aqueous humor lactic acid dehydrogenase in retinoblastoma. Am J Ophthalmol 78:612, 1974
13. Spaulding AG: Persistent hyperplastic primary vitreous humor: a finding in a 71-year-old man. Surv Ophthalmol 12:448, 1967
14. Spaulding AG, Naumann GOH: Persistent hyperplastic primary vitreous in an adult. Arch Ophthalmol 77:666, 1967
15. Bach L, Seefelder R: Atlas zur Entwicklungsgeschichte des Menschlichen Auges. Leipzig, Engelmann, 1914
16. Barber AN: Embryology of the Human Eye. St. Louis, Mosby, 1955
17. Mann I: The Development of the Human Eye. London, Butler and Tanner, 1964
18. Duke-Elder S, Cooke C: Normal and abnormal development: embryology. In Duke-Elder S (ed): System of Ophthalmology, vol 3, pt 1. St. Louis, Mosby, 1963
19. Cairns JE: Normal development of the hyaloid and retinal vessel in the rat. Br J Ophthalmol 43:485, 1959
20. Gloor BP: Zur Entwicklung des Glaskorpers und der Zonula, I und II. Albrecht von Graefes Arch Klin Exp Ophthalmol 186:299, 1973
21. Braekevelt CR, Hollenberg MJ: Comparative electron microscopic study development of hyaloid and retinal capillaries in albino rats. Am J Ophthalmol 69:1032, 1970
22. Mann IC: The relations of the hyaloid canal in the foetus and in the adult. J Anat 62:290, 1928
23. Hamming NA, Apple DJ, Gieser DK, Vygantas CM: Ultrastructure of the hyaloid vasculature in primates, in press
24. Hamming NA, Apple DJ, Gieser DK, Vygantas CM: Developmental anatomy of the sheath of the hyaloid artery in primates: Special reference to the developing vitreous and its relation to Cloquet's canal. Submitted for publication
25. Mittendorf WF: On the frequency of posterior capsular opacities at the place of attachment of the hyaloid artery. Trans Am Ophthalmol Soc 6:413, 1892
26. Mittendorf WF: Punctate or hyaline opacities of the posterior lens capsule. Ophthalmol Record 15:489, 1906

27. Reese AB: Persistent hyperplastic primary vitreous. Am J Ophthalmol 40:317, 1955
28. Font RL, Yanoff M, Zimmerman L: Intraocular adipose tissue and persistent hyperplastic primary vitreous. Arch Ophthalmol 82:43, 1969
29. Acers TE, Coston TO: Persistent hyperplastic primary vitreous. Am J Ophthalmol 63:734, 1967
30. Gass JDM: Surgical excision of persistent hyperplastic primary vitreous. Arch Ophthalmol 82:163, 1970
31. Van Selm J: Surgery for retinal dysplasia and hyperplasia of the persistent primary vitreous. Trans Ophthalmol Soc UK 89:545, 1970
32. Smith RE, Maumenee AE: Persistent hyperplastic primary vitreous: results of surgery. Trans Am Acad Ophthalmol Otolaryngol 78:OP911, 1974
33. Peyman GA, Sanders DR, Nagpal KC: Management of persistent hyperplastic primary vitreous by pars plana vitrectomy. Br J Ophthalmol 11:756, 1976
34. Manschot WA: Persistent hyperplastic primary vitreous. Arch Ophthalmol 59:188, 1958
35. Wolter JR, Flaherty NW: Persistent hyperplastic vitreous. Am J Ophthalmol 47:491, 1959
36. Francois J: Prepapillary cyst developed from remnants of the hyaloid artery. Br J Ophthalmol 34:365, 1950
37. Tower P: Congenital prepapillary cyst. Arch Ophthalmol 48:433, 1952
38. Bisland T: Vascular loops in the vitreous. Arch Ophthalmol 49:514, 1953
39. Petersen HP: Persistence of the Bergmeister papilla with glial overgrowth. Acta Ophthalmol 46:430, 1968
40. Pruett RC, Schepens CL: Posterior hyperplastic primary vitreous. Am J Ophthalmol 69:534, 1970
41. Hamada S, Ellsworth RM: Congenital retinal detachment and the optic disc anomaly. Am J Ophthalmol 71:460, 1971
42. Blodi FC: Preretinal glial nodules in persistence and hyperplasia of primary vitreous. Arch Ophthalmol 87:531, 1972
43. Joseph M, Ivry M, Oliver M: Persistent hyperplastic primary vitreous at the optic nerve head. Am J Ophthalmol 73:580, 1973
44. Bullock JD: Developmental vitreous cysts. Arch Ophthalmol 91:83, 1974
45. Mann IC: A case of congenital abnormality of the retina. Trans Ophthalmol Soc UK 48:383, 1928
46. Mann IC: Congenital retinal fold. Br J Ophthalmol 19:641, 1935
47. Mann IC: Developmental Abnormalities of the Eye, 2nd ed. London, British Medical Society, 1967
48. Warburg M: Norrie's disease and falciform detachment of the retina. In Goldberg MF (ed): Genetic Diseases in Ophthalmology. Boston, Little, Brown, 1974, p 430
49. Weve H: Über "Ablatio falciformis cong." Arch Augenheilkd 109:371, 1936
50. Weve H: Congenital aphakia with hyaloid artery and retinal fold. Ophthalmologica 97:7908, 1939
51. Coats G: Forms of retinal disease with massive exudation. R Lond Ophthalmol Hosp Rep 17:440, 1908
52. Reese AB: Telangiectasia of the retina and Coats' disease. Am J Ophthalmol 42:1, 1956
53. Tripathi R, Ashton N: Electron microscopical study of Coats' disease. Br J Ophthalmol 55:289, 1971
54. Gieser DK, Apple DJ, Goldberg MF: Pathologic findings of adult Coats' syndrome. Read before the Central Section of the Association for Research in Vision and Ophthalmology, Milwaukee, Wisc, 1973
55. Archer DB: Leber's miliary aneurysms. Ophthalmol Dig 33:8, 1971
56. Wise GN, Dollery CT, Henkind P: The Retinal Circulation. New York, Harper & Row, 1971
57. Font RL, Ferry AP: The phakomatoses. Int Ophthalmol Clin 12:1, 1972

58. Goldberg MF, Duke JR: Von Hippel-Lindau disease: histopathologic findings in a treated and an untreated eye. Am J Ophthalmol 66:693, 1968
59. Apple DJ, Goldberg MF, Wyhinny GJ: Treatment of von Hippel-Lindau disease by argon laser photocoagulation: II. Histopathologic evaluation of treated angiomata. Arch Ophthalmol 92:126, 1974
60. Terry TL: Extreme prematurity and fibroblastic overgrowth of persistent vascular sheath behind each crystalline lens: I. Preliminary report. Am J Ophthalmol 25:203, 1942
61. Reese AB, Blodi FC: Retrolental fibroplasia. In: Acta XVI Concilium Ophthalmologicum Britannia 1950. London, British Medical Association, 1951, p 445
62. Reese AB: Retrolental fibroplasia. Am J Ophthalmol 34:1, 1951
63. Reese AB, King MJ, Owens WC: A classification of retrolental fibroplasia. Am J Ophthalmol 36:1333, 1953
64. Ashton N, Ward B, Serpell G: Role of oxygen in the genesis of retrolental fibroplasia: a preliminary report. Br J Ophthalmol 37:513, 1953
65. Patz A: Oxygen studies in retrolental hyperplasia: IV. Clinical and experimental observations. Am J Ophthalmol 38:291, 1954
66. Owens WC, Friedenwald JA, Silverman WA, et al: Symposium: retrolental fibroplasia (retinopathy of prematurity). Trans Am Acad Ophthalmol Otolaryngol 59:7, 1955
67. Patz A: Retrolental fibroplasia. Trans Am Ophthalmol Soc 66:940, 1968
68. Beaver PC, Snyder CH, Correra GM, Dent JG, Lafferty JW: Chronic eosinophilia due to visceral larva migrans: report of three cases. Pediatrics 9:7, 1952
69. Zinkham WH: Visceral larva migrans due to Toxocara as a cause of eosinophilia. Johns Hopkins Med J 123:41, 1968
70. Wilkinson CP, Welsh RB: Intraocular Toxocara. Am J Ophthalmol 71:921, 1971
71. Wilder HC: Nematode endophthalmitis. Trans Am Acad Ophthalmol Otolaryngol 55:99, 1950
72. Duguid IM: Chronic endophthalmitis due to Toxocara. Br J Ophthalmol 45:705, 1961
73. Duguid IM: Features of ocular infestation by Toxocara. Br J Ophthalmol 45:789, 1961
74. Rey A: Nematode endophthalmitis due to Toxocara. Br J Ophthalmol 46:616, 1962
75. Brown DH: Ocular Toxocara canis. J Pediatr Ophthalmol 7:182, 1970
76. Ashton N: Larval granulomatosis of the retina due to Toxocara. Br J Ophthalmol 44:129, 1960
77. Irvine WC, Irvine AR Jr: Nematode endophthalmitis: Toxo cara canis: report of one case. Am J Ophthalmol 47:185, 1959
78. Welsh RB, Maumenee AE, Wahlen HE: Peripheral posterior segment inflammation, vitreous opacities, and edema of the posterior pole: pars planitis. Arch Ophthalmol 64:540, 1960
79. Reese AB, Blodi FC: Retinal dysplasia. Am J Ophthalmol 33:23, 1950
80. Reese AB, Straatsma BR: Retinal dysplasia. Arch Ophthalmol 45:199, 1958
81. Hunter WS, Zimmerman LE: Unilateral retinal dysplasia. Arch Ophthalmol 74:23, 1965
82. Holmes LB: Norrie's disease: an X-linked syndrome of retinal malformation, mental retardation and deafness. N Engl J Med 284:367, 1971
83. Fradlin AH: Norrie's disease: congenital progressive oculo-acoustico-cerebral degeneration. Am J Ophthalmol 72:947, 1971
84. Brini A, Sacrez P, Levy JP: Maladie de Norrie. Ann Oculist 205:1, 1972
85. Townes P, Roca PD: Norrie's disease (hereditary oculo-acoustic-cerebral degeneration): report of a United States family. Am J Ophthalmol 76:797, 1973
86. Apple DJ, Fishman GA, Goldberg MF: Ocular histopathology of Norrie's disease. Am J Ophthalmol 78:196, 1974

87. Apple DJ: Chromosome induced ocular disease. In Goldberg MF (ed): Genetic Diseases in Ophthalmology. Boston, Little, Brown, 1974, p 257
88. Bloch B: Eigentümliche bisher nicht beschriebene Pigmentaffektion. Schweiz Med Wochenschr 56:404, 1926
89. Sulzberger MB: Über eine bisher nicht beschriebene congenitale Pigment anomalie (Incontinentia pigmenti). Arch Dermatol Syphilol 154:19, 1928
90. Sulzberger MB: Incontinentia pigmenti (Bloch-Sulzberger). Arch Dermatol Syphilol 38:57, 1938
91. Lenz W: Zur Genetik der Incontinentia pigmenti. Ann Paediatr 196:149, 1961
92. Lever WF: Histopathology of the Skin, 4th ed. Philadelphia, Lippincott, 1967
93. McCrary JA, Smith JL: Conjunctival and retinal incontinentia pigmenti. Arch Ophthalmol 79:417, 1968
94. Scott JG, Friedmann AI, Chitters M, Pepler WJ: Ocular changes in the Bloch-Sulzberger syndrome (incontinentia pigmenti). Br J Ophthalmol 39:276, 1955
95. Wollensak J: Charakteristische Augenbefunde beim Syndroma Bloch-Sulzberger Incontinentia pigmenti). Klin Monatsbl Augenheilkd 134:692, 1959
96. Best W, Rentsch F: Über das "Pseudogliom" bei der Incontinentia pigmenti. Klin Monatsbl Augenheilkd 164:19, 1974
97. Miller RJ, Anderson RE: A retrolental mass in incontinentia pigmenti. Surv Ophthalmol 11:41, 1966
98. Benedikt O, Ehalt H: Familär auftretendes Bloch-Sulzberger-Syndrom (Incontinentia pigmenti) mit Augenbeteiligung. Klin Monatsbl Augenheilkd 157:652, 1970
99. Findlay GH: On the pathogenesis of incontinentia pigmenti. Br J Dermatol 64:141, 1952
100. Cole JG, Cole HG: Incontinentia pigmenti. Am J Ophthalmol 47:321, 1959
101. Watzke RC, Stevens TS, Carney RG: Retinal vascular changes of incontinentia pigmenti. Arch Ophthalmol 94:743, 1976
102. Deutman AF: The Hereditary Dystrophies of the Posterior Pole of the Eye. Springfield, Ill, Thomas, 1971
103. Yanoff M, Kertesz E, Zimmerman LE: Histopathology of juvenile retinoschisis. Arch Ophthalmol 79:49, 1968
104. Zimmerman LE, Naumann G: Pathology of retinoschisis. In McPherson A (ed): Transactions of the International Symposium on New and Controversial Aspects of Retinal Detachment. St. Louis, Mosby, 1968, p 400
105. Friedenwald JS: Massive gliosis of the retina. In: Contributions of Ophthalmic Science: Dedicated to Dr. Edward Jackson. Menasha, Wisc, Banta, 1926, p 23
106. Reese AB: Massive retinal fibrosis in children. Am J Ophthalmol 19:576, 1936
107. Yanoff M, Davis RL, Zimmerman LE: Massive gliosis of the retina. Int Ophthalmol Clin 11:211, 1971
108. Boniuk M, Zimmerman LE: Spontaneous regression of retinoblastoma. Int Ophthalmol Clin 2:525, 1962
109. Zimmerman LE: Verhoeff's "terato-neuroma": a critical reappraisal in light of new observations and current concepts of embryonic tumors. Am J Ophthalmol 72:1039, 1971

Delia N. Sang
Daniel M. Albert

18 Recent Advances in the Study of Retinoblastoma

Retinoblastoma was until the late nineteenth century a uniformly fatal neoplasm of childhood. The recommendations of the Scottish surgeon James Wardrop in 1809[1] (Figs. 18.1–18.3) to treat this disease with early enucleation became widely accepted with the practice of chloroform and ether general anesthesia in the 1840s. As von Helmholtz's ophthalmoscope, which was introduced in 1851, became extensively used, tumors were diagnosed at an earlier age. Von Graefe's cautions to excise a long segment of optic nerve[2] and Hilgartner's[3] application of radiation therapy to retinoblastoma in 1903 resulted in an increasing number of cured patients.[4] More sophisticated advances in diagnosis and therapy, such as Reese's classification of retinoblastoma and the institution of protocol therapy,[5] and Kupfer's initiation to the use of chemotherapy in addition to radiotherapy[6] contributed to the progressive decrease in mortality. Current survival rates have been improved from the 5 percent reported in 1869[4] to recent figures of at least 80 percent in most series,[7] and up to 90 percent or more in favorable cases.[8, 9]

Retinoblastoma remains the most common intraocular tumor of childhood and the second most common primary intraocular tumor in any age group. This tumor is responsible for approximately 1 percent of all deaths from cancer in the age group of newborns to 15 years.[10] Because of the high incidence of spontaneous regression, the high incidence of second primary tumors, the unusual mode of inheritance, and the epidemiologic and biochemical characteristics of retinoblastoma, this disease may serve as a model for other neoplasms in terms of its immunopathology, genetics, and possible viral oncogenesis. The modalities of treatment of retinoblastoma, at present, are effective in saving lives and, through the efforts of Reese, Ellsworth and others, offers an increased chance of preserving vision. Unfortunately, these methods, as with all cancer therapy at the present time, remain destructive to normal as well as neoplastic cells. The determination of the basic processes governing the cause and pathogenesis of retinoblastoma, and elucidation of the immunologic response of the host to this tumor, will hopefully serve as a basis for the development of a specific tumor-directed therapy of cancer.

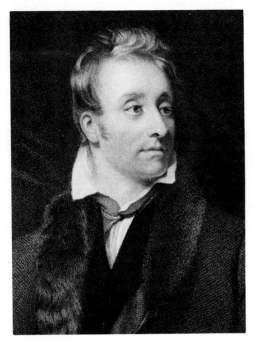

FIG. 18.1. James Wardrop (1738–1830), Scottish surgeon who first described retinoblastoma as a distinct entity and advised enucleation as a method of attempting a cure.

FIG. 18.2. Wardrop's illustration showing typical appearance of child with retinoblastoma in the preophthalmoscopic era. (From Wardrop: Observations on Fungus Haematodes, 1809. Courtesy of Constable)

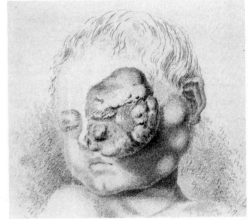

GENERAL CONSIDERATIONS

Epidemiology

The frequency of occurrence of retinoblastoma has been estimated in the past as 1:17,000 to 1:34,000 live births.[11] Of extreme concern is the marked rise in frequency over the past 30 to 40 years:[12-15] Hemmes[13] and Schappert-Kimmijser et al[14] reported studies in Holland reflecting an incidence of 1:34,000 in 1927 to 1929, rising to an incidence of 1:15,000 in the same population in the period 1952 to 1955. Tarkkanen et al,[15] in their series, documented a marked rise in Finland, with incidences of 1:82,000 from 1912 to 1919, 1:30,000 from 1935 to 1939, and finally

1:16,000 from 1960 to 1964. The reasons for these trends have been interpreted to be multifactorial: they include the decrease in mortality rate and the subsequent increase in numbers of progeny. These factors alone, however, do not fully account for this increase. Other considerations include a cumulative progressive exposure to nonspecific ambient radiation as well as other possible exogenous influences which may result in a greater spontaneous mutation rate both in the general population and in a particularly susceptible subgroup.

The average age of diagnosis has been in the range of 18 months in most past reports.[11] More recently there has been evidence that the mean age of diagnosis for the hereditary group, which is characteristically bilateral, is earlier[16] (ie, at approximately 12 to 14 months of age) than that for the sporadic group, which is usually unilateral (at approximately 24 to 30 months of age).[17, 18] At large referral centers, there is early diagnosis made in the group of patients followed closely and diagnosed early while asymptomatic because of a previously known positive family history. A number of case reports of spontaneously regressed lesions have documented the diagnosis of retinoblastoma in the older age groups;[19-21] we assume that the actual occurrence was much earlier than the time of diagnosis.

There has been either no sex predilection in past series[7] or a slight male preponderance.[8, 22] Jensen and Miller,[7] in their epidemiologic review of 269 deaths

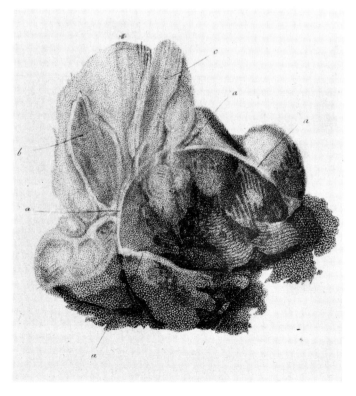

FIG. 18.3. One of Wardrop's dissections. He concluded that the tumor arose from the retina. (From Wardrop: Observations on Fungus Haematodes, 1809. Courtesy of Constable)

secondary to retinoblastoma, discovered a peak in mortality at 2 to 3 years of age which was 2½ times greater in blacks than in whites. Newell et al[23] found that more than 50 percent of whites with the disease were diagnosed at less than 2 years of age, while less than 25 percent of blacks were diagnosed in the same age group. From these data, it appears that the higher mortality rate among blacks is at least in large part due to delayed diagnosis and delayed treatment. The clinical impression that case clustering occurs has been noted,[24] with large differences in incidence based on geographic location, possible racial predilection, or other uncharacterized local factors, eg, the high number of new cases of retinoblastoma seen in Haiti (Fig. 18.4) where the estimated frequency is as high as 1:3300 live births and the estimated incidence rate is 11:100,000.[25] Various other reports in the literature have documented a higher incidence of retinoblastoma in some black populations: Kodilinye[26] found 1:192 patients in Nigeria over a 2½-year period; Bras et al[27] found an annual incidence of 24:100,000 in Jamaica in the 0–4-year age group; and Macklin[28] has found a higher mutation rate for retinoblastoma in blacks versus whites in Ohio.

Genetics

The genetic factors in retinoblastoma have been extensively reported and detailed reviews are available.[29, 30] The heritable form of retinoblastoma appears to involve a single rare autosomal dominant gene of high but incomplete penetrance that has been estimated to be 60 to 95 percent by some authors,[5, 31] and as low as 20 percent by others.[28] This picture of incomplete penetrance may be further clini-

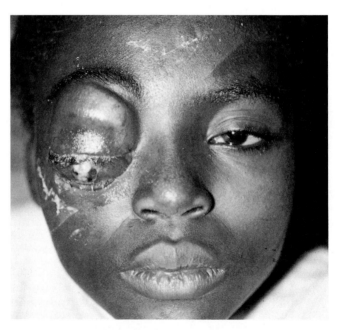

FIG. 18.4. Retinoblastoma with orbital invasion in a Haitian child.

cally complicated by gonadal mosaicism in a parent. Approximately 20 to 30 percent of cases overall have been estimated to be bilateral,[5, 11, 30, 32, 33] with bilaterality occurring in 58 to 65 percent of the hereditary group and 15 to 32 percent of the sporadic nonhereditary group.[28, 33] Thirty-five to 45 percent of cases are estimated to be hereditary, and 55 to 65 percent nonhereditary. Twenty-five to 30 percent of cases are bilateral and hereditary; 70 to 75 percent of cases are unilateral.[30] An estimated 5 to 10 percent of the unilaterals may also be hereditary but characterized by incompletely expressed germinal mutations for bilateral retinoblastoma.[34] Knudson[30] hypothesizes that this is a cancer caused by two mutational events: in the hereditary or prezygotic form, the first mutation is germinal and the second is somatic; in the sporadic (nonhereditary) or postzygotic form, both mutations are somatic. Each of these mutations is estimated to occur at an approximately equivalent rate of about 2×10^{-7} per year or 2.3 to 5×10^{-5} per generation,[30, 35] an unusually high mutation rate.

The unilateral sporadic case of retinoblastoma has low heritability with 4 to 9 percent of offspring affected;[14, 34, 36] the bilateral "sporadic" case will have approximately 50 percent affected.[11] In some series, hereditary retinoblastoma is detected up to one year earlier than the nonhereditary type, and the distribution of the ages at which the two forms are first diagnosed and first present corresponds well to Knudson's "two-hit" hypothesis. In these instances, the hereditary cases would only require one somatic mutation, ie, most likely one postnatal event, rather than two, and thereby would exhibit tumor involvement earlier.

Clinically it may be difficult to distinguish multicentric foci of origin from areas of seeding; 84 percent of tumors in one series were estimated to be multicentric.[11] By the two-mutation hypothesis, the prezygotic group would have a predisposition for primaries within the same organ in addition to second primaries in other organ systems.[17] The explanation for this is that all cells would be affected by the germinal event except for those cases with mosaicism. The probability that a carrier of the retinoblastoma gene will develop at least one retinal tumor is calculated at approximately 0.95; the probability that a non-gene carrier will develop at least one retinal tumor is estimated at 1:30,000. By Knudson's application of the Poisson distribution, the mean number of tumors in the hereditary case in either one or both eyes per individual is three to four, and the likelihood of a patient with unilateral nonheritable retinoblastoma developing a second focus is exceedingly small. The mean number of tumors per genetically susceptible individual has been developed as a function of age, with the change in the mean number of tumors with time interpreted in terms of the maturation and development of retinal cells.[37] These speculations need confirmation with clinicohistopathologic correlation.

Second Tumors

According to the chromosomal theory of carcinogenesis, chromosomal aberration may be the etiology of generalized vulnerability of various tissues of the body to exogenous as well as endogenous carcinogenic factors.[38] Approximately one percent[7] of patients with malignancies in the age group 0–19 years develop another primary tumor elsewhere, and approximately 15 percent of all deaths in retinoblastoma in one series have been secondary to these lesions.[7] This appears to be particularly true of patients with the bilateral, presumably genetic, form of retinoblastoma who receive radiotherapy.[39–43] Strong et al[44] have hypothesized that any carcinogenic agent, for example ambient atmospheric radiation as well as local radiation treatment to the eye, may increase the incidence of a second mutational event in any susceptible cell in the body. This would raise the occurrence of second primary tumors in this disease from 1 percent to as high as 30 percent. Up to 75 percent of second tumors in hereditary retinoblastoma are estimated to be found in previously irradiated areas,[7, 45] and there is some evidence that there is no particular correlation with the dose of radiation received.[46, 47] The shorter the latent period, the greater the likelihood that the second tumor will be a mesenchymal tumor; the longer the latent period, the more likely it is to be an epithelial type of lesion.[43] The latent period from the time of diagnosis of the retinoblastoma to the time of diagnosis of the second tumor has ranged from 4 to 26 years.[42] Osteogenic sarcoma[48, 49] is by far the most common second primary malignancy reported, and constitutes more than 50 percent of second tumors. Other second tumors reported include fibrosarcoma, malignant mesenchymoma, undifferentiated sarcoma, chondrosarcoma, carcinoma, angiosarcoma, acute leukemia, and melanoma.[7, 44, 50] Of particular interest is evidence suggestive of tumor specfiic antigen[51] and C-type particles in osteosarcomas,[52] and the finding that there may be a high incidence of malignancies in non-affected family members: 9.6 percent of relatives of patients with bilateral retinoblastoma in a Mayo clinic series.[53]

Chromosomal Studies

There have been isolated studies reporting unusually high intelligence in children with retinoblastoma.[54–57] In contradistinction, Jensen and Miller[17] and others have also described an unexpected incidence of mental retardation: 21 cases of mental retardation in 1623 cases of retinoblastoma, much in excess of the anticipated incidence of 4.7. Concurrent congenital malformations occurring in a small minority of retinoblastoma patients has stimulated a search for chromosomal abnormalities which have been recently reviewed.[29] The vast majority of patients whose karyotypes have been examined, both by routine chromosome studies[29, 58, 59] and by scanning electron microscopy,[60] in both bilateral and unilateral patients, hereditary and sporadic cases, have shown no evidence of chromosomal aberration.

A number of reports in the literature have, however, reflected a high incidence of this intraocular tumor in patients with documented chromosomal defects. To date, 13 of 45 patients with the D-deletion syndrome variously described by a number of authors have been found to have retinoblastoma.[29, 61–64, 64A] In general, most reported cases have been associated with a characteristic malformation syndrome of varying extent, including such signs as mental or developmental retardation, hypertelorism, protruding maxilla, hypoplasia or aplasia of the thumb, short fingers, pelvic girdle anomalies, anogenital malformations. The associated ocular malformations may include microphthalmos, iris colobomata, choroidal abnormalities and ptosis. Abnormalities may be minimal or absent, although some degree of mental retardation has been present in all cases.[64A]

With refined techniques, including autoradiography, quinacrine fluorescence, and analysis of the DNA d-r Giemsa pattern, the involved area on the D group chromosome in affected patients has consistently been the long arm of chromosome 13. This association of retinoblastoma with the syndrome involving a deletion of this particular chromosome might suggest the absence of a locus which normally suppresses a retinoblastoma gene, or the unmasking of some mechanism which may allow increased tumor susceptibility. There may be a morphologically undetectable, single consistently deleted area on the 13 chromosome; however, in each of the published reports thus far an apparently different set of regions of the D chromosome appears to be involved. Orye[62] described the missing portion as the broadest of the three bands normally present on the distal portion of the long arm; Wilson's studies[65] show the abnormality to be distal to the midportion of the long arm and different from that in Orye's patient; and Taylor[64] speculates that the proximal part of the long arm near the centromere may be responsible for a "retinoblastoma locus" in D-ring cases.

The association of retinoblastoma with trisomy 21, or Down's syndrome, has been reported by a number of authors;[66-68] the combination of trisomy 21, XXX, and retinoblastoma has also been reported, with an extrapolated incidence of 1:12.5 billion births.[69] Overall, it appears thus far that chromosomal abnormalities are not present in those cases which do not present with other associated developmental defects. No familial cases of retinoblastoma with chromosomal abnormalities have been reported. Only in the case of a patient with mental or developmental retardation or other abnormalities is investigation of the karyotype indicated.

It should be noted here that retinoblastoma is seen not only in the normal sized eye, but may also be found in (1) the phthisical eye with a spontaneously regressed lesion, (2) in the microphthalmic eye associated with a chromosomal syndrome, and (3) on rare occasions in the congenitally microphthalmic eye: A. R. Irvine, Jr. presented to the Verhoeff Society a case of retinoblastoma occurring in an eye with persistent hyperplastic primary vitreous (PHPV).[70]

A study of eyes of embryos with chromosomal defects has revealed cases of triploidy associated with a higher incidence of retinal dysplasia and rosette formation,[71] but no instances of retinoblastoma.

DIAGNOSIS OF RETINOBLASTOMA: NEW TECHNIQUES

The clinical manifestations and differential diagnosis of retinoblastoma have been widely reviewed elsewhere,[11, 72-74] with most patients presenting classically with signs including leukocoria (Fig. 18.5), strabismus, and decreased visual acuity. There have been multiple case reports in the literature describing less common modes of presentation,[75-78] including a sizeable number of patients with ocular inflammations, hyphema, glaucoma, or a concurrent history of trauma to the eye, and a nonvisualizable fundus.[79, 80] In Stafford's series,[81] there were a total of 14.9 percent misdiagnoses in 618 cases of retinoblastoma initially felt clinically to be either primary ocular inflammations or diseases other than ocular inflammation. In the majority of cases, the diagnosis can be made with information provided by the clinical history and presentation and through ophthalmoscopic examination including scleral indentation.[82]

Early diagnosis of retinoblastoma is of great consequence in the treatment of

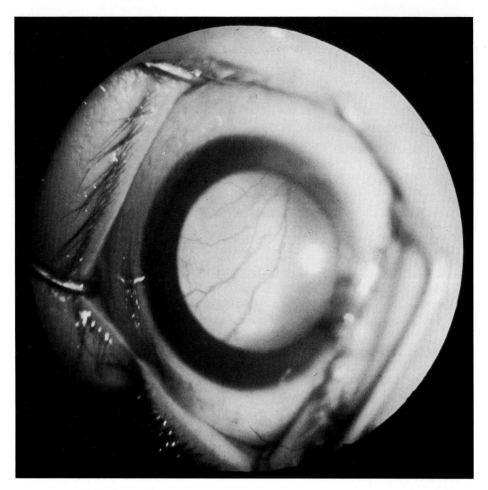

FIG. 18.5. "White pupil," the classic presenting sign of retinoblastoma.

the disease, and several noninvasive techniques are helpful: 75 percent of 20 laboratory specimens of retinoblastoma exhibited calcification within the orbit on x-ray.[83] Intraocular calcification is occasionally seen in other conditions including Coats' disease, toxacara endophthalmitis, toxoplasmosis, cysticercosis, tuberculosis, and lues. B-scan ultrasonography may replace x-ray examination as the most sensitive diagnostic tool for the demonstration of intraocular calcification. Shields et al[84] have documented four retinoblastoma patients with atypical presentations and questionable diagnoses in whom there was histologic confirmation of intraocular calcifications found on ultrasound study; in three out of the four cases, calcification had not been detected on skull x-ray. Ultrasound studies have proved useful in the evaluation of patients with atypical presentations of retinoblastoma. Sterns et al,[85] in a series of 20 patients, have described two ultrasonic types—"solid" and "cystic." They suggest that the solid type may represent the early lesion while the cystic type may be characteristic of more advanced tumor with necrosis and islands of tumor free in the vitreous. This may also be consistent with cysts that have been described histopathologically[85] (Fig. 18.6). The "cystic" type of ultrasound recordings may also occur in eyes with vitreous hemorrhage and debris. B-scan examinations at this time are helpful in following changes in size of intraocular masses in the eye with opaque media.

Anterior chamber paracenteses hold a definite though undefined risk to the retinoblastoma patient, but have been performed occasionally and have been described in patients with this tumor whose presenting signs included uveitis[87, 88] and hypopyon[89] (Fig. 18.7). Electron microscopic studies of tumor cells in anterior chamber fluid were used in one case to differentiate anterior chamber involvement of medulloepithelioma from suspected retinoblastoma.[190]

Considerable attention has been given to the presence of aqueous lactic dehydrogenase (LDH) in the diagnosis of retinoblastoma. In the normal eye, the major intraocular sources of LDH activity are: corneal endothelium, lens epithelium, ciliary body nonpigmented epithelium, and outer neurosensory retina.[91] In addition, LDH is presumably released by blood and tumor cells as they undergo necrosis. Dias et al[92] have reported a total aqueous humor LDH activity of 0–350 U/100 ml in 46 patients with nonneoplastic ocular conditions, as compared with levels of 1800–3250 U/100 ml in 4 patients with retinoblastoma. Swartz et al[91] evaluated 33 patients, of whom 7 patients with retinoblastoma had aqueous humor LDH levels significantly higher than those in patients with non-tumorous ocular disease or ocular melanoma. In 6 out of these 7 patients, $LDH_{aq} : LDH_{serum}$ ratios were de-

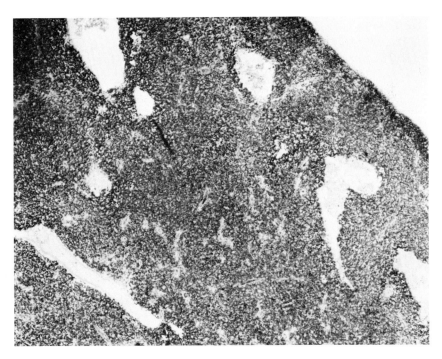

FIG. 18.6. "Cystic" retinoblastoma lesion: cystic spaces in degenerating retinoblastoma.

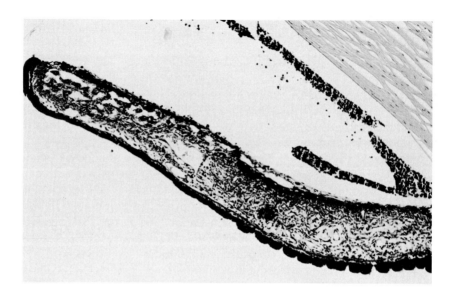

FIG. 18.7. Pseudohypopyon, rubeosis, and ectropion uveae in eye with retinoblastoma.

scribed and classified into three groups (1) ratio of $LDH_{aq}:LDH_{serum}$ greater than 1.50 (all retinoblastoma patients), (2) ratio of 1.03 (one case of nematode endophthalmitis), (3) ratio less than 0.60 (five malignant melanomas plus twenty nontumors). It has been noted[192] that a ratio of less than 1.00 does not necessarily exclude the possibility of retinoblastoma, and that a ratio of greater than 1.5 does not necessarily rule out diseases other than retinoblastoma; the aqueous humor: serum LDH ratios are suggestive but not diagnostic.

Kabak and Romano,[93] in a recent small series of seven patients with nonneoplastic ocular disease and three patients with bilateral retinoblastoma, found no consistent correlation between aqueous humor and serum LDH activity. In the retinoblastoma group, the total aqueous humor LDH level was not consistently elevated, but, in examining the LDH isoenzymes, it appeared that in all of the retinoblastoma cases, the $LDH_5:LDH_1$ ratio was greater than 5, as compared with values of less than or equal to 1.4 in the controls. Preliminary studies by Russell[94] indicate that retinoblastoma may produce significant levels of a heat stable fraction of LDH separable from LDH fractions that result directly from necrosis. At this point, it is doubtful that paracentesis for LDH levels is justified prior to enucleation except in extraordinary situations.

The radioactive phosphorus uptake test has been useful in the diagnosis of posterior uveal melanoma.[95] Notably, there have been no known false positive tests in Shields' series and only extremely rare false negative tests with appropriate techniques,[96] contributing to the marked decrease in the number of enucleations for lesions simulating melanoma.[97] The test has been felt to give characteristic results in retinoblastoma,[11] but has been generally unattractive because of potential hazardous side effects which may occur in the developing bones of the young patient.

Carcinoembryonic antigen (CEA) may be most useful where there is the suspicion of GI metastasis to the choroid. In one series,[151] 60 patients were studied, including 56 with uveal melanoma, two with metastases from GI tract carcinomas, one from breast carcinoma, and one from a cutaneous malignant melanoma. Within the uveal melanoma group, there was no clearcut relationship between the plasma CEA level and extent or prognosis of disease. Of interest was the fact that the two cases of metastatic disease from GI tract sources had elevations to greater than 18.7 ng/ml; all controls and other tumors gave rise to CEA levels less than 10 ng/ml. CEA levels were subsequently studied in retinoblastoma in Michelson's second series,[98] with distinct elevations of the CEA in four out of five patients, all of whom responded to a decrease in the tumor burden by enucleation with a decrease in the CEA level. No CEA was found to be present in the retinoblastoma tissue itself. Abnormal alpha-feto protein (αFP) values have hitherto only been reported in three childhood malignancies: teratoma, seminoma, and hepatoblastoma. Alpha-feto protein was also found to be elevated in four out of five retinoblastoma patients in Michelson's series.[98] Both serial CEA and serial αFP levels may have diagnostic significance in following the occurrence of metastatic disease and the response to therapy in those patients where it is initially found to be abnormal.

The clinical and histologic similarities between neuroblastoma and retinoblastoma have long been appreciated. In view of the fact that there is increased urinary excretion of vanilmandelic acid (VMA) and homovanillic acid (HVA) in children with neuroblastoma, Brown[99] working with Reese inconclusively examined the urine of 12 patients with retinoblastoma for excretion of these catecholamine metabolites. Subsequent studies, which have included patients with extensive metastatic disease from retinoblastoma,[100] have shown no evidence for elevated urinary levels of these compounds.

A search for other compounds in the aqueous humor or urine of these patients, such as (1) other catecholamine-related compounds, as suggested by the presence of neuro-secretory granules which have been found in retinoblastoma,[101] (2) cystathionine, which has been found in the urine of patients with neuroblastoma, ganglioneuroblastoma, and hepatoblastoma,[102, 103] and (3) desmosterol,[104] which has been demonstrated in human and experimental neuronal brain tumors in tissue culture, may have some potential as diagnostic tests.

HISTOPATHOLOGY

Clinically and grossly, retinoblastoma has been said to exhibit two modes of macroscopic growth: (1) exophytic, with tumor growing in the subretinal space, producing retinal detachment, (2) endophytic, with tumor growing into the vitreous space, producing masses on the surface of the retina, readily seen with the ophthalmoscope. This distinction is of questionable significance since most tumors,

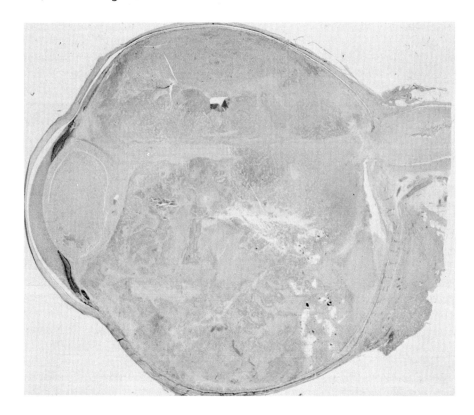

FIG. 18.8. Eye filled with retinoblastoma as seen under low power.

on pathologic examination (Fig. 18.8), are found to contain both endophytic and exophytic areas. There has been no concrete evidence to substantiate the hypothesis that this form of growth indicates the site of origin of the tumor in the retina. Neither tumor responsiveness to irradiation nor prognosis has been related to these descriptive categories. In addition to the endophytic and exophytic growth patterns, there is an infiltrating type,[105] in which the retina itself appears to be replaced but only slightly thickened by tumor cells. The latter has been described as a rare variant, occurring in 1.4 percent of 720 cases,[89] characteristically presenting in childhood at a later age than usual, frequently with a hypopyon, and with a relatively good prognosis in this series.

In discussing the origin and differentiation of retinoblastoma, it is necessary to first consider the retina. The retina is derived from the primitive medullary epithelium. The neural type develops into three major groups of cells: (1) the ependymal cells, (2) the spongioblasts, which later differentiate further into astrocytes, and (3) the germinal cells, which differentiate further into medulloblasts (glial cell precursors) and neuroblasts (precursors of photoreceptors, bipolar cells and ganglion cells). Retinoblastoma is generally believed to arise from the neuroblastic cells of the retina, called "retinoblasts" by Verhoeff. This is consistent with the presence of inner and outer photoreceptor cell elements which Ts'o et al described in well-differentiated retinoblastoma.[106] On light microscopic examination, undifferentiated areas of these tumors are composed of small round cells with large hyperchromatic nuclei and scanty cytoplasm.

Certain organized arrangements of cells may be found: (1) Flexner-Wintersteiner rosettes (Fig. 18.9), were first described by Flexner and then Wintersteiner in the 1890's: these structures were composed of cuboidal or short columnar cells, radially arranged around a lumen; the nuclei are displaced away from the lumen which is demarcated by a fine limiting "membrane," resembling the external limiting membrane of the retina. Through this membrane-like structure protrude blunt processes resembling photoreceptor cell elements, some of which taper into fine filaments.[106] Acid mucopolysaccharides resistant to hyaluronidase similar to that normally surrounding rods and cones[107] have been found in the rosette lumen. These rosettes may bear certain similarities to the primitive unilayer type of rosette of retinal dysplasia.[108–110]

(2) Homer Wright rosettes are radial arrangements of cells around a tangle of fibrils, similar to those which may be found in neuroblastoma.

(3) Fleurettes[111] (Fig. 18.10) are structures interpreted to represent photoreceptor differentiation, found in areas of pale-appearing cells with abundant eosinophilic cytoplasm and smaller, only slightly hyperchromatic nuclei. The fleurettes under light microscopy are fleur-de-lis–like arrangements of cells with long cytoplasmic processes extending for 15 to 20 microns and traversing a fenestrated membrane. Eighteen out of 300 consecutive cases of retinoblastoma contained fleurettes,

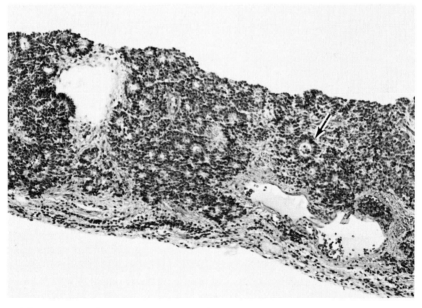

FIG. 18.9. Area of well-differentiated retinoblastoma containing Flexner-Wintersteiner rosettes and sinusoidal blood vessels.

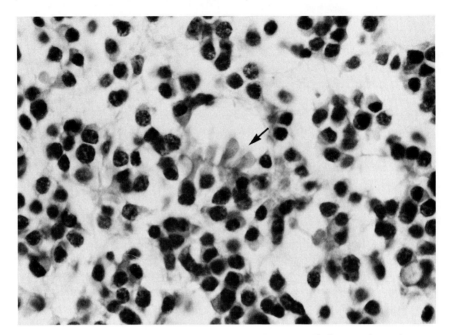

FIG. 18.10. Well-differentiated area of retinoblastoma with fleurette formation.

with evidence of transition areas where both Flexner-Wintersteiner rosettes and fleurettes were present. We have seen occasional tumors composed entirely of well differentiated fleurette-containing areas.

Other characteristic histologic findings include: perivascular cuffing surrounded by areas of extensive necrosis (Fig. 18.11) and extensive calcification, occasionally with osseous formation; basophilia in areas of blood vessels has been characterized as deposits of DNA.[112]

Electron microscopic studies have demonstrated the presence of organelles and other subcellular structures in retinoblastoma cells which are also characteristic of normal photoreceptor cells. Popoff[113, 114] et al studied retinoblastoma cells from in vivo and in vitro sources and showed a strong resemblance of these cells to normal human fetal retina. The following cytologic features were present in both: rosettes composed of cells with basally placed nuclei and mitochondria present in the luminal apex of the cell; cilia with the characteristic 9+0 configuration; desmosomes; and nuclear triple membrane structures with the central dense layer of either granular or fibrillar chromatin bounded on both sides by membrane. Characteristic microtubules have been described by Albert et al[115] from both in vivo tumor and in vitro tissue culture samples. Most microtubules are fixed only by glutaraldehyde, but those found in retinoblastoma are preserved by both chrome osmium and glutaraldehyde, behaving like microtubules previously observed in normal photoreceptor axons and rods.[116, 117]

Ts'o et al[106, 111] further described Flexner-Wintersteiner rosettes as having: (1) terminal bars of the luminal limiting membrane, (2) cytoplasmic microtubules, (3) cilia of the 9+0 configuration, (4) lamellated membranous structures in

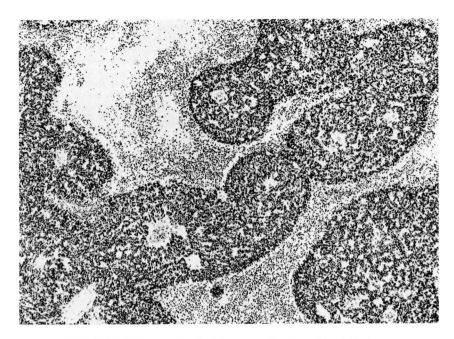

FIG. 18.11. Pale necrotic retinoblastoma cells adjacent to viable tumor.

the lumen, and (5) acid mucopolysaccharides resistant to hyaluronidase in the lumen. Analogously, the photoreceptor cells of normal control retina were noted to have: (1) terminal bars of the external limiting membrane, (2) cytoplasmic microtubules, (3) cilia with the 9+0 pattern, (4) lamellated structures in the rods and cones, and (5) acid mucopolysaccharides resistant to hyaluronidase surrounding the outer segments of rods and cones.

In a review of the ultrastructural findings in retinoblastoma, Albert et al[25] noted additional features that were studied in both freshly removed tumor tissue and in tissue culture cells: in addition to zonula adherens-like intercellular attachments, macula adherens, triple membrane structures, 9+0 cilia, and microtubules most abundant in the Golgi area, other characteristic structures present consistently in retinoblastoma cells but not necessarily unique in these were: bristle coated vesicles, dense core secretory granules, and annulate lamellae. Annulate lamellae were felt to be a variation and extension of cytomembranes resembling the nuclear membrane. The bristle coated vesicles may have a function in protein transport and have been observed in photoreceptor cells. The dense core secretory granules are thought to be neurosecretory vesicles, and are morphologically consistent with catecholamine-containing organelles in adrenergic[118] and retinal amacrine cells.[101, 119]

Tsukahara,[120] from studies of survival rates in retinoblastoma correlated with histopathologic material, concluded that there is an equivalent degree of differentiation in the two eyes of a bilaterally involved patient. However, in an examination of 18 cases with fleurette photoreceptor differentiation, Ts'o et al[111] found dissimilar histology when comparing parts of eyes in four out of five bilateral cases: only one of these bilaterally involved patients in this series exhibited photoreceptor differentiation in the tumors of both eyes.

It was speculated at one time that the tumor in the unilateral, hereditary group might be histologically distinguishable from the sporadic unilateral cases, or that bilateral tumors might be histologically distinguishable from the unilateral ones.[121] There has been little documented clinical or pathologic evidence to support this.[122] There appears to be a clinical impression among some ophthalmologists, however, that a difference in macroscopic presentation exists.[123] Sporadic cases are thought to occur more commonly with a single, large, retinal based lesion which may have vitreous seeding but no evidence of true multicentricity, and genetic cases with multifocal, small to moderate-sized lesions (Fig. 18.12).

Prognosis is associated with degree of differentiation: the presence of rosettes and fleurettes offers the best prognosis for survival, although the tumor itself may

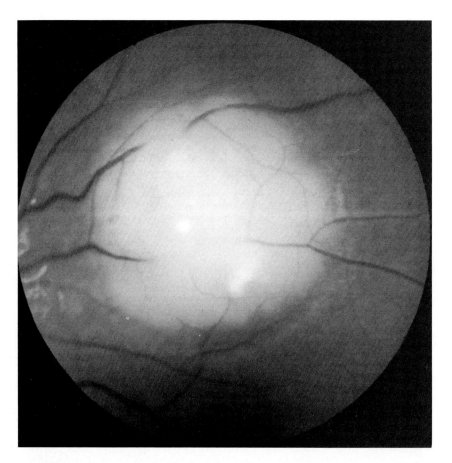

FIG. 18.12. Small lesion of retinoblastoma occurring in an eye of a patient with multiple, bilateral retinoblastomas.

be more radioresistant. Tsukahara,[120] in a review of 150 cases, classified retinoblastoma into three groups according to the degree of rosette formation, and interpreted the well-differentiated group to have had an increased resistance to radiotherapy as well as a lower mortality rate in spite of that increased resistance. In a study by Ts'o et al,[124] 42 out of 54 eyes contained viable tumor after irradiation. Of this group, 40 percent of the eyes containing viable tumor had evidence of photoreceptor differentiation (fleurettes), compared with a much lower frequency of photoreceptor differentiation, six percent, in eyes containing retinoblastoma that were not treated with radiation.[111] The implication is that in eyes enucleated for a clinical suspicion of viable tumor remaining after radiotherapy, a greater proportion of tumors containing fleurettes is present because those are the more radioresistant cells. In the follow-up of those patients, 12 out of 13 patients with photoreceptor differentiation survived. It was concluded that retinoblastoma containing fleurettes was a less anaplastic type of tumor with relative benignity and a better prognosis for life.

Metastatic disease in retinoblastoma usually occurs primarily secondary to spread via the optic nerve or by hematogenous dissemination. Choroidal invasion (Fig. 18.13) is frequently accompanied by blood-borne metastases. Carbajal[125] studied 20 fatal cases of retinoblastoma, and found that six out of seven cases with choroidal involvement developed metastases. Brown[126] noted a 60 to 62 percent

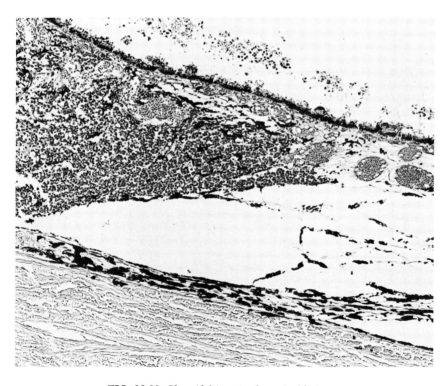

FIG. 18.13. Choroidal invasion by retinoblastoma.

mortality rate with choroidal "whole thickness" involvement, 72 to 80 percent mortality in patients with scleral involvement, and 43 to 85 percent mortality in patients with epibulbar involvement. Howard's studies[127] have suggested that patients who have received several light coagulation treatments develop breaks in Bruch's membrane in the treated areas, hyaline necrosis of the inner scleral layers, and direct invasion of the sclera with massive choroidal involvement by active tumor in five out of five patients. Ellsworth has commented that "in all cases seen personally, there was definite evidence of choroidal extension prior to the light coagulation."[11] Subsequently, Redler and Ellsworth[128] found that a large proportion, 62 percent, of enucleated eyes in their series had at least some evidence of choroidal invasion and suggested that invasion of the choroidal circulation does not necessarily occur early in the course of invasion of the choroid. They noted that only massive involvement appears to affect prognosis, stressing that the volume of choroid occupied by tumor correlated better with prognosis than did simply the presence or absence of choroidal extension.

Tumor growing into the optic nerve (Fig. 18.14) occurs with malignant cells extending into and through the lamina cribrosa until there is dissemination into the vasculature or subarachnoid space. Invasion of the optic nerve more than 3mm posterior to the nerve head raises the mortality rate in this disease to 60 to 70 percent or higher. With involvement of the optic nerve up to the lamina cribrosa but not beyond it, there is approximately a 15 percent mortality; with invasion beyond the lamina cribrosa, there is approximately a 44 percent mortality; and with tumor extending to the line of resection, a 65 percent mortality is found.[129] There may be

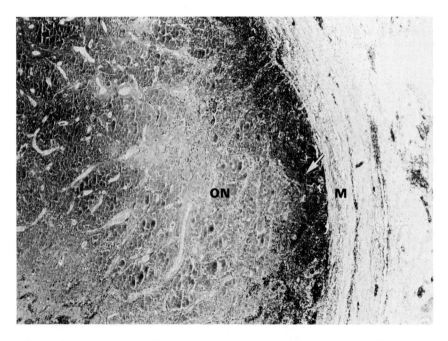

FIG. 18.14. Retinoblastoma infiltrating optic nerve in enucleated eye (ON: optic nerve. M: meninges). Arrow indicates area of particularly dense tumor infiltration.

considerable crush artifact at the line of transection, and possibly many of the surviving cases in the latter category did not actually have residual tumor.

The prognosis for orbital retinoblastoma (Fig. 18.4) is grim and various studies have confirmed this.[64, 130] Histologic findings based on examination of the enucleated globe have been grouped by Ellsworth according to risk for orbital extension: (1) unequivocal: here tumor is present at the line of resection; (2) equivocal: (a) highly suspect: in these patients tumor cells are present in the choroid and scleral emissary canals, or tumor extends into the choroid and border tissue of the nerve, or scleral necrosis is present; (b) less suspect: examination reveals either marked choroidal extension alone or scattered tumor cells in the epibulbar tissue. In this series, 88 percent of 74 retinoblastoma deaths had biopsy-documented evidence of orbital extension.

The most common sites of distant metastasis are: the central nervous system, skull, distal bones, lymph nodes, and spinal cord; occasionally these may occur many years after the last evidence of tumor activity in the retina is noted.[131, 132]

Distant metastases in bones outside of the skull have been found in about 50 percent of deaths.[133] The histologic pattern of metastases is usually of the undifferentiated type and is difficult to distinguish from other small round cell tumors of childhood. Bony metastases from retinoblastoma closely resemble Ewing's sarcoma on light microscopy and routine histologic studies.

On bone marrow aspiration, malignant cells may be similar to certain atypical cells,[134] such as abnormal mononuclear cells which are commonly found circulating in patients with a malignancy without bone marrow invasion or infiltration.[135] Tissue culture techniques and electron microscopy may become extremely useful in the differentiation of late metastases to bone from second primary tumors involving bone in these children.

RECENT OBSERVATIONS AND RESEARCH DIRECTIONS

Possible Viral Etiology

The three groups of viruses thought to have a possible role in oncogenesis are: (1) the oncogenic DNA viruses, including polyoma virus, simian viruses such as SV 40, and the adenoviruses; (2) the herpes virus; and (3) the oncorna RNA tumor viruses, A-, B-, and C-type.

Virally caused cancer is a biologic phenomenon that is widespread among most species of animals. There have been studies demonstrating viral induction of tumors even in primates,[136] and there is increasing suspicion of an association between human cancer and viruses,[137] although Koch's postulates have not been fulfilled in this regard for any type of human cancer. Arguments in favor of a viral etiology for cancers include: (1) the finding of certain virus-like particles in tumor cells, (2) the finding of tumor specific antigens and antibodies,[52] and (3) analogy to animal models.[138, 139] Viruses have been implicated in acute leukemia, Burkitt's lymphoma, and cervical carcinoma, and structures resembling virus particles have been described in leukemia, sarcomas, and breast carcinoma.[140–143]

There are no convincing models of spontaneous retinoblastoma in animals, but experimental ocular tumors have been produced by transformation by viruses. Albert et al[144] have performed studies inducing tumors morphologically resembling certain human ocular tumors by infecting explant cultures of adult hamster retina, choroid, and iris, and then injecting the transformed cells into homologous hosts, utilizing four oncogenic DNA viruses: (1) simian virus 40 (SV 40), (2) adenovirus 7 – LLE46 strain, (3) polyoma virus, (4) adenovirus 12. All tissues underwent malignant transformation with SV 40, and choroid and iris were transformed by LLE46; the resultant tumors were composed of epithelioid and spindle-shaped cells with large nuclei. Retina transformed by LLE46 gave rise to neoplasms which were dimorphic, containing epithelioid and spindle-shaped SV 40-like areas, as well as areas resembling the small, round cells of adenovirus-induced lesions. Two of the viruses transformed only retina: polyoma virus and adenovirus 12. Of note was the fact that the adenovirus 12-transformed retina gave rise to neoplasms resembling undifferentiated retinoblastoma, composed of small cells with scanty cytoplasm and large hyperchromatic nuclei, with no rosettes or other evidence of formed neural elements. The morphology of adenovirus-induced tumors is largely determined by the viral genome, although variations in morphology are described.

Kobayashi and Mukai[145] subsequently induced similar retinoblastoma-like undifferentiated intraocular tumors in rats with adenovirus 12, and Mukai et al[146] using immunofluorescent studies of T-antigens[147] in cells transformed by adenovirus, reported that adenovirus 12 oncogenesis in the developing retina appears to involve sensory ganglioneuronic cell precursors and not differentiating photoreceptor cells. In more recent studies, Albert et al[101] have induced ocular tumors with rosette-like structures by injecting newborn fetal cats with feline leukemia virus. Kobayashi et al,[148] using human embryo kidney cells infected with adenovirus 12 which are then inoculated into the vitreous of newborn rats, found tumors in 3 out of 35 animals, with evidence of perivascular cuffing by tumor cells and "a marked tendency to form rosettes" without the characteristics of Flexner-Wintersteiner rosettes.

Lens epithelium, a tissue with no apparent malignant potential under normal circumstances, has also been demonstrated to have the potential to undergo neoplastic transformation[149] under certain conditions: hamster lens epithelium, infected with SV 40 and then injected into irradiated 4-week-old hamsters, produced tumors consisting of undifferentiated polygonal or spindle-shaped cells, similar to the other sarcomatous tumors previously derived from SV 40-transformed ocular tissue. The tumor contained basement membrane material resembling lens capsule.[101]

Studies of the relationships of chromosomal and pathologic findings in Rous sarcoma virus-induced tumors in the mouse suggest a correlation between the histology of the tumor and the karyotype of the tumor cells themselves. It appears that in the evaluation of these Rous tumors, polyploidy and frequent chromosomal structural variation were found in immature, large, rapidly growing tumors, whereas the normal diploid karyotype without apparent chromosomal structural variation was found in the mature, small, slowly growing lesions.[150] Examination of retinoblastoma cells in tissue culture has shown variable numbers of minute chromosomes in these cells,[151] the etiology of which is not clear.

Burkitt's lymphoma is an undifferentiated sarcoma extensively studied because of its association with a herpes-like virus, the Epstein-Barr virus (EB virus). This tumor is of particular importance in the study of the viral etiology of tumors for several reasons, foremost of which are: (1) it is the single human tumor to date consistently associated with a virus; (2) EB virus is also associated with infectious mononucleosis, a non-neoplastic condition, and its occurrence in both diseases raises the question of what the circumstances and conditions are for neoplastic versus infectious transformation by a virus; (3) the geographic distribution of Burkitt's lymphoma appears to be associated with that of chronic malaria. It is speculated by Burkitt that this may be a determining factor in the epidemiology of the disease. An exogenous factor such as malaria or other infection may alter the reticuloendo-thelial system; this in turn may allow a virus, which may or may not occur ubiqui-tously, and which may or may not normally be nonpathogenic, to induce non-malignant or malignant transformation.[152]

There has recently been increasing interest in retinoblastoma as a virally in-duced or virally associated tumor. Among the reasons for this is the resemblance to Burkitt's lymphoma, with respect to epidemiologic, genetic, clinical, and tissue culture features. Evidence for a viral etiology in Burkitt's cited by Zimmerman[122] are: (1) case clustering in space and time, (2) high incidence of survival even in cases with minimal therapy, (3) remissions with convalescent serum, (4) tumor specific antigen, (5) viral particles in tissue culture, (6) antibodies to the virus in Burkitt's patients. Retinoblastoma is noted to present with: (1) a clinical impres-sion of case clustering in space and time, (2) long term survival in most cases, with short term therapy, (3) cases of spontaneous regression, (4) discrete multifocality, and (5) in vitro growth characteristics which are similar to those of Burkitt's lymphoma and unlike those of most other solid tumors.

The possible role of viruses in the pathogenesis of ocular tumors has been reviewed.[153] A viral factor may well be involved in the etiology of retinoblastoma at any of a number of levels, including the hypothesized initial genetic mutation of the hereditary cases in Knudson's two mutation hypothesis,[30] accounting in part for the erratic picture of incomplete penetrance occasionally presenting as horizontal rather than vertical transmission. A viral factor could be involved in the second somatic mutation as a postnatal event. Also, it may be influential in an event prior to one of the two mutations, by providing an altered, more susceptible substrate, predisposing the retinal cell to the effects of exogenous mutagens.

In 1970, Temin and Mizutani[154] and Baltimore[155] independently published their discoveries of an RNA-directed DNA polymerase, or "reverse transcriptase;" apparently, such a DNA polymerase exists in the virions of essentially all oncogenic RNA tumor viruses. This enzyme allowed the virus to utilize its viral RNA as a template for the synthesis of DNA when it is in the transformed cell, thus permit-ting the incorporation of the viral genetic information into the host cell in a heri-table form which may, generations later, become the template for the production of progeny viral RNA. Replication of RNA tumor viruses within the host cell may result in cell death or neoplastic transformation.

Two major models for viral-induced neoplasia have been proposed, involving either activation of information of an RNA tumor virus, or creation of new infor-mation for transformation.[156] By the latter "protovirus hypothesis,"[157] only part of the information is transmitted and there is new production of information, pre-sumably by recombination with host genome information. By the former "oncogene hypothesis," the entire information of the virus is transmitted in the germ cells, and is later activated, possibly by de-repression of the pre-existing information. Todaro and Huebner[139, 158] suggest that endogenous virogenes and oncogenes are repressed in normal cells. Various carcinogens such as chemicals, radiation, or superinfection by other viruses may de-repress incorporated viral information and allow full expression of either the virogene, allowing for production of progeny virus, or the oncogene, allowing for transformation into tumorous host cells.

There has been no demonstrable evidence of virus-like particles on electron microscopic studies of retinoblastoma as yet. The detection of RNA-directed DNA polymerase activity may be an important indicator of the presence of viral infection, particularly when the virus exists in the form of genetic material incorporated into the host cell without overt production of progency virons that can be morphologically detected. This enzyme has been reported in all of the animal RNA tumor viruses analyzed thus far. Ross[159] and Goodman[160] showed that the relative activity toward different synthetic templates may make it possible to separate nontumor related DNA polymerases from animal RNA tumor virus DNA polymerase, and Gallo[161] has reviewed the criteria for the demonstration of the latter enzyme.

Reid et al,[162] using a poly(A)oligo(dT) and a poly(A)poly(dT) template in various tumors, detected RNA-directed DNA polymerase activity in medulloblastoma, retinoblastoma, neuroblastoma, and ocular melanoma, with no activity found in normal human ocular connective tissue, cerebellum, or retina. Albert et al[163] further assayed ten specimens of retinoblastoma for this reverse transcriptase with three different polymerase templates, poly(rA)poly(dT), poly(A)oligo(dT), poly(dA)oligo(dT), and found resulting patterns of responses parallel to those exhibited by RNA oncogenic viruses. Similar results were found in two neuroblastoma specimens, two medulloblastomas, choroidal melanoma, and experimentally induced feline retinal tumors, with the following controls: normal adult adrenal, brain and fetal tissue. The enzyme was not found in two breast carcinoma samples, one ovarian carcinoma, two gastrointestinal tract carcinomas, one ependymoma, or one reticulum cell sarcoma. In this particular study, of especial significance is the evidence presented that, in one of the retinoblastoma cases examined for enzyme activity, the tumor and retina immediately adjacent to it were positive for the presence of RNA-directed DNA polymerase, while a sample of retina at a distance from the tumor was negative. In melanoma, it appears that use of $_{32}$P prior to enucleation prevents subsequent detection of the enzyme.[101]

In tissue culture studies, it has also been shown that retinoblastoma cell lines grown for more than 30 months still continue to have readily detectable levels of RNA-directed DNA polymerase activity similar to that described for the RNA oncogenic viruses. It is stressed that this activity may also be found in certain fetal tissues, and may be interpreted to be associated with either viral or fetal components in the retinoblastoma cell.[164]

Other Enzyme Studies

Other specific enzymes in the retinoblastoma cell lines have been evaluated to examine the degree of similarity between retinoblastoma cells and embryonic retinal cells: glutamine transferase appears during the development of the retina and, although its precise role is as yet uncharacterized, it is of importance in that there is far higher activity in the retina than elsewhere in the body. There is a sharp rise in levels coincidental with the final phase of maturation of retinal cells.[165] The activity of glutamine transferase can be induced with cortisol by eight-fold in the developing chick embryo retina[166] and appears to require that cells grow either in the intact retina or in aggregates of retinal cells and not in monolayers of cells.[167, 168] In studies of retinoblastoma tissue culture cell lines that retained rosette formation, Reid et al[164] have found induction of enzyme activity with steroids, consistent with a significant degree of differentiation in this tumor, including the retention of certain functions of normal developing retinal cells.

Tissue Culture

Because of the relative scarcity of fresh retinoblastoma cells for research purposes, it has been of importance to set up continuous in vitro cell lines of retinoblastoma. There have been a number of attempts in the literature with varying results.[169, 170] Popoff et al[113] have used a Maximow double coverslip system for their short term in vitro studies. Albert et al[25] and Reid et al[151] have successfully maintained retinoblastoma cell lines resembling the in vivo tumor for periods of up to four years (Fig. 18.15). The tissue culture techniques used are described in detail elsewhere.[115] The growth pattern is characteristic, with the tumors growing in vitro in a diphasic manner: the first phase is noted at 24 to 96 hours after explant cultures are started when migration of cells is seen, with predominantly spindle-shaped

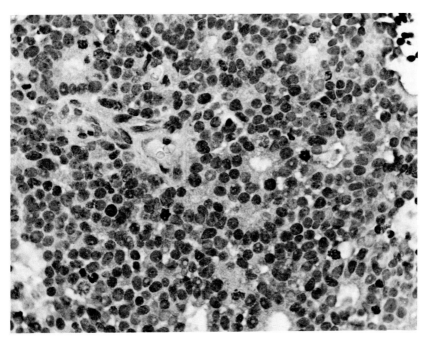

FIG. 18.15. Section cut through clump of retinoblastoma cells developing in vitro. Note Flexner-Wintersteiner-like rosettes. ×400.

forms and some small epithelioid cells, polygonal cells, and neuron-like cells; the spindle-shaped cells continue to predominate, attached to the surface of the tissue culture flask. The second phase is generally noted at 2 to 12 weeks, when clusters of smaller round cells appear, arising from the fibroblast-like stroma (Figs. 18.16, 18.17) and then separate away and grow as a suspension culture (Fig. 18.18). RNA-directed DNA polymerase activity has been demonstrated in the cultured cells, and studies of a cell line (Y79) have shown characteristics of the original tumor, both by light microscopy and electron microscopy.[151] Light microscopic findings revealed typical Flexner-Wintersteiner rosettes and foci of necrotic-appearing cells, and electron microscopic findings have included frequent nuclear envelope infoldings, triple membrane structures, microtubules, coated vesicles, annulate lamellae, and macula adherens-type junctions previously described.[25, 171]

Nerve growth factor, a protein capable of inducing differentiation of normal sympathetic cells, both in vitro and in vivo,[172] has been characterized as a 30,000 molecular weight compound with structural similarities to insulin or proinsulin,[173] and appears to produce outgrowth of neurites from sensory and sympathetic cells

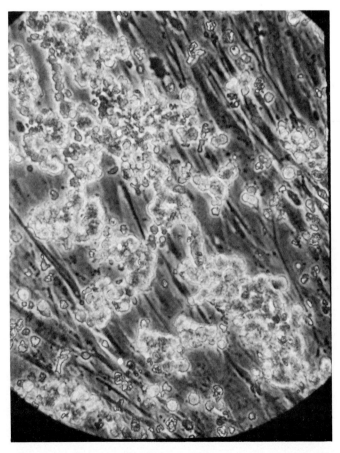

FIG. 18.16. Diphasic pattern of retinoblastoma grown in tissue culture. Note the fibroblast-like cells in background and round cells overlying them. ×240.

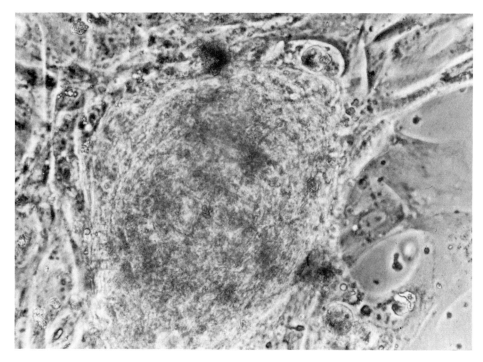

FIG 18.17. High power view of retinoblastoma in tissue culture showing mound-like appearance of tumor cells.

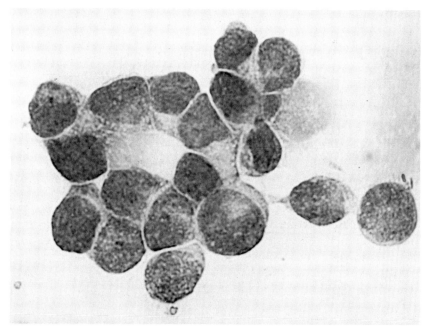

FIG. 18.18. High power view of retinoblastoma cells from continuous cell line Y-79 maintained in vitro for four years. ×1100.

only during certain periods in embryonic development.[174] C1300 murine neuroblastoma cells in tissue culture have been shown to have binding sites for the nerve growth factor molecule on the cell surface membrane,[175, 176] and the development of cytoplasmic processes filled with microtubules has been described as a response to this protein factor.[177] Similarly, nerve growth factor may prove useful in the tissue culture of retinoblastoma cells, in order to elicit neuronal differentiation, especially in the tissue culturing of biopsied specimens of suspected metastatic lesions in retinoblastoma patients. Such a response, if present, may aid in the differentiation of retinoblastoma metastatic to bone, a neuronal tumor, from such tumors as Ewing's sarcoma in these patients.

Evidence of neurosecretory granules in retinoblastoma is of particular significance in terms of further characterization of the cell of origin of the tumor. In addition, it is important in terms of a continued search for catecholamine metabolites other than vanilmandelic acid (VMA) and homovanillic acid (HVA) in aqueous humor or urine, such as have been found in other neural tumors of childhood;[178] such compounds may have diagnostic and clinical usefulness.

On electron microscopic studies, neurosecretory granules have been found in a tissue culture line as well as in two retinoblastoma tumors,[101] some measuring approximately 1100 to 1300 A, and others measuring 400 to 600 A. Studies of normal retina revealed neurosecretory granules of a diameter of 1000 to 1300 A present within amacrine cells. These structures are morphologically characteristic of storage sites for biogenic amines, and cells treated with formaldehyde vapor using the histochemical technique of Falck et al[179] showed fluorescence, presumably secondary to 3,4-dihydroisoquinolines formed from condensation with catecholamines present in neurotransmitter deposits within the cell. Dopamine may act as an inhibitory retinal neurotransmitter in the normal retina, and dopaminergic neurons at the junction of the retinal inner nuclear and inner plexiform layers have been reported;[180] which neurotransmitter is present in these tumor cell vesicles is not as yet well defined. Evidence of fluorescence in retinoblastoma tissue culture cells is similar to findings in the C1300 murine neuroblastoma cells,[181] where it was found to be localized to the terminations of the cell processes. These experiments showed a negative result in control cells, in this case, Burkitt's lymphoma cell cultures.

Tennyson et al[182, 183] have observed that some large granular vesicles morphologically appearing like catecholamine storage sites in the rat neostriatum and cat caudate nucleus may be biogenic amine-containing organelles. Other similar vesicles could not be documented as catecholamine-containing by cytochemical evaluation, and Tennyson et al speculate that these structures may have a heterogeneous function. Further experimentation with retinoblastoma cells is in progress in order to better define the functional characteristics of these "neurosecretory granules" in tissue culture: (1) electron microscopic techniques with histochemical characterization, depletion, and repletion of these neurosecretory vesicles, as has been done in sympathetic nerves of rat iris and pineal gland[184]; (2) autoradiographic localization of tritiated catecholamines in the retinoblastoma cells, such as has been done in cultured neuroblastoma cells[185]; (3) permanganate and false transmitter tagging of vesicles, as has been studied in catecholamine-containing structures in rat neostriatum[32]; and (4) incubation of cells in thorium dioxide to determine the extent of pinocytotic activity, as has been used in evaluation of the neurosecretory axon terminals of the crustacean sinus gland.[186]

Tumor Angiogenesis Factor

Two major stages in the growth and establishment of a solid tumor have been described[181]: The first is an avascular state in which a spheroidal growth of cells occurs. This is probably self-regulating, whether by accumulation of toxins or a deficiency of nutrients, and/or oxygen deficiency. The first stage may be divided into three phases: (1) initial exponential growth; (2) linear growth with concurrent central necrosis, which is probably secondary to a decreased surface area-to-volume ratio and the resulting decreased oxygen diffusion to the center; and (3) a dormant phase occurring at a maximal diameter of about 3 to 4 mm and approximately 10^6 cells. At this point there is no further expansion in size of the spheroid, although the cells on the surface continue to divide and proliferate, replacing the cells in the center which are necrosing. Clinical examples of the avascular phase cited by Folkman include cervical carcinoma in situ and early cutaneous malignant melanomas. Early vitreous seeding of retinoblastoma represents an additional example. Experimental examples include various tumors implanted into the anterior chamber which have experimentally been maintained in a state of dormancy.[188, 189] In the second vascular stage, blood vessel formation, or "tumor angiogenesis,"[190] enables a tumor to reinitiate exponential growth, and a diffusable "tumor angiogenesis factor" is stated to be responsible for the capacity to vascularize.

According to Folkman's work,[190] endothelial cell stimulation and capillary proliferation may be induced by some types of inflammation, including responses to local trauma secondary to such sources as intense heat, delayed hypersensitivity reactions, and some wounds. Such capillary growth may be mediated by various prostaglandins and vasoactive or inflammatory amines including serotonin, bradykinin, or histamine. Algire and Chalkey[191] have studied the vascular reactions of mice to wounds and to normal and neoplastic transplants in transparent chambers inserted into skin flaps. They observed that transplants of normal tissue gave rise to new capillary formation at approximately six days, with progressive differentiation into arterioles and venules, and subsequent slowing of the vascular proliferative activity. Transplants of sarcomas and mammary gland carcinomas, in contrast, gave rise to proliferation of capillaries at three days without differentiation into arterioles or venules, and without any slowing of activity, but with continued vigorous growth of the abnormal vessels.

Folkman[192] has shown evidence of tumor angiogenesis in the following models: the chorioallantoic membrane, hamster cheek pouch, intracorneal pockets for tumor implants, and the rat dorsal air sac.[193] Vascularization induced by the presence of tumor is reported to be distinguishable from that associated with overt inflammation,[193] documented delayed hypersensitivity reactions, or trauma. Gimbrone,[194] using high tumor incidence strains of mice, has demonstrated that such "tumor angiogenesis" may be induced also by preneoplastic tissue. Using normal and abnormal mouse mammary tissue implanted into rabbit iris, 4 percent of normal implants gave rise to angiogenesis, 39 percent of nontransplantable hyperplastic tissue, 60 percent of transplantable hyperplastic tissue, and 97 percent of mammary carcinomatous tissue.

The work of Greenblatt and Shubik[195] has suggested that tumor angiogenesis factor is a diffusable factor and undergoes humoral transmission without overt cell-to-cell interaction. Evidence for this is found in which angiogenesis was induced through a millipore filter in the hamster cheek pouch system.[195] In addition, Gimbrone demonstrated activity over distances of about 2.5mm[196] to about 6 to 8 mm[197] with intracorneal tumor implants. Neovascularization was documented by various methods: slit-lamp study, histology, autoradiography of tritiated thymidine in endothelial cells, and preparations in which the entire microvascular system of the iris was outlined with colloidal carbon.

Tumor angiogenesis factor is mitogenic to endothelial cells, appears to be responsible for angiogenesis, and has been isolated and partially characterized.[198] It has been isolated from Walker 256 ascitic carcinoma cells, mouse B-16 melanoma, human neuroblastoma, Wilms' tumor, and hepatoblastoma, and has been found in a fraction containing tumor nonhistone proteins.[199] It is now described as a molecule of approximately 100,000 molecular weight, and is a compound which is rapidly destroyed by ribonuclease and by heating to 56 degrees, but which is unharmed by trypsin. TAF is composed of 25 percent ribonucleic acid, 10 percent protein, and 50 percent carbohydrate.[200]

If, as Folkman and co-workers suggest, tumor angiogenesis factor plays a critical role in the vascularization and proliferation of neoplasms, inhibition of angiogenesis based on suppression or inhibition of TAF may be of great importance in the treatment of such diseases. In the search for an inhibitor of such angiogenesis, uncalcified cartilage has been noted to appear to have some potential. Eisenstein et al[201] evaluated the resistance of various tissues to invasion by proliferating vascular mesenchyme in the chorioallantoic membrane system: hyaline cartilage was impenetrable to such vascularization, while calcified cartilage was readily penetrable. Brem et al[202] more recently showed that such cartilage appears not only to resist invasion, but actually may inhibit tumor angiogenesis over distances of up to 2 mm. This finding suggests that there exists a diffusable material in hyaline cartilage which inhibits capillary proliferation induced by tumors. Cartilage which was treated with lyophilization for two days, boiled in distilled water for ten minutes, and reconstituted in Ringer's solution, did not appear to have this inhibiting property.

The blood vessels of retinoblastomas have been interpreted to arise from retinal vessels and generally they appear incompletely developed, with thin walls and saccular microaneurysmal dilatations[203] when examined in trypsin digestion preparations.[204] There may be other abnormalities in their endothelial appearance similar to the changes demonstrated with histochemical staining in brain tumors.[205] Tumor cell death may be a result of multiple thromboses in abnormally structured vessels, and the high incidence of spontaneous regression has been suggested as being related to this factor. It is also possible that spontaneous regression may be related to some "tumor angiogenesis" inhibitory effect arising from host immune interactions with the new and anomalous tumor vasculature.

Tumor seeds in the vitreous do not appear to become vascularized until they are virtually in contact with the retina. The possibility that some inhibitory property of the vitreous may affect a "tumor angiogenesis factor" warrants consideration. This is particularly pertinent in view of the similarities between the vitreous and hyaline cartilage: both tissues have a common mesodermal origin; similar biochemical constituents are present in both, including high levels of mucopolysaccharides, hydroxyprolines, and hyaluronic acid; and both are vascularized during early fetal development, only later becoming avascular structures.

Walton and Grant[206] have noted an increased incidence of iris neovascularization in eyes with posterior retinoblastomas. In 56 eyes studied with rubeosis iridis, 38 had retinoblastoma, and 18 were associated with retinal detachments of other etiologies. Out of 88 eyes with retinoblastoma examined, 44 percent had iris neovascularization. The occurrence of rubeosis may be associated with choroidal invasion by the tumor: 45 percent of eyes with both retinoblastoma and iris neovascularization had choroidal infiltration versus 15 percent of eyes with retinoblastoma and no evidence of iris neovascularization. If rubeosis were a reflection of the level of tumor angiogenesis factor in the anterior chamber, it may be that identification and quantitation of TAF in the aqueous humor would correlate with the extent of choroidal tumor involvement in the eye. The work of Stafford and co-workers,[81] however, suggests that inflammation is not a rare occurrence in retinoblastoma, and this factor may in large measure account for the rubeosis in many of these patients.

Preliminary data by Albert et al,[101] using retinoblastoma tumor tissue itself, inoculated into the anterior chamber of a variety of animals, have shown no evidence of a neovascular response in local tissues such as the iris. It is entirely possible that retinoblastoma itself contains or produces no tumor angiogenesis factor under these experimental conditions, or that TAF is a result of some complex host cell–tumor interaction, immune or otherwise, which is inoperative in this system.

As noted above, one experimental biologic assay for TAF is the corneal pocket, where tumor is placed within the corneal stroma. Studies of the inhibition of tumor angiogenesis showed that, in this intracorneal pocket system, a vascular endothelial response was significantly reduced by prior irradiation of the animal, glutaraldehyde treatment, and indomethacin treatment.[101] This suggests that the tumor angiogenesis response in this situation may possibly involve: (1) the reticuloendothelial system without causing overt inflammation, which would have been suppressed by radiation; (2) the histocompatibility antigen sites on the tumor cell constituents, which were presumably shielded from the host immune mechanism by glutaraldehyde covalent binding[207]; and (3) prostaglandin mediators,[208–210] the synthesis of which is classically inhibited by such agents as indomethacin, both in extraocular[211] and intraocular[212] tissues.

Spontaneous Regression

Tumor growth in general is limited by loss of functional capillaries as a result of vascular stasis and thromboses, and the relative rates of proliferation of parenchymal, stromal, and endothelial cells in relation to the mass of tumor.[213]

Retinoblastomas are unusual in their high incidence of spontaneous regression, and abnormalities of the tumor vasculature may be at least partially responsible. This phenomenon has been reported by many authors,[19, 20, 214, 215] with examples of spontaneous regression diagnosed in a variety of age groups, including older children, the asymptomatic adult presenting with affected offspring, and adults with phthisis bulbi.[5, 216] Boniuk and Zimmerman[217] have reported 13 phthisical eyes among 14 enucleated eyes with regressed retinoblastoma, and stressed the importance of the finding of the presence of large nests of calcified tumor cells. Diagnosis of a regressed retinoblastoma has been made on the basis of such additional data as the characteristic ophthalmoscopic picture with elevated chalk white areas of calcification and focal areas of chorioretinal atrophy, the presence of viable tumor in the opposite eye, and a positive family history for retinoblastoma.[217, 218]

The pathogenesis of spontaneous regression has not as yet been fully studied, but speculation about its cause has focused on ischemia within the tumor and immunologic protection by the host. Scanty stromal vascularization may account for areas of ischemia, and this relative avascularity may be secondary to a lack of tumor angiogenesis factor or the inhibition of such a factor, either by some environmental chemical component or by an immune response. Regressions have been associated with acute febrile illnesses and other nonspecific Freund's adjuvant-type of stimuli to the immune system. Cole[219] describes such examples in his reports of spontaneous regression in other tumors, including regression in melanomas following fever associated with administration of blood transfusions, and resolution of colonic carcinomas following abscess formation. Other immune mechanisms involving antigen-antibody complexes are suggested in a report of an eye with a partially regressed retinoblastoma associated with necrosis of the central retinal artery and vein, in addition to severe choroidal arteriolar sclerosis in the tumor which may have been the result of immune complex involvement.[220] The possibility that a causative virus may be associated with spontaneous regression in this tumor has been referred to by Zimmerman.[122]

Calcification in Retinoblastoma

Calcium deposition is common in retinoblastoma and is generally in evidence in lesions undergoing spontaneous or induced regression.[5] Dystrophic calcification, occurring in particular tissues in the absence of a generalized abnormality in calcium metabolism, is a common reaction of the body to injury secondary to various types of granulomatous inflammation and various types of tumor. A similar process may occur in retinoblastoma. Calcific deposition, however, does not usually accompany other degenerative or inflammatory processes in the eye, although it occasionally does occur. In sympathetic ophthalmia and in necrotic melanomas, calcium is absent in the face of such processes.[221] Ocular calcification is occasionally seen in Coats' disease and other abnormalities in the eyes of children.

In retinoblastoma, calcific deposits are almost invariably located in areas of tumor necrosis within the neoplasm (Fig. 18.19), and calcification appears to be absent in areas of photoreceptor differentiation where no necrosis is found. In considering the role of calcification in spontaneous regression, the following questions must yet be answered: (1) Is the tumor especially sensitive to calcification? (2) Is

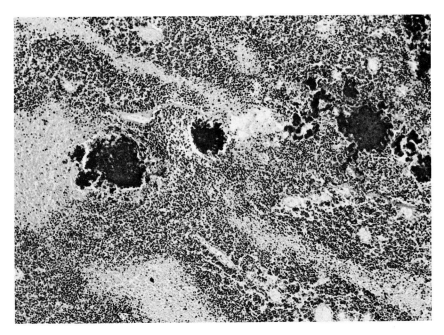

FIG. 18.19. Areas of calcium in necrotic retinoblastoma.

the local calcium concentration in cases of spontaneous regression sufficiently high to inhibit growth? (3) Is calcium deposition a purely secondary process which follows the stages which actually determine tumor retrogression?

"Calciphylaxis," a term coined by Selye,[222] has been proposed as a possible mechanism in the pathogenesis of some types of dystrophic calcification in both soft tissues and blood vessels, involving the concept of local or generalized calcinosis followed by inflammation, sclerosis, and cell death. Selye has suggested that dystrophic calcification of various soft tissues and subsequent destruction of the involved tissue in experimental animals may be produced with: (1) prior tissue sensitization by a "sensitizing calcifier," ie, a systemic calcifying factor such as parathormone, vitamin D, or hypercalcemia, followed by (2) a critical period between the sensitizer and treatment with a second agent, the challenger, and (3) the challenging agent, which may be a chemical adjuvant or a number of other stimuli, including trauma and injections of various compounds.

In his last paper in 1966, Verhoeff[223] emphasized the possibility that retinoblastoma cells may be particularly sensitive to calcification, and suggested the use of calcifying agents such as vitamin D in these patients: "My age of more than 91 years and my retirement from practice years ago prevent me from trying this treatment. To ascertain its efficacy I urge ophthalmologists observing suitable patients with this dreadful affliction to treat their patients with large doses of vitamin D for a long period."

The presence of atopic calcium may predispose the involved tissues to other processes, possibly including immunologic ones, and may subsequently lead to spontaneous regression of the tumor. Prostaglandins have been thought to be involved in the transfer of calcium across various surfaces and membranes, and PGB_1, which has been found in calf growth cartilage, may play a role in the regulation of calcium metabolism and mineralization.[224] Tashjian et al[225] have documented high levels of a bone resorption stimulating factor in the mouse fibrosarcoma, $HSDM_1$, which is found to be PGE_2, a prostaglandin responsible for hypercalcemia. It is possible that various other tumors, including retinoblastoma, may be capable of producing a localized hypercalcemia.

DNA Deposition in Retinoblastoma

At least some areas of hematoxyphilia, especially those around blood vessels, have been demonstrated to contain precipitated DNA (desoxyribonucleic acid). Mullaney[112] reported the finding of DNA deposits around venules, comparable to the areas of "calcified" material in oat cell carcinoma of the lung, which also appears to contain DNA. Mullaney subsequently[226] found that the deposits occurred (1) in the vascular walls, both with and without association with calcium deposits; (2) occasionally free of vessels in globular form; and (3) in one instance, on non-neoplastic iris blood vessel walls. These DNA deposits did not appear to necessarily parallel the degree of necrosis or calcification in the tumor. There was some evidence, however, that this is not found in tumors containing well-formed rosettes. Datta[227] has further reported, in a study of six specimens, the demonstration of DNA in examples of non-neoplastic areas of the eye that had come into contact with necrotic tumor—the posterior surface of a lens capsule, and a portion of internal membrane of the retina in one case.

The precipitated DNA may represent precipitation with circulating anti-DNA antibodies, and have been studied by ultrastructural examination in oat cell carcinomas,[228] where the material appears to consist of a fine fibrillar substance surrounding nuclear fragments. It will be important to determine (1) whether these DNA deposits in the vessel walls of retinoblastoma tumor are in fact antibody–antigen complexes, (2) whether they are simply the end-product of tumor necrosis, (3) at what point they occur in the course of tumor necrosis or spontaneous regression, and (3) whether calcium deposition in retinoblastoma is associated with calcium binding to anti–DNA–DNA complexes.

Immunologic Considerations in Retinoblastoma

The suspicion that host immune mechanisms play an important role in retinoblastoma stems from various observations. Foremost among these are the occurrence of spontaneous regression, although it has been commonly observed that spontaneous regressions may occur in one lesion and not others in the same eye at any given time, and the finding of DNA deposits around blood vessels.

Tumor-specific antigens, or tumor-specific transplantation antigens,[229] are macromolecules which are present in tumor cells and absent in normal cells, against which immune reactions may be directed. Humoral antibodies to specific antigens of animal tumors have been demonstrated in vitro,[230] and claims for similar antibodies against human tumor-specific transplantation antigens have been made for Burkitt's lymphoma,[231] malignant melanoma,[232, 233] gastrointestinal tract carcinoma,[234] and osteosarcoma.[51] Tumor-specific antigens have also been implicated in neuroblastoma.[235] In the course of anaplastic change associated with malignant transformation, certain antigens present in fetal life reappear as tumor specific antigens, possibly by derepression. This is referred to as "antigenic reversion." Examples of these are the carcinoembryonic antigen (CEA) and alpha-feto protein, both of which have been described in retinoblastoma,[98] placental alkaline phosphatase, α_2H ferroprotein, fetal sulphoglycoprotein antigen, and heterophile fetal antigen.[236]

The cell-mediated immune response to tumor antigens presumably plays a major role in the host's defense against the tumor. Many believe that it has a more significant role here than does humoral immunity. Tests of cutaneous delayed hypersensitivity responses have been performed and studied in patients with such conditions as acute leukemia,[237] Burkitt's lymphoma,[238] and ocular malignant melanoma.[239] In in vitro studies performed by Char et al,[240] evaluating cell-mediated immunity to a retinoblastoma tissue culture line in patients with retinoblastoma, 11 of 14 patients with retinoblastoma had high levels of cytotoxicity against labeled retinoblastoma cells as measured by an ^{125}I-iododeoxyuridine assay system. The lymphocytotoxicity may well be directed toward: (1) tumor-associated transplantation antigens of retinoblastoma, (2) common tissue antigens, (3) de-repressed fetal antigens, since retinoblastoma cells do bear certain similarities to developing retinal cells, or (4) viral antigens. The latter possibility is included in view of the evidence suggestive of a viral role in the oncogenesis of this tumor. Subsequently, Char and Herberman[241] reported the skin testing of eight of these patients with retinoblastoma with crude membrane extracts of retinoblastoma tissue culture cells. They described a positive response in eight out of eight nonanergic patients with retinoblastoma tested with the crude membrane extract, prepared by a method which apparently generally yields a large fraction of HLA antigens. In contrast, five out of five nonanergic control patients with other types of malignancy, including ocular melanoma, systemic melanoma, and metastatic breast carcinoma, had a negative response. The antigen eliciting this cutaneous delayed hypersensitivity response has not as yet been characterized.

Cellular immunity to tumor specific transplantation antigens has been demonstrated in animal experiments in a variety of ways. These include neutralization tests with animal tumors and tissue culture experiments with animal tumors. Neutralization tests with human tumors have been inconclusive. Tissue culture studies of human tumors have suggested that neuroblastomas may possess tumor specific antigens toward which lymphocyte mediated immune reactions can be detected with the colony inhibition bioassay. In this test, lymphocytes from neuroblastoma patients appear to inhibit colony formation by neuroblastoma cells as compared to control lymphocytes.[230, 242] A similar tumor specific response has been noted in four patients with retinoblastoma.[243] Our knowledge of details of cell-mediated lymphocytotoxicity in retinoblastoma and lymphocyte blastogenic responses against the retinoblastoma tissue culture lines, including evaluation of the separate responses of the T-cell and B-cell systems, must await future studies in this field.

A weak or early immunologic response to tumors may stimulate rather than repress tumor growth.[244] It appears that many patients have serum factors which are able to inhibit or depress the effect of cell-mediated responses to tumor antigens. This effect, referred to as the "blocking phenomenon," has recently been reviewed by Hellström and Hellström.[245] Blocking serum factors are thought to be (1) antigenic tumor material complexed to an antibody component from the host cell, (2) free tumor antigens, or (3) less likely, they may be antibodies to the receptor sites of the host's own cytotoxic lymphocytes. Clinically, there appears to be a correlation between tumor growth in vivo and the presence of a blocking serum activity in vitro.[246] From a therapeutic point of view, it would be important to know whether blocking serum activity could be separated and distinguished from the rest of the anti-tumor cell-mediated or humoral immune response. If this were feasible, it might then be possible to devise a method for increasing the anti-tumor response while decreasing the blocking activity. Further complicating the picture of the immune reaction to tumors is the presence of other serum factors in tumor-free patients which may "unblock" the blocking mechanism;[247] it has been speculated that "unblocking" factor may be free antibody.

Tissue typing of retinoblastoma may reveal further genetic factors which may influence the penetrance of the gene for retinoblastoma. These would include histocompatibility antigens, the "SD HLA" antigens (serologically detectable HLA antigens) and the "LC MLC" loci (lymphocyte depleted mixed lymphocyte culture loci). Animal studies have indicated that correlations between such antigens and susceptibility to virus-induced leukemias and tumors may exist,[248, 249] perhaps with parallel implications for human tumors.[250]

Studies of Rogentine et al[251] in acute lymphocytic leukemia (ALL) suggest that HLA_2 in this disease is not necessarily associated with an increased susceptibility to ALL, as was previously thought. Rather, it may be associated with an improved prognosis and resistance to this disease in patients who suffer from it, and Rogentine has hypothesized that HLA_2 may be linked with an immune response to tumor associated antigens.

Various aspects of the human histocompatibility system have been studied in cases of Hodgkin's disease[252] and retinoblastoma,[253] in addition to acute lymphocytic leukemia.[251] Bertrams et al[253] have looked at 21 HLA antigens of the first and second HLA series in a total of 122 children with retinoblastoma in 64 families. They found evidence of an increased frequency of the antigen W5 and a decreased frequency of the antigen HLA_{12}, without any apparent significant difference between the unilaterally and bilaterally affected groups. In a study of a three-generation family,[254] there was no clearcut association between HLA, MLR, and the occurrence of retinoblastoma.

SUMMARY

Retinoblastoma, the most common intraocular tumor of children, remains an area of challenge to visual science. The preceding review has touched upon many diverse areas and attempted to put these into perspective for retinoblastoma with regard to other tumors. Some of the highlights are noted below, with particular regard to areas of promise for further research:

I. Epidemiology and genetics
   a. role of genetic inheritance, perhaps best defined in the work of Knudson
   b. high incidence of second primary tumors, increasingly apparent
   c. multifocality of retinoblastoma in the genetic group of patients, possibly representing, in addition to bilaterality, a difference between sporadic and inherited presentations of retinoblastoma
   d. chromosomal studies, primarily important in those patients with other congenital anomalies or mental or developmental retardation
II. New techniques in diagnosis
   a. evaluation of recent claims regarding the findings of aqueous humor LDH and serum CEA and alpha feto-protein levels, potentially diagnostically helpful
   b. histopathology of retinoblastoma, both by light and electron microscopy, yielding new findings in recent years
III. Recent research efforts in retinoblastoma
   a. viral induction of retinoblastoma-like tumors in experimental animals
   b. detection of RNA-dependent DNA polymerase and glutamine transferase activity
   c. tissue culture and electron microscopic studies, offering fresh insights into the cause and pathogenesis of this tumor
   d. the finding of neurosecretory granules on electron microscopic evaluation
   e. role of tumor angiogenesis factor in the growth of retinoblastoma and in its spontaneous regression
   f. calcification in this tumor
   g. reported DNA deposition in vessel walls
   h. immunopathologic considerations

In summary, we have considered a variety of clinical and experimental aspects of retinoblastoma. All represent areas for further investigation for the understanding of the nature of this tumor. Immunotherapy holds promise for the control of cancers such as retinoblastoma by active or passive immunization, adjuvant therapy, or by blocking the blocking antibodies. Continued research efforts which elucidate the basic biochemical, epidemiologic, and immunopathologic characteristics of retinoblastoma offer us hope of uncovering features of this tumor that will permit the development of more specific and nondestructive methods of diagnosis and treatment.

ACKNOWLEDGMENTS

The photographic assistance of Mr. Andrew Levin and the secretarial assistance of Ms. Jeanne Reardon are appreciated.

REFERENCES

1. Wardrop J: Observations on the Fungus Haematodes. Edinburgh, Constable, 1809
2. Von Graefe, cited by LaGrange F: Traite des tumeurs de l'oeil, de l'orbite et des annexes. Paris, Steinheil, 1901
3. Hilgartner HL: Report of a case of double glioma treated with x-ray. Texas Med J 18:322, 1903
4. Dunphy EB: The story of retinoblastoma. Trans Am Acad Ophthalmol Otolaryngol 68:249, 1964
5. Reese AB: Tumors of the Eye. New York, Harper & Row, 1963
6. Kupfer C: Retinoblastoma treated with intravenous nitrogen mustard. Am J Ophthalmol 36:1721, 1953
7. Jensen RD, Miller RW: Retinoblastoma: epidemiologic characteristics. N Engl J Med 285:307, 1971
8. Bedford MA, Bedotto C, MacFaul PA: Retinoblastoma: a study of 139 cases. Br J Ophthalmol 55:19, 1971
9. Ellsworth RM: Treatment of retinoblastoma. Am J Ophthalmol 66:49, 1968
10. Miller RW: Fifty-two forms of childhood cancer: United States mortality experience, 1960–66. J Pediatr 75:685, 1969
11. Ellsworth RM: The practical management of retinoblastoma. Trans Am Ophthalmol Soc 67:462, 1969
12. Barry G, Mullaney J: Retinoblastoma in the Republic of Ireland. Trans Ophthalmol Soc UK 91:839, 1971
13. Hemmes GD: Untersuchung nach dem Vorkommen von Glioma retinae bei Verwandten von mit dieser Krankheit Behafteten. Klin Monatsbl Augenheilkd 86:331, 1931
14. Schappert-Kimmijser J, Hemmes GD, Nijland R: The heredity of retinoblastoma. Ophthalmologica 151:197, 1966
15. Tarkkanen A, Tuovinen E: Retinoblastoma in Finland 1912–64. Acta Ophthalmol 49:293, 1971
16. Aherne G, Roberts DF: Retinoblastoma: a clinical survey and its genetic implications. Clin Genet 8:275, 1975
17. Knudson AG Jr: The genetics of childhood cancer. Cancer 35:1022, 1975
18. Höpping W, Renelt P: The treatment of retinoblastoma. Mod Probl Ophthalmol 12:580, 1974
19. Karsgaard AT: Spontaneous regression of retinoblastoma: a report of two cases. Can J Ophthalmol 6:218, 1971
20. Morris WE, LaPiana FG: Spontaneous regression of bilateral multifocal retinoblastoma with preservation of normal visual acuity. Ann Ophthalmol 6:1192, 1974
21. Pearce WG, Gillan JG: Bilateral spontaneous regression of retinoblastoma. Can J Ophthalmol 7:234, 1972
22. Howard GM, Ellsworth RM: Differential diagnosis of retinoblastoma: a statistical survey of 500 children: II. Factor relating to the diagnosis of retinoblastoma. Am J Ophthalmol 60:618, 1965
23. Newell GR, Roberts JD, Baranovsky A: Retinoblastoma: presentation and survival in Negro children compared with whites. J Natl Cancer Inst 49:989, 1972
24. Ellsworth, cited by Zimmerman LE: Changing concepts concerning the pathogenesis of infectious diseases. Am J Ophthalmol 69:947, 1970
25. Albert DM, Lahav M, Lesser R, et al: Recent observations regarding retinoblastoma: I. Ultrastructure, tissue culture growth, incidence, and animal models. Trans Ophthalmol Soc UK 94:909, 1974
26. Kodilinye HC: Retinoblastoma in Nigeria: problems of treatment. Am J Ophthalmol 63:469, 1967
27. Bras G, Cole H, Ashmeade-Dyer A, et al: Report on 151 childhood malignancies observed in Jamaica. J Natl Cancer Inst 43:417, 1969
28. Macklin MT: A study of retinoblastoma in Ohio. Am J Hum Genet 12:1, 1960

29. Francois J, Matton MT, DeBie S, et al: Genesis and genetics of retinoblastoma. Ophthalmologica 170:405, 1975
30. Knudson AG Jr: Mutation and cancer: statistical study of retinoblastoma. Proc Natl Acad Sci 68:820, 1971
31. Ellsworth RM: Hereditary and preventive aspects of retinoblastoma. Sight Sav Rev 39:17, 1969
32. Hökfelt T, Jonsson G, Lidbrink P: Electron microscopic identification of monoamine nerve ending particles in rat brain homogenates. Brain Res 22:147, 1970
33. Griffith AD, Sorsby A: The genetics of retinoblastoma. Br J Ophthalmol 28:279, 1944
34. Sorsby A: Bilateral retinoblastoma: a dominantly inherited affection. Br Med J 2:580, 1972
35. Falls HF, Neel JV: Genetics of retinoblastoma. Arch Ophthalmol 46:367, 1951
36. Smith SM, Sorsby A: Retinoblastoma: some genetic aspects. Ann Hum Genet 23:50, 1958
37. Knudson AG Jr, Hethcote HW, Brown BW: Mutation and childhood cancer: a probabilistic model for the incidence of retinoblastoma. Proc Natl Acad Sci 72:5116, 1975
38. Porter IH, Benedict WF, Brown CD, et al: Recent advances in molecular pathology: a review: some aspects of chromosome changes in cancer. Exp Mol Pathol 11:340, 1969
39. Thompson RW, Small RC, Stein JJ: Treatment of retinoblastoma. Am J Roentgenol Radium Ther Nucl Med 114:16, 1972
40. Shah IC, Arlen M, Miller T: Osteogenic sarcoma developing after radiotherapy for retinoblastoma. Am Surg 40:485, 1974
41. Yoneyama T, Greenlaw RH: Osteogenic sarcoma following radiotherapy for retinoblastoma. Radiology 93:1185, 1969
42. Forrest AW: Tumors following radiation about the eye. Trans Am Acad Ophthalmol Otolaryngol 65:694, 1961
43. Soloway HB: Radiation-induced neoplasms following curative therapy for retinoblastoma. Cancer 19:1984, 1966
44. Strong LC, Knudson AG Jr: Second cancers in retinoblastoma. Lancet 2:1086, 1973
45. The changing pattern of retinoblastoma, editorial. Lancet 2:1016, 1971
46. Sang DN, Ellsworth RM: Unpublished data
47. Abramson DH, Ellsworth RM, Zimmerman LE: Nonocular cancer in retinoblastoma survivors. Trans Am Acad Ophthalmol Otolaryngol 81:454, 1976
48. Aherne G: Retinoblastoma associated with primary malignant tumours. Trans Ophthalmol Soc UK 94:938, 1974
49. Schimke RN, Lowman JT, Cowan GAB: Retinoblastoma and osteogenic sarcoma in siblings. Cancer 34:2077, 1974
50. Lennox EL, Draper GJ, Sanders BM: Retinoblastoma: a study of natural history and prognosis of 268 cases. Br Med J 3:731, 1975
51. Morton DL, Malmgren RA: Human osteosarcomas: immunologic evidence suggesting an associated infectious agent. Science 162:1279, 1968
52. Morton DL, Malmgren RA, Hall WT, et al: Immunologic and virus studies with human sarcomas. Surgery 66:152, 1969
53. Gordon H: Family studies in retinoblastoma. In Bergsma D (ed): Medical Genetics Today. Baltimore, Johns Hopkins Press, 1974
54. Levitt EA, Rosenbaum AL, Willerman L, et al: Intelligence of retinoblastoma patients and their siblings. Child Dev 43:939, 1972
55. Eldridge R, O'Meara K, Kitchin D: Superior intelligence in sighted retinoblastoma patients and their families. J Med Genet 9:331, 1972
56. Thurrell RJ, Josephson TS: Retinoblastoma and intelligence. Psychosomatics 7:368, 1966

57. Williams M: Superior intelligence of children blinded from retinoblastoma. Arch Dis Child 43:204, 1968
58. Wiener S, Reese AB, Hyman GA: Chromosome studies in retinoblastoma. Arch Ophthalmol 69:311, 1963
59. Mark J: Chromosomal analysis of a human retinoblastoma. Acta Ophthalmol 48: 124, 1970
60. Pruett RC, Atkins L: Chromosome studies in patients with retinoblastoma. Arch Ophthalmol 82:177, 1969
61. Howard RO, Breg WR, Albert DM, et al: Retinoblastoma and chromosome abnormality. Arch Ophthalmol 92:490, 1974
62. Orye E, Delbeke MJ, Vandenabeele B: Retinoblastoma and D-chromosome deletions. Lancet 2:1376, 1972
63. Lele KP, Penrose LS, Stallard HB: Chromosome deletion in a case of retinoblastoma. Ann Hum Genet 27:171, 1963
64. Taylor AI: Dq-, Dr and retinoblastoma. Humangenetik 10:209, 1970
64A. Knudson AG Jr, Meadows AT, Nichols WW, Hill R: Chromosomal deletion and retinoblastoma. N Engl J Med 295:1120, 1976
65. Wilson MG, Towner JW, Fujimoto A: Retinoblastoma and D-chromosome deletions. Am J Hum Genet 25:57, 1973
66. Taktikos A: Association of retinoblastoma with mental defect and other pathological manifestations. Br J Ophthalmol 48:495, 1964
67. Miller RW: Neoplasia and Down's syndrome. Ann NY Acad Sci 171:637, 1970
68. Cernea P, Teodorescu F, Angheloni T: Retinoblastome a mosaicisme chromosomien 46,XX/47,XX;G+. Ann Ocul 206:607, 1973
69. Day RW, Wright SW, Koons A, et al: XXX 21-trisomy and retinoblastoma. Lancet 2:154, 1963
70. Irvine AR Jr, Albert DM, Sang DN: Retinal neoplasia and dysplasia: II. Retinoblastoma occurring with persistence and hyperplasia of the primary vitreous. Invest Ophthalmol, in press
71. Howard RO, Boue J, Deluchat C, et al: The eyes of embryos with chromosome abnormalities. Am J Ophthalmol 78:167, 1974
72. Bedford MA: Treatment of retinoblastoma. Adv Ophthalmol 31:2, 1975
73. Howard GM, Ellsworth RM: Differential diagnosis of retinoblastoma: a statistical survey of 500 children: I. Relative frequency of the lesions which simulate retinoblastoma. Am J Ophthalmol 60:610, 1965
74. Bishop JO, Madson EC: Retinoblastoma: review of current status. Surv Ophthalmol 19:342, 1975
75. Binder PS: Unusual manifestations of retinoblastoma. Am J Ophthalmol 77:674, 1974
76. Schuster SAD, Ferguson EC III: Unusual presentations of retinoblastoma. South Med J 63:4, 1970
77. Andrew JM, Smith DR: Unsuspected retinoblastoma. Am J Ophthalmol 60:536, 1965
78. Friendly DS, Parks MM: Concurrence of hereditary congenital cataracts and hereditary retinoblastoma. Arch Ophthalmol 84:525, 1970
79. Weizenblatt S: Differential diagnostic difficulties in atypical retinoblastoma. Arch Ophthalmol 58:699, 1957
80. Spaulding AG, Naumann G: Unsuspected retinoblastoma. Arch Ophthalmol 76: 575, 1966
81. Stafford WR, Yanoff M, Parnell BL: Retinoblastoma initially misdiagnosed as primary ocular inflammations. Arch Ophthalmol 82:771, 1969
82. Howard GM, Ellsworth RM: Findings in the peripheral fundi of patients with retinoblastoma. Am J Ophthalmol 62:243, 1966
83. Pfeiffer RL: Roentgenographic diagnosis of retinoblastoma. Arch Ophthalmol 15: 811, 1936

84. Shields JA, Leonard BC, Michelson JB, et al: B-scan ultrasonography in the diagnosis of atypical retinoblastoma. Can J Ophthalmol 11:42, 1976
85. Sterns GK, Coleman DJ, Ellsworth RM: The ultrasonographic characteristics of retinoblastoma. Am J Ophthalmol 78:606, 1974
86. Ginsberg J, Spaulding AG, Asbury T: Cystic retinoblastoma. Am J Ophthalmol 80:930, 1975
87. Hogan MJ, Wood I, Godfrey W: Aqueous humor cytology in uveitis. Arch Ophthalmol 89:217, 1973
88. Richards WW: Retinoblastoma simulating uveitis. Am J Ophthalmol 65:427, 1968
89. Morgan G: Diffuse infiltrating retinoblastoma. Br J Ophthalmol 55:600, 1971
90. Jakobiec FA, Howard GM, Ellsworth RM, et al: Electron microscopic diagnosis of medulloepithelioma. Am J Ophthalmol 79:321, 1975
91. Swartz M, Herbst RW, Goldberg MF: Aqueous humor lactic acid dehydrogenase in retinoblastoma. Am J Ophthalmol 78:612, 1974
92. Dias PLR, Shanmuganathan SS, Rajaratnam M: Lactic dehydrogenase activity of aqueous humour in retinoblastoma. Br J Ophthalmol 55:130, 1971
92A. Romano PE, Kabak J: Aqueous humor lactic acid dehydrogenase in retinoblastoma. Am J Ophthalmol 79:697, 1975
93. Kabak J, Romano PE: Aqueous humour lactic acid dehydrogenase isoenzymes in retinoblastoma. Br J Ophthalmol 59:268, 1975
94. Russell P: Personal communication, 1977
95. Hagler WS, Jarrett WH II, Humphrey WT: The radioactive phosphorus uptake test in diagnosis of uveal melanoma. Arch Ophthalmol 83:548, 1970
96. Shields JA, Hagler WS, Federman JL, et al: The significance of the P32 uptake test in the diagnosis of posterior uveal melanomas. Trans Am Acad Ophthalmol Otolaryngol 79:297, 1975
97. Shields JA, McDonald PR: Improvements in the diagnosis of posterior uveal melanomas. Arch Ophthalmol 91:259, 1974
97A. Michelson JB, Felberg NT, Shields JA: Carcinoembryonic antigen. Arch Ophthalmol 94:414, 1976
98. Michelson JB, Felberg NT, Shields JA: Fetal antigens in retinoblastoma. Cancer 37:719, 1976
99. Brown DH: The urinary excretion of vanilmandelic acid (VMA) and homovanillic acid in children with retinoblastoma. Am J Ophthalmol 62:239, 1966
100. Renelt P, Trieschmann W: Vanilmandelic acid urinary excretion in the diagnosis of retinoblastoma. Albrecht von Graefes Arch Klin Exp Ophthalmol 188:281, 1973
101. Albert DM, Lahav M, Colby ED, Shadduck JA, Sang DN: Retinal neoplasia and dysplasia: I. Induction by feline leukemia virus. Invest Ophthalmol, in press
102. Geiser CF, Efron ML: Cystathioninuria in patients with neuroblastoma or ganglioneuroblastoma. Cancer 22:856, 1968
103. Mullaney J: Retinoblastoma: a review and some new aspects. Irish J Med Sci 8:57, 1969
104. Weiss JF, Cravioto H, Bennett K, et al: Desmosterol in human and experimental brain tumors in tissue culture. Arch Neurol 33:180, 1976
105. Schofield PB: Diffuse infiltrating retinoblastoma. Br J Ophthalmol 44:35, 1960
106. Ts'o MOM, Fine BS, Zimmerman LE: The Flexner-Wintersteiner rosettes in retinoblastoma. Arch Pathol 88:664, 1969
107. Zimmerman LE: Applications of histochemical methods for the demonstration of acid mucopolysaccharides to ophthalmic pathology. Trans Am Acad Ophthalmol Otolaryngol 62:697, 1958
108. Andersen SR: Differentiation features in some retinal tumors and in dysplastic retinal conditions. Am J Ophthalmol 71:231, 1971

109. Lahav M, Albert DM, Wyand S: Clinical and histopathologic classification of retinal dysplasia. Am J Ophthalmol 75:648, 1973
110. Lahav M, Albert DM, Craft JL: Light and electron microscopic study of dysplastic rosette-like structures occurring in the disorganized mature retina. Albrecht von Graefes Archiv Klin Exp Ophthalmol 195:57, 1975
111. Ts'o MOM, Zimmerman LE, Fine BS: The nature of retinoblastoma: I. Photoreceptor differentiation: a clinical and histopathologic study. Am J Ophthalmol 69:339, 1970
112. Mullaney J: DNA in retinoblastoma. Lancet 2:918, 1968
113. Popoff N, Ellsworth RM: The fine structure of nuclear alterations in retinoblastoma and in the developing human retina: in vivo and in vitro observations. J Ultrastruct Res 29:535, 1969
114. Popoff N, Ellsworth RM: The fine structure of retinoblastoma: in vivo and in vitro observations. Lab Invest 25:389, 1971
115. Albert DM, Dalton AJ, Rabson AS: Microtubules in retinoblastoma. Am J Ophthalmol 69:296, 1970
116. Fine BS: Observations on the axoplasm of neural elements in the human retina. In Proceedings of the Third European Regional Conference on Electron Microscopy, Vol B. Prague, Publishing House of the Czechoslovak Academy of Science, 1964, p 319
117. Sheffield JB: Microtubules in the outer nuclear layer of rabbit retina. J Microsc (Oxf) 5:173, 1966
118. Geffen LB, Livett BG: Synaptic vesicles in sympathetic neurons. Physiol Rev 51:98, 1971
119. Laties AM, Jacobowitz D: A comparative study of the autonomic innervation of the eye in monkey, cat, and rabbit. Anat Rec 156:383, 1966
120. Tsukahara I: A histopathological study on the prognosis and radiosensitivity of retinoblastoma. Arch Ophthalmol 63:1005, 1960
121. Cummings JN, Sorsby A: Unilateral and bilateral retinoblastoma: a possible histological difference. Br J Ophthalmol 28:533, 1944
122. Zimmerman LE: Changing concepts concerning the pathogenesis of infectious diseases. Am J Ophthalmol 69:947, 1970
123. Bedford MA: Personal communication, 1976
124. Ts'o MOM, Zimmerman LE, Fine BS, et al: A cause of radioresistance in retinoblastoma: photoreceptor differentiation. Trans Am Acad Ophthalmol Otolaryngol 74:959, 1970
125. Carbajal UM: Metastasis in retinoblastoma. Am J Ophthalmol 48:47, 1959
126. Brown DH: The clinicopathology of retinoblastoma. Am J Ophthalmol 61:508, 1966
127. Howard GM: Ocular effects of radiation and photocoagulation. Arch Ophthalmol 76:7, 1966
128. Redler LD, Ellsworth RM: Prognostic importance of choroidal invasion in retinoblastoma. Arch Ophthalmol 90:294, 1973
129. Yanoff M, Fine BS: Ocular Pathology. New York, Harper & Row, 1975
130. Ellsworth RM: Orbital retinoblastoma. Trans Am Ophthalmol Soc 72:79, 1974
131. Jafek BW, Lindford R, Foos RY: Late recurrent retinoblastoma in the nasal vestibule. Arch Otolaryngol 94:264, 1971
132. Ytteborg J, Arnesen K: Late recurrence of retinoblastoma. Acta Ophthalmol 50:367, 1972
133. Merriam GR: Retinoblastoma: analysis of 17 autopsies. Arch Ophthalmol 44:71, 1950
134. Salsbury AJ, Bedford MA, Dobree JH: Bone marrow appearances in children suffering from retinoblastoma. Br J Ophthalmol 52:388, 1968
135. Alexander RF, Spriggs AI: The differential diagnosis of tumor cells in circulating blood. J Clin Pathol 13:414, 1960

136. Munroe JS, Windle WF: Tumors induced in primates by chicken sarcoma virus. Science 140:1415, 1963
137. Todaro GJ, Zeve V, Aaronson SA: Virus in cell culture derived from human tumor patients. Nature 226:1047, 1970
138. Berman LD: Comparative morphologic study of the virus-induced solid tumors of Syrian hamsters. J Natl Cancer Inst 39:847, 1967
139. Todaro GJ, Huebner RJ: NAS Symposium: new evidence as the basis for increased efforts in cancer research. The viral oncogene hypothesis: new evidence. Proc Natl Acad Sci USA 69:1009, 1972
140. Dmochowski L, Taylor HG, Grey CE, et al: Viruses and mycoplasma (PPLO) in human leukemia. Cancer 18:1345, 1965
141. Dmochowski L, Yumoto T, Grey CE, et al: Electron microscopic studies of human leukemia and lymphoma. Cancer 20:760, 1967
142. Chopra HC, Feller WF: Viruslike particles in human breast cancer. Texas Rep Biol Med 27:945, 1969
143. Henle W: Evidence for viruses in acute leukemia and Burkitt's tumor. Cancer 21:580, 1968
144. Albert DM, Rabson AS, Dalton AJ: In vitro neoplastic transformation of uveal and retinal tissue by oncogenic DNA viruses. Invest Ophthalmol 7:357, 1968
145. Kobayashi S, Mukai N: Retinoblastoma-like tumors induced in rats by human adenovirus. Invest Ophthalmol 12:853, 1973
146. Mukai N, Murao T: Retinal tumor induction by ocular inoculation of human adenovirus in 3-day-old rats. J Neuropathol Exp Neurol 34:28, 1975
147. Pope JH, Rowe WP: Detection of specific antigen in SV 40-transformed cells by immunofluorescence. J Exp Med 120:121, 1964
148. Kobayashi S, Mukai N: Retinoblastoma-like tumors induced by human adenovirus type 12 in rats. Cancer Res 34:1646, 1974
149. Albert DM, Rabson AS, Grimes PA, et al: Neoplastic transformation in vitro of hamster lens epithelium by simian virus 40. Science 164:1077, 1969
150. Mark J: Relationship of chromosomal and pathological findings in Rous sarcoma virus-induced tumours in the mouse. Int J Cancer 3:663, 1968
151. Reid TW, Albert DM, Rabson AS, et al: Characteristics of an established cell line of retinoblastoma. J Natl Cancer Inst 53:347, 1974
152. Burkitt DP: Etiology of Burkitt's lymphoma: an alternative hypothesis to a vectored virus. J Natl Cancer Inst 42:19, 1969
153. Albert DM, Rabson AS: The role of viruses in the pathogenesis of ocular tumors. Int Ophthalmol Clin 12:195, 1972
154. Temin HM, Mizutani S: RNA-dependent DNA polymerase in virions of Rous sarcoma virus. Nature 226:1211, 1970
155. Baltimore D: RNA-dependent DNA polymerase in virions of RNA tumour viruses. Nature 226:1209, 1970
156. Temin HM: The RNA tumour viruses: background and foreground. Proc Natl Acad Sci USA 69:1016, 1972
157. Temin HM: On the origin of the genes for neoplasia: GHA Clowes Memorial Lecture. Cancer Res 34:2835, 1974
158. Todaro GJ: Evolution and modes of transmission of RNA tumor viruses. Am J Pathol 81:590, 1975
159. Ross J, Scolnick EM, Todaro GJ, et al: Separation of murine cellular and murine leukemia virus DNA polymerases. Nature (New Biol) 231:163, 1971
160. Goodman NC, Spiegelman S: Distinguishing reverse transcriptase of an RNA tumor virus from other known DNA polymerases. Proc Natl Acad Sci USA 68:2203, 1971
161. Gallo RC: Summary of recent observations on the molecular biology of RNA tumor viruses and attempts at application to human leukemia. Am J Clin Pathol 60:80, 1973

162. Reid TW, Albert DM: RNA-dependent DNA polymerase activity in human tumors. Biochem Biophys Res Commun 46:383, 1972
163. Albert DM, Reid TW: RNA-directed DNA polymerase activity in retinoblastoma: report of its presence and possible significance. Trans Am Acad Ophthalmol Otolaryngol 77:630, 1973
164. Reid TW, Russell P: Recent observations regarding retinoblastoma: II. An enzyme study of retinoblastoma. Trans Ophthalmol Soc UK 94:929, 1974
165. Moscona AA, Kirk DL: Control of glutamine synthetase in the embryonic retina in vitro. Science 148:519, 1965
166. Reif-Lehrer L, Coghlin J: Conversion of glutamic acid to glutamine by retinal glutamine synthetase. Exp Eye Res 17:321, 1973
167. Morris JE, Moscona AA: Induction of glutamine synthetase in embryonic retina: its dependence on cell interactions. Science 167:1736, 1970
168. Reif-Lehrer L: Glutamine synthetase activity in human retinal tissue. Arch Ophthalmol 86:72, 1971
169. Yoneda C, VanHerick W: Tissue culture cell strain derived from retinoblastoma. Am J Ophthalmol 55:987, 1963
170. Huang LH, Sery TW, Chen MM, et al: Experimental retinoblastoma: I Morphology and behavior of cells cultivated in vitro. Am J Ophthalmol 70:771, 1970
171. Albert DM, Rabson AS, Dalton AJ: Tissue culture study of human retinoblastoma. Invest Ophthalmol 9:64, 1970
172. Levi-Montalcini R, Angeletti PU: Essential role of the nerve growth factor in the survival and maintenance of dissociated sensory and sympathetic embryonic nerve cells in vitro. Dev Biol 7:653, 1963
173. Frazier WA, Angeletti RH, Bradshaw RA: Nerve growth factor and insulin. Science 167:482, 1972
174. Levi-Montalcini R, Angeletti PU: Nerve growth factor. Physiol Rev 48:534, 1968
175. Revoltella R, Bertolini L, Pediconi M, et al: Specific binding of nerve growth factor (NGF) by murine C1300 neuroblastoma cells. J Exp Med 140:437, 1974
176. Revoltella R, Bosman C, Bertolini L: Detection of nerve growth factor binding sites on neuroblastoma cells by rosette formation. Cancer Res 35:890, 1975
177. Bosman C, Revoltella R, Bertolini L: Phagocytosis of nerve growth factor-coated erythrocytes in neuroblastoma rosette-forming cells. Cancer Res 35:896, 1975
178. Voorhees ML, Gardner LI: Studies of catecholamine excretion by children with neural tumors. J Clin Endocrinol Metab 22:126, 1962
179. Falck B, Hillarp NA, Thieme G, et al: Fluorescence of catecholamines and related compounds condensed with formaldehyde. J Histochem Cytochem 10:348, 1962
180. Kramer SG: Dopamine: a retinal neurotransmitter: I. Retinal uptake, storage, and light-stimulated release of H3-dopamine in vivo. Invest Ophthalmol 10:438, 1971
181. DeLellis RA, Rabson AS, Albert DM: The cytochemical distribution of catecholamines in the C1300 murine neuroblastoma. J Histochem Cytochem 18:913, 1970
182. Tennyson VM, Heikkila R, Mytilineou C, et al: 5-hydroxy-dopamine "tagged" neuronal boutons in rabbit neostriatum: inter-relationship between vesicles and axonal membrane. Brain Res 82:341, 1974
183. Tennyson VM, Marco LA: Intrinsic connections of caudate neurons: II. Fluorescence and electron microscopy following chronic isolation. Brain Res 53:307, 1973
184. Tennyson VM, Cohen G, Mytilineou C, et al: 6-7-dihydroxytetrahydroisoquinoline: electron microscopic evidence for uptake into the amine-binding vesicles in sympathetic nerves of rat iris and pineal gland. Brain Res 51:161, 1973
185. Goldstein MN: Incorporation and release of H3-catecholamines by cultured fetal human sympathetic nerve cells and neuroblastoma cells. Proc Soc Exp Biol Med 125:993, 1967
186. Bunt AH: Formation of coated and "synaptic" vesicles within neurosecretory axon terminals of the crustacean sinus gland. J Ultrastruct Res 28:411, 1969

187. Folkman J, Hochberg M: Self-regulation of growth in three dimensions. J Exp Med 138:745, 1973
188. Gimbrone MA Jr, Leapman SB, Cotran RS, et al: Tumor dormancy in vivo by prevention of neovascularization. J Exp Med 136:261, 1972
189. Greene HSN, Arnold H: The homologous and heterologous transplantation of brain and brain tumors. J Neurosurg 2:315, 1945
190. Folkman J: The vascularization of tumors. Sci Am 234:59, 1976
191. Algire GH, Chalkey HW: Vascular reactions of normal and malignant tissues in vivo: I. Vascular reactions of mice to wounds and to normal and neoplastic transplants. J Natl Cancer Inst 6:73, 1945
192. Folkman J: Tumor angiogenesis: a possible control point in tumor growth. Ann Intern Med 82:96, 1975
193. Cavallo T, Sade R, Folkman J, et al: Tumor angiogenesis rapid induction of endothelial mitoses demonstrated by autoradiography. J Cell Biol 54:408, 1972
194. Gimbrone MA Jr, Gullino PM: Neovascularization induced by intraocular xenografts of normal, preneoplastic and neoplastic mouse mammary tumors. Fed Proc 33:596, 1974
195. Greenblatt M, Shubik P: Tumor angiogenesis: transfilter diffusion studies in the hamster by the transparent chamber technique. J Natl Cancer Inst 41:111, 1968
196. Gimbrone MA Jr, Cotran RS, Leapman SB, et al: Tumor growth and neovascularization: an experimental model using the rabbit cornea. J Natl Cancer Inst 52:413, 1974
197. Gimbrone MA Jr, Leapman SB, Cotran RS, et al: Tumor angiogenesis: iris neovascularization at a distance from experimental intraocular tumors. J Natl Cancer Inst 50:219, 1973
198. Folkman J, Merler E, Abernathy C, et al: Isolation of a tumor factor responsible for angiogenesis. J Exp Med 133:275, 1971
199. Tuan D, Smith S, Folkman J, et al: Isolation of the nonhistone proteins of rat Walker carcinoma 256: their association with tumor angiogenesis. Biochemistry 12:3159, 1973
200. Folkman J: Tumor angiogenesis: therapeutic implications. N Engl J Med 285:1182, 1971
201. Eisenstein R, Sorgente N, Soble LW, et al: The resistance of certain tissues to invasion: penetrability of explanted tissues by vascularized mesenchyme. Am J Pathol 73:765, 1973
202. Brem H, Folkman J: Inhibition of tumor angiogenesis mediated by cartilage. J Exp Med 141:427, 1975
203. Wolter JR: The blood vessels of retinoblastomas. Arch Ophthalmol 66:545, 1961
204. Kuwabara T, Cogan DG: Studies of retinal vascular patterns: I. Normal architecture. Arch Ophthalmol 64:904, 1960
205. O'Connor JS, Laws ER Jr: Changes in histochemical staining of brain tumor blood vessels associated with increasing malignancy. Acta Neuropathol 14:161, 1969
206. Walton DS, Grant WM: Retinoblastoma and iris neovascularization. Am J Ophthalmol 65:598, 1968
207. Schechter I: Prolonged survival of glutaraldehyde-treated skin homografts. Proc Natl Acad Sci USA 68:1590, 1971
208. Perkins ES: Prostaglandins and the eye. Adv Ophthalmol 29:2, 1975
209. Eakins KE, Whitelocke RAF, Perkins ES, et al: Release of prostaglandins in ocular inflammation in the rabbit. Nature (New Biol) 239:248, 1972
210. Waitzman MB: Possible new concepts relating prostaglandins to various ocular functions. Surv Ophthalmol 14:301, 1970
211. Vane JR: Inhibition of prostaglandin synthesis as a mechanism of action for aspirin-like drugs. Nature (New Biol) 231:232, 1971
212. Bhattacherjee P, Eakins KE: Inhibition of the prostaglandin synthetase systems in ocular tissues by indomethacin. Br J Pharmacol 50:227, 1974

213. Tannock IF: Population kinetics of carcinoma cells, capillary endothelial cells, and fibroblasts in a transplanted mouse mammary tumor. Cancer Res 30:2470, 1970
214. Lindley J, Smith S: Histology and spontaneous regression of retinoblastoma. Trans Ophthalmol Soc UK 94:953, 1974
215. Nehen JH: Spontaneous regression of retinoblastoma. Acta Ophthalmol 53:647, 1975
216. Stewart JK, Smith JLS, Arnold EL: Spontaneous regression of retinoblastoma. Br J Ophthalmol 40:449, 1956
217. Boniuk M, Zimmerman LE: Spontaneous regression of retinoblastoma. Int Ophthalmol Clin 2:525, 1962
218. Boniuk M. Girard LJ: Spontaneous regression of bilateral retinoblastoma. Trans Am Acad Ophthalmol Otolaryngol 73:194, 1969
219. Cole WH: Spontaneous regression of cancer: the metabolic triumph of the host? Ann NY Acad Sci 230:111, 1974
220. Andersen SR, Jensen OA: Retinoblastoma with necrosis of central retinal artery and vein and partial spontaneous regression. Acta Ophthalmol 52:183, 1974
221. Zeiter HJ: Calcification and ossification in ocular tissue. Am J Ophthalmol 53:265, 1962
222. Selye H: Calciphylaxis. Chicago, University of Chicago Press, 1962
223. Verhoeff FH: Retinoblastoma undergoing spontaneous regression: calcifying agent suggested in treatment of retinoblastoma. Am J Ophthalmol 62:573, 1966
224. Wong PYK, Wuthier RE: Isolation and identification of prostaglandin PGBI in growth cartilage. Prostaglandins 8:125, 1974
225. Tashjian AH, Voelkel EF, Goldhaber P, et al: Prostaglandins, calcium metabolism and cancer. Fed Proc 33:81, 1974
226. Mullaney J: Retinoblastoma with DNA precipitation. Arch Ophthalmol 82:454, 1969
227. Datta BN: DNA coating of blood vessels in retinoblastoma. Am J Clin Pathol 62:94, 1974
228. Ahmed A: Some ultrastructural observations of hematoxyphil vascular change in oat-cell carcinoma. J Pathol 112:1, 1974
229. Klein G: Tumor-specific transplantation antigens: GHA Clowes Memorial Lecture. Cancer Res 28:625, 1968
230. Hellström KE, Hellström IE: Cellular immunity against tumor antigens. Adv Cancer Res 12:167, 1969
231. Klein G, Clifford P, Klein E, et al: Membrane immunofluorescence reactions of Burkitt lymphoma cells from biopsy specimens and tissue cultures. J Natl Cancer Inst 39:1027, 1967
232. Lewis MG, Ikonopisov RL, Nairn RC, et al: Tumor-specific antibodies in human malignant melanoma and their relationship to the extent of the disease. Br Med J 3:547, 1969
233. Morton DL, Malmgren RA, Holmes EC, et al: Demonstration of antibodies against human malignant melanoma by immunofluorescence. Surgery 64:233, 1968
234. Gold P, Gold M, Freedman SO: Cellular location of carcino-embryonic antigens of the human digestive system. Cancer Res 28:1331, 1968
235. Hellström IE, Hellström KE, Pierce GE, et al: Demonstration of cell-bound and humoral immunity against neuroblastoma cells. Proc Natl Acad Sci USA 60:1231, 1968
236. Gold P: Antigenic reversion in human cancer. Ann Rev Med 22:85, 1971
237. Char DH, Lepourhiet A, Leventhal B, et al: Cutaneous delayed hypersensitivity responses to tumor-associated and other antigens in acute leukemia. Int J Cancer 12:409, 1973
238. Bluming AZ, Ziegler JL, Fass L, et al: Delayed cutaneous sensitivity reactions to autologous Burkitt lymphoma protein extract: results of a prospective 2½ year study. Clin Exp Immunol 9:713, 1971
239. Char DH, Hollinshead A, Cogan DG, et al: Cutaneous delayed hypersensitivity

reactions to soluble melanoma antigen in patients with ocular malignant melanoma. N Engl J Med 291:274, 1974

240. Char DH, Ellsworth RM, Rabson AS, et al: Cell-mediated immunity to a retinoblastoma tissue culture line in patients with retinoblastoma. Am J Ophthalmol 78:5, 1974

241. Char DH, Herberman RB: Cutaneous delayed hypersensitivity responses of patients with retinoblastoma to standard recall antigens and crude membrane extracts of retinoblastoma tissue culture cells. Am J Ophthalmol 78:40, 1974

242. Hellström IE, Hellström KE, Pierce GE, et al: Cellular and humoral immunity to different types of human neoplasms. Nature 220:1352, 1968

243. Hellström IE, Hellström KE: Personal communication, 1976

244. Prehn RT: Immunomodulation of tumor growth. Am J Pathol 77:119, 1974

245. Hellström KE, Hellström IE: Lymphocyte-mediated cytotoxicity and blocking serum activity to tumor antigens. Adv Immunol 18:209, 1974

246. Hellström IE, Sjögren HO, Warner G, et al: Blocking of cell-mediated tumor immunity by sera from patients with growing neoplasms. Int J Cancer 7:226, 1971

247. Hellström IE, Hellström KE, Sjögren HO, et al: Serum factors in tumor-free patients cancelling the blocking of cell-mediated tumor immunity. Int J Cancer 8:185, 1971

248. Lilly F, Boyse EA, Old LJ: Genetic basis of susceptibility to viral leukemogenesis. Lancet 2:1207, 1964

249. McDevitt HO, Bodmer WF: Histocompatibility antigens, immune responsiveness and susceptibility to disease. Am J Med 52:1, 1972

250. Günther E, Albert E, Kueppers F, et al: The biological significance of the histocompatibility antigens. Humangenetik 14:173, 1972

251. Rogentine GN, Trapani RJ, Yankee RA, et al: HL-A antigens and acute lymphocytic leukemia: the nature of the HL-A2 association. Tissue Antigens 3:470, 1973

252. Bertrams J, Kuwert E, Böhme U, et al: HL-A antigens in Hodgkin's disease and multiple myeloma: increased frequency of W18 in both diseases. Tissue Antigens 2:41, 1972

253. Bertrams J, Schildberg P, Höpping W, et al: HL-A antigens in retinoblastoma. Tissue Antigens 3:78, 1973

254. Jones AL: Immunogenetics of retinoblastoma. Trans Ophthalmol Soc UK 94:945, 1974

Mano Swartz

19 Aqueous Humor Lactic Acid Dehydrogenase in Retinoblastoma

In 1971, Dias and associates reported elevated levels of aqueous humor LDH in patients with retinoblastoma.[1] This test has appeal because it is easy to obtain fluid by anterior chamber paracentesis and because laboratories are already equipped to determine LDH levels.

PROCEDURE

To test this observation, we studied the patients with leukocoria at the University of Illinois Eye and Ear Infirmary during 1973 and 1974.[2] Aqueous humor specimens were collected at examination under anesthesia from only those patients who had no evidence of anterior segment involvement. The paracentesis was performed with a 25-gauge needle on a tuberculin syringe, obtaining 0.2 ml of fluid. The paracentesis was done prior to scleral depression in order to prevent secondary aqueous production, and blood in the specimen was avoided, since red blood cells are rich in LDH. The anterior chamber was allowed to re-form spontaneously. Simultaneous serum specimens were drawn because clinical laboratories may report LDH levels in different units. We determined an aqueous-to-serum LDH ratio to eliminate the units and to facilitate the comparison of results from other laboratories.

In our series we assayed aqueous humor specimens from 7 eyes with histologically proved retinoblastoma, 16 eyes with nonretinoblastoma leukocoria, 5 eyes with uveal melanoma, and 6 eyes with senile cataract (Table 19.1, Fig. 19.1).

Our pediatric age group comparisons included eyes in which retinoblastoma was suspected, and eight were actually enucleated because retinoblastoma could not be excluded on clinical grounds. The highest aqueous-to-serum LDH ratio in this group occurred in an eye with active nematode endophthalmitis. We found relatively low values in five malignant melanomas, one examined immediately after enucleation. An eye tested immediately after enucleation for absolute glaucoma had a ratio of 0.23. In six cases of senile cataract where paracentesis was performed through the limbal groove at the time of cataract extraction, the aqueous LDH was also low.

RESULTS AND COMMENT

Aqueous-to-serum LDH ratios in six retinoblastoma-affected eyes ranged from 1.56 to 9.47. For all nonretinoblastoma cases the range of ratios was 0 to 1.03. The range of the ratios does not overlap, and the separation is therefore highly sig-

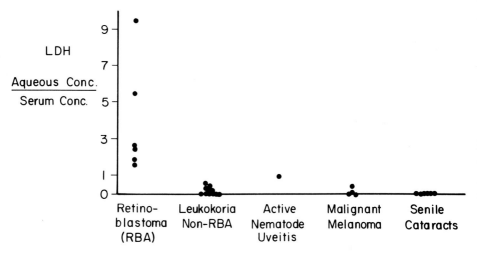

FIG. 19.1. Distributions of LDH ratios by diagnostic category. (From Swartz et al: Am J Oph-thalmol 78:612, 1974)

nificant. Kabak and Romano,[3] however, reported contradictory results with aqueous-to-serum ratios of LDH at less than one in four eyes with retinoblastoma. Although the total aqueous LDH was not elevated, Kabak and Romano[3] and others[4] have demonstrated variable increases in certain LDH isoenzymes. Albert has noted that cultured retinoblastoma cells liberate LDH into the media while other tumor cells such as malignant melanoma cells do not.[5]

Although the LDH assay has been used in an investigative manner, the following case report may indicate how the aqueous LDH assay may be used in the future as a clinical tool.

Case Report: A 14-month-old white girl had developed a right esotropia at the age of 12 months. In June 1971, examination under anesthesia confirmed the clinical diagnosis of bilateral retinoblastoma. The right eye was enucleated and the left eye was treated with 3850 rads of cobalt over one month. The patient also received intraarterial triethylenemelamine. In October 1971 she was found to have a total retinal detachment. An LDH assay was not done since the test was not being performed at this time. In January 1972 all lesions had enlarged, and in February she received intravenous cyclophosphamide and cryotherapy to the 9 o'clock lesion over a five-day period. In August 1972 cryotherapy was repeated, and she continued to take oral cyclophosphamide. In 1973 all lesions had regressed.

In January 1974 there was a questionable change in the inferotemporal lesion, but her aqueous LDH level was 0 compared with a serum value of 65. By May she was developing a progressive posterior subcapsular cataract, and no change was seen in her lesions. In December 1974 she had a discission and aspiration of the lens, and the cyclophosphamide treatment was stopped. By June 1975 she had developed a dense vitreous hemorrhage totally obscuring the view of the posterior segment. Her aqueous LDH level was 24 units. In July 1975 the eye was enucleated.

Table 19.1

*Summary of Cases Studied**

Diagnosis and Case No.	LDH Concentration (IU)		Aqueous Humor/ Serum LDH Ratio
	Aqueous Humor	Serum	
Retinoblastoma stage			
1 II	135	73	1.85
2 III	205	—	—
3 V	235	97	2.42
4 V	180	115	1.56
5 V	270	107	2.52
6 V	590†	102	5.78
7 V	900†	95	9.47
Nematode endophthalmitis			
1 Active	70	68	1.03
2 Inactive	20	68	0.29
3 Inactive	15	73	0.21
Trauma			
1 Intraretinal and intravitreal hemorrhage	3	90	0.03
2 Retinal detachment and rubeosis iridis	54	89	0.61
Choroidal hemangioma	2	54	0.04
PHPV	184‡	855‡	0.21
Retrolental fibroplasia with vitreous hemorrhage	7	79	0.09
Tuberous sclerosis			
1 Right eye	24	216	0.11
2 Left eye	17	216	0.09
Pediatric anterior segment surgery			
1 Pupillary membrane	0	74	0
2 Subluxated lens	0	76	0
3 Rubella cataract	0	—	0
4 Rubella cataract	5	88	0.06
5 Congenital cataract	0	—	0
6 Traumatic cataract	30	71	0.42
Malignant melanoma			
1 Ciliary body	30†	65	0.46
2 Ciliary body and choroid	36	—	—
3 Choroid	10	62	0.16
4 Choroid	0	65	0
5 Choroid	0.9	56	0.02
Senile cataract			
1	4.0	51	0.08
2	2.3	49	0.05
3	0	62	0
4	2.8	50	0.06
5	6.0	53	0.01
6	0	47	0

* *Adapted from Swartz et al: Am J Ophthalmol 78:612, 1974.*
† *Paracentesis performed immediately after enucleation.*
‡ *LDH was determined using a 184 duPont Automatic Clinical Analyzer (ACA units); normal serum values are 120 to 210 ACA units.*

Histopathologic examination revealed the posterior capsule to be intact in front of a dense vitreous hemorrhage. Examination of the tumors revealed dense calcification and necrosis with no viable tumor cells.

The use of LDH and other chemical substances in the diagnosis of retinoblastoma is still in the investigative stage. By following cases such as these longitudinally, we hope to learn at what point the LDH value becomes significant with respect to small volumes of active tumor cells. When we can accurately fingerprint the LDH from the retinoblastoma, for example, by isoenzymes, and can recognize false-positive results, then the decisions concerning treatment in children with leukocoria may be made more accurately without unnecessary delays.

REFERENCES

1. Dias PLR, Shanmuganthan SS, Rajaratnam M: Lactic dehydrogenase activity of aqueous humor in retinoblastoma. Br J Ophthalmol 55:130, 1971
2. Swartz M, Herbst RW, Goldberg MF: Aqueous humor lactic acid dehydrogenase in retinoblastoma. Am J Ophthalmol 78:612, 1974
3. Kabak J, Romano PE: Aqueous humor lactic dehydrogenase isoenzymes in retinoblastoma. Br J Ophthalmol 59:268, 1975
4. Keneko A: Lactic acid dehydrogenase activity and isoenzyme in the retinoblastoma. Acta Soc Ophthalmol Jap 76:672, 1972
5. Albert D: Personal communication, 1976

Robert M. Ellsworth

20 Current Concepts in the Treatment of Retinoblastoma

The treatment of retinoblastoma depends greatly on the extent of disease at the time treatment is contemplated. Thus we have developed a classification of intraocular retinoblastoma that indicates the chance of successfully treating an eye by a variety of methods depending on the size and location of the tumor (Table 20.1). This classification is not based on prognosis for life but for ocular survival.

Table 20.1

Prognosis for Successful Treatment

Group 1—Very favorable
Solitary tumor smaller than 4 disk diameters, at or behind the equator
Multiple tumors, none larger than 4 disk diameters, all at or behind the equator
Group 2—Favorable
Solitary tumor 4 to 10 disk diameters in size, at or behind the equator
Multiple tumors 4 to 10 disk diameters in size, all behind the equator
Group 3—Doubtful
Any lesion anterior to the equator
Solitary tumor larger than 10 disk diameters, behind the equator
Group 4—Unfavorable
Multiple tumors, some larger than 10 disk diameters
Any lesion extending anteriorly to the ora serrata
Group 5—Very unfavorable
Massive tumors involving over half the retina
Vitreous seeding

CLASSIFICATION OF RETINOBLASTOMA

Group 1 retinoblastomas (Fig. 20.1) are small tumors of less than 4 disk diameters. In analyzing our series, it seemed that tumors smaller than this size almost invariably did well, but larger tumors presented more difficulty. Multiplicity does not seem to alter the outcome, as long as the tumors are in the back part of the eye where irradiation treatment can be applied more directly.

Group 2 retinoblastomas measure 4 to 10 disk diameters (Fig. 20.2). These tumors, which occur either singly or in groups, have a slightly less favorable treatment prognosis because of an increased overall tumor mass.

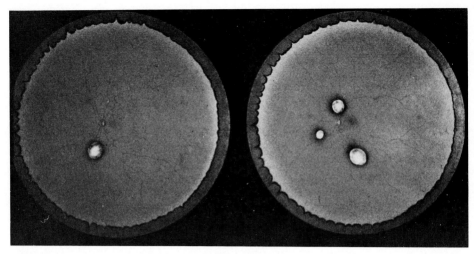

FIG. 20.1. Group 1 retinoblastoma. Left, Small single tumor. Right, Multiple small tumors.

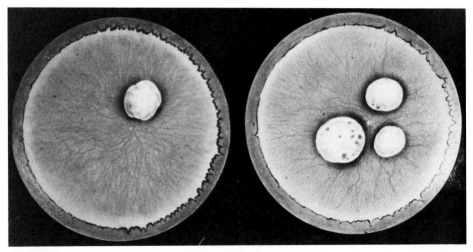

FIG. 20.2. Group 2 retinoblastoma. Left, Single tumor between 4 and 10 disk diameters. Right, Multiple tumors of 4 to 10 disk diameters.

Problems begin when the tumor is larger than 10 disk diameters or when it is located anterior to the equator. Tumors with these characteristics are classified in group 3 (Fig. 20.3). In analyzing a group of treatment failures some years ago, it appeared that an anterior location near the ora serrata, especially on the nasal side of the eye, seemed to be the common denominator. We thought there were a number of possible reasons. First, this series goes back to the 1930s, long before the day of the indirect ophthalmoscope, and lesions anterior to the equator simply were not seen. With the binocular indirect ophthalmoscope and scleral depression this detection is no longer a problem. The second problem is the difficulty in photo-

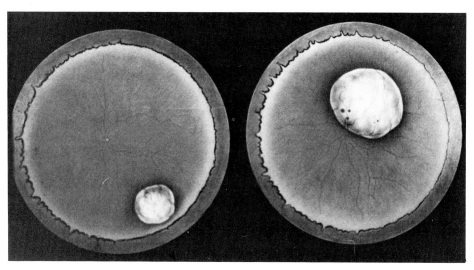

FIG. 20.3. Group 3 retinoblastoma. Left, Tumors located anterior to the equator. Right, Tumors larger than 10 disk diameters.

coagulating lesions near the ora serrata. This subject will be examined in further detail in the discussion of photocoagulation. The third difficulty in treating anterior tumors is the positioning of an x-ray beam. Irradiation at the ora serrata is within 1 mm of the lens. In attempts to avoid the lens and to prevent cataract formation, some of these anterior tumors may not receive a homogeneous dose of radiation.

Retinoblastoma seems to have a predilection for the ora serrata. There are several theoretical reasons for this tendency. First, the tumor cells may spread in the potential subretinal space until they reach the ora, where they are mechanically trapped and then grow (Fig. 20.4). Another explanation is that this area of the retina is not fully differentiated in young children. More mitotic change may occur in the anterior retina. Difficulties with anteriorly located tumors also occur when the tumor acquires a direct blood supply from the uvea, which seems to happen especially often if there is tumor adjacent to the ciliary body (Fig. 20.5). Once a retinoblastoma has a good choroidal blood supply, controlling its growth is very difficult.

Group 4 consists of multiple large tumors and lesions extending to the ora serrata (Fig. 20.6). These are more extreme examples of group 3 problems and anterior tumors often extend into the oral teeth.

Group 5 is comprised of massive tumors and vitreous seeding. Seeding is a bad prognostic sign and, in general, is a reflection of large tumor size (Fig. 20.7). Occasionally a small, highly pedunculated lesion begins to seed off the crown of the tumor. Under these circumstances, seeding is not as bad a sign as it may be when it is associated with larger tumors.

In addition to the intraocular manifestations of retinoblastoma, a child may present with exophthalmos and orbital disease (Fig. 20.8) or with widespread metastatic disease. Indeed, these are the most common signs of retinoblastoma in many parts of the world.

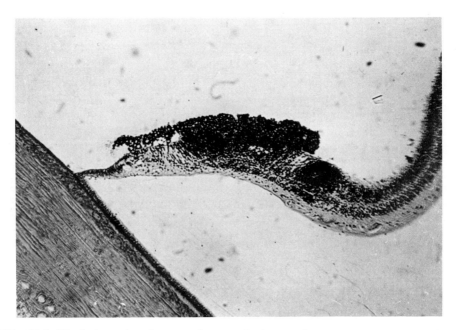

FIG. 20.4. Histologic section demonstrating spread of retinoblastoma cells into the potential subretinal space, where they travel to the ora serrata, are trapped, and grow.

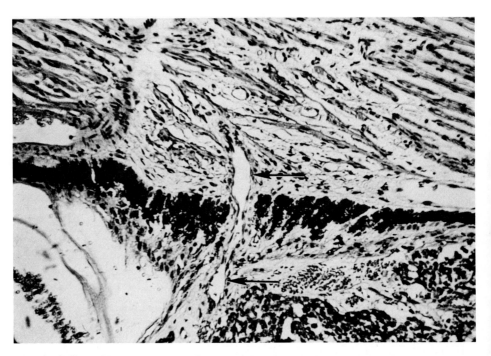

FIG. 20.5. Retinoblastoma growing adjacent to the ciliary body with a large blood vessel from the uveal tract to supply the tumor (arrows).

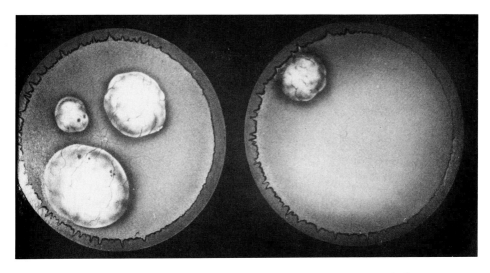

FIG. 20.6. Group 4 retinoblastoma. Left, Multiple large tumors. Right, Single large tumor extending to the ora serrata.

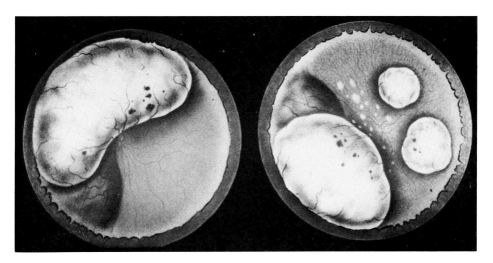

FIG. 20.7. Group 5 retinoblastoma. Left, Massive tumors. Right, Vitreous seeding.

GENERAL PRINCIPLES IN THE TREATMENT OF RETINOBLASTOMA

In general, patients with tumors in groups 1, 2, and 3 and perhaps the smaller, more posterior tumors in group 4 may be treated with irradiation alone. Desperate cases with massive tumors in an only remaining eye are treated with irradiation and chemotherapy, either triethylenemelamine or combined cyclophosphamide (Cytoxan) and vincristine for a year. Photocoagulation or cryotherapy may be used to

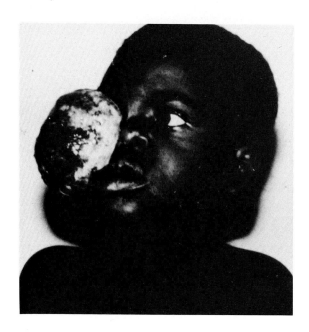

FIG. 20.8. Orbital retinoblastoma.

destroy any remaining tumor that does not disappear, especially in the anterior portion of the retina.

If the tumor recurs or a new tumor arises (if the patient is followed carefully, the tumor should not be very big when it is first seen), photocoagulation or freezing usually works. If the recurrence is bigger, a cobalt 60 plaque may be applied. A second dose of external beam irradiation is administered only as a last resort.

Although the prognosis for orbital tumors is poor, these cases can be cured. In reviewing our series of over 100 cases of orbital retinoblastomas, the five-year survival rate with treatment was 9 percent, compared with an overall patient survival rate of 82 percent in our total series of about 1300 cases. Some of these orbital cases were treated a number of years ago before the advent of modern chemotherapy; thus, the survival of patients with biopsy-proved orbital retinoblastoma should be better than 9 percent in the future.

In the past, we felt that exenteration was the best first step in orbital disease. In the past three or four years we have turned to irradiation and chemotherapy without exenteration, largely because we felt the outlook was worse than it is and we hated to put the child through a mutilating operation. The rationale for exenteration is to remove the principle tumor mass, with the hope that irradiation and chemotherapy will have a better chance of destroying remaining tumor cells. Experimental evidence indicates that chemotherapeutic agents are more effective against sheets of cells and isolated cells than they are against large masses of cells. Retinoblastoma in the eye is a relatively avascular, necrotic tissue whose blood supply may not be good enough to allow the chemotherapeutic agents access to the tumor.

The histologic characteristics of retinoblastoma growing outside the eye are entirely different. There are no areas of necrosis and no rosette formation. When the tumor has a good blood supply it blooms and grows rapidly. Our current treatment is irradiation, with a dose of 5000 rads calculated at the orbital apex, and chemotherapy using up to 500 mg of adriamycin as an inducing drug, followed by cyclophosphamide and vincristine for a year.

Cells that resemble tumor cells commonly appear in the orbit after enucleation. It is very difficult to identify tumor cells outside the eye. We hope to develop a fluorescent antibody slide technique to identify cells of retinal origin if they are seen in the orbit or in bone marrow, for example. Unfortunately, we cannot make such an identification at present. When the evidence for remaining tumor in the orbit is equivocal, we do not recommend exenteration. These children are treated with cyclophosphamide, vincristine, and radiation, but not with adriamycin, the long-term effects of which are unknown. Adriamycin may be necessary in certain desperate situations, but not when the indications are equivocal. When tumor cells remain in the proximal end of the cut optic nerve, the survival rate has been 60 percent; obviously this is an entirely different situation.

The mortality for metastatic retinoblastoma is 100 percent. This is tacit evidence that the stage of the disease at the time the child is first seen is the single most important factor in the outcome of treatment. There has never been a cure, and we aim for six months to a year of palliation, although lately we have been obtaining even better results. We think adriamycin is a very good inducing drug, and perhaps the combination of adriamycin, vincristine, and cyclophosphamide will enable these children to survive for longer periods. These children have all kinds of problems, but a lot can be done for them. If they have lesions in the mandible and cannot chew, irradiation of the jaw eliminates the pain and helps their alimentation. In addition, we try to learn something from these children while we make them as comfortable as possible. For example, several children had convulsions after intrathecal administration of new chemotherapeutic agents, and we went back to using methotrexate.

ENUCLEATION

We are basically concerned with the treatment of intraocular disease. Once or twice a year we see a patient who has bilateral, symmetric disease so advanced that bilateral enucleation is the only reasonable treatment. This is a terrible price to pay to cure a cancer, but sometimes it is the only alternative. More commonly, the presentation is asymmetric, with the disease far advanced in one eye, the eye that led to the detection of the disease, and the tumors in the other eye much smaller and more treatable.

The term "conservative treatment" has come to mean something short of removing the eye; while such treatment may be conservative as far as the eye is concerned, it certainly is not conservative in terms of the patient's life. It must always be kept in mind when treating retinoblastoma that the wager is sight for life; the decision to try to preserve sight is all right, as long as it is a reasonable gamble. But there sometimes comes a point when the risk to life is greater than the possible visual gain, and at that time the remaining eye must be removed.

What we are treating then, in most cases, is the eye remaining after the more advanced eye has been removed. In general, we treat any eye that has one quadrant of retina uninvolved with tumor even though that retina may be detached at the time of treatment. These detachments go back into place spontaneously over a period of 6 to 18 months if the tumor is controlled. We have seen several patients who had retinal breaks, but most of these have been exudative detachments that reattached spontaneously.

If both eyes are involved with small tumors (groups 1, 2, or 3), we treat both eyes. We have treated a large number of cases in this manner, but have not publicized this approach. We are concerned that clinicians will begin to treat advanced retinoblastoma in patients with a favorable fellow eye and that this practice will increase mortality.

In the presence of a normal fellow eye, treatment requires extreme care; however, our results have been so good in recent years, we feel that such treatment is justified. We occasionally treat both eyes in advanced, symmetric cases, eg, large tumors that threaten the macula in each eye. These tumors are often highly pendunculated and may overhang the nerve and macular area; the examiner may not be able to guess whether or not the fovea might be spared as the tumor shrinks down. We treat both eyes through crossed temporal portals with a tumor dose of 4500 rads in both eyes, and then watch them very carefully. About half of the patients treated in this way have ultimately lost one eye and had the other eye spared; one-fourth of these patients ultimately lost both eyes; and about one-fourth retained both eyes. This approach probably does not alter the prognosis for life, but one can never be certain.

IRRADIATION

Any of a variety of methods may be used to treat small tumors, but, unfortunately, most cases are so far advanced by the time we see them that only some type of irradiation will solve the problem. Retinoblastoma is an exquisitely radiosensitive tumor. Malignant melanoma is a highly radioresistant tumor, which explains in part why the treatment of these two diseases is so different.

Irradiation technique has varied widely over the years. We have tried using a great variety of procedures. Generally, no sedation is necessary, although once in a while a "tiger" requires sedation. Before the first treatment, the child may be acclimated to the equipment by putting him under the machine, turning it on without radiation, letting him listen to it hum, and having him realize that he is not going to be hurt. The Flexicast, made by the Picker X-Ray Corporation, is a very clever device, necessary to efficient execution of radiation therapy. It is a large pillow with two arms, made of heavy plastic, connected to a vacuum pump. The pillow is bunched up around the child's head with an arm of the pillow swung around the neck. Once the child's head is in place, the vacuum pump is turned on and the air is evacuated; the pillow becomes absolutely rigid and the child cannot move the head at all.

For a while, we had the children look at fixation devices to keep their eyes stationary: mobiles for little children and movies projected on the ceiling for older children. Then we watched these eyes on closed-circuit television and found that the plane of the ora serrata does not move very much and that there is no real need for any type of fixation. We have sutured the eyes so they would not move at all, but this practice added to the difficulty. We have found that we can irradiate these eyes without producing cataracts using only the Flexicast type of head fixation.

There are many advantages of supervoltage over orthovoltage irradiation, and two of them are highly significant. One is the sharp edge of the high-energy beam. With ordinary 220 to 280 kV irradiation and the beam directed through a temporal portal up to the back of the lens, the lens itself receives about 40 percent of the tumor dose. With a supervoltage beam, for example, the 22½ Mev Betatron beam that we use, the dose is less than 1 mm off the edge of the beam. The knife-edge beam can be moved up to the lens without producing a cataract. Since there are no cells in the back of the lens, I think that one can irradiate the back of the lens, the posterior 1 or 2 mm, without producing cataract. Even a resultant cataract is not too serious a complication because it does not occur immediately.

The second important advantage of supervoltage irradiation is an isodose curve, which indicates that the dose is greater at a depth than it is at the surface (Fig. 20.9). With the 200 kV orthovoltage irradiation that was used in the past, a beam directed to the right temple delivered a 100 percent dose to the skin. If we wanted to deliver 3500 rads to the main tumor mass from the temporal side (the tumor is usually 3 to 5 cm deep to the skin and bone), the skin received almost twice the dose the tumor did. This exposure explains why these patients developed bone deformities and skin changes. With the Betatron supervoltage beam, the dose is low at the surface and, due to tissue ionization, as the beam penetrates the tissue, the dose increases until, at a depth of about 4 or 5 cm, it is maximal. The tumor receives 100 percent of the dose, the surface skin receives about 40 percent, and the exit skin receives about 60 percent.

We have also experimented with various types of fractionation patterns. At one time we put the children to sleep and gave them 1000 rads at each of three sessions one week apart. A lot of hemorrhagic complications resulted, so we stopped that routine. The children are now treated three times a week, on Monday,

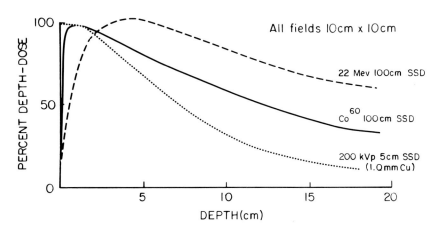

FIG. 20.9. Depth–dose curves for orthovoltage and supervoltage irradiation. Percentage depth-dose versus depth for orthovoltage x-rays, Cobalt 60 γ-rays, and 22 Mev x-rays.

Wednesday, and Friday. We try to keep the daily dose below 400 rads and the total weekly dose below 1200 rads; consequently, the average favorable cases in groups 1, 2, and 3 receive 3500 rads in nine treatments over three weeks. When the tumors are further advanced, we increase the dose to 4500 rads because we think we have one shot at these advanced eyes and the increased radiation exposure is a reasonable expedient.

Investigators around the country have urged us to increase our dose, others to decrease it. Dr. Henry Kaplan at Stanford, one of the world's leading radiobiologists, has suggested that since nervous tissue is highly resistant to radiation, we should go up to 5500 or 6000 rads. We have had occasion to use this dose and the vascular complications in the retina have been much greater. Dr. Richard Galbraith in Melbourne and Dr. Gil Cleasby in San Francisco have suggested that since certain of these tumors can be cured by 800 or 1000 rads, we should lower the dose. Certain tumors are so responsive that they can be controlled by less radiation. Dr. Galbraith has treated some patients with lower doses, but the recurrence rate was much higher. With a second course of irradiation, the cumulative dose is in the range of 8000 rads, where the complications are very high. We are certain that a dose in the range of 3500 to 4500 rads cures most retinoblastomas and does not irreparably damage most normal retinas. We use a single 3 × 4-cm temporal portal.

Regression Patterns Following Irradiation

One of the most difficult parts of the treatment of retinoblastoma is the interpretation of regression patterns. Unfortunately, these tumors do not all respond in the same way.

Years ago, Reese termed the first type of pattern "cottage cheese," because that is exactly what these regressions look like (Fig. 20.10). About two or three weeks after irradiation, over a period of several days, the tumor breaks down into this mass of cottage cheese-appearing material. We originally thought that this material was calcium, but we wondered how this calcification could happen so suddenly. A certain sequence of calcium and phosphate ions and enzymes is required and we could not imagine this process occurring in the eye. Then it was suggested that when DNA is put in suspension it takes on this appearance; we are now speculating that this cottage cheese material is largely DNA or a mixture of DNA and calcium.

The type 1 or cottage cheese pattern is the response of the anaplastic, undifferentiated areas of the tumor. It is easy to interpret because it happens very quickly and very dramatically, and it does not change thereafter. There is a terrific decrease in volume and this glistening white material remains. If the tumors are small, they may be entirely absorbed. A few patients—one of whom had six tumors in one eye —have no trace of tumor after radiation.

The type 2 pattern is entirely different; it does not present this cottage cheese material at all. The tumor simply shrinks down and becomes slightly less vascular (Fig. 20.11). We call this type 2 pattern the "differentiated" pattern because these tumors have Flexner-Wintersteiner rosettes and fleurettes, and they do not respond as dramatically to irradiation. After irradiation the tumor decreases in volume and

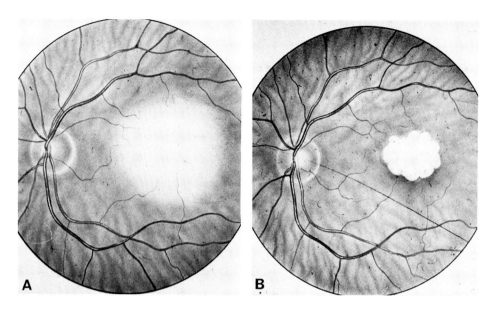

FIG. 20.10. Type 1 regression pattern. **A.** Before irradiation. **B.** After irradiation. Note cottage cheese-like appearance.

loses its pink color and capillary injection, but it remains elevated and the normal retinal vessels sweep over the surface. Irradiation does not change the original appearance very much, and we follow them much more closely because their course is unpredictable. We believe that these tumors do not have as much growth potential as those with large areas of undifferentiated or anaplastic cells. We have had occasion to examine one of these regressions histologically when a child was killed in an automobile accident, and the tumor cells looked viable. However, microscopic examination does not reveal whether tumor cells are capable of multiplying and spreading. These tumors seem to be in a state of suspended animation. We have followed some of these patients for 20 or 30 years and the irradiation seems to have sterilized their tumors.

The third or mixed type of regression pattern is the most common one: foci of cottage cheese material represent the anaplastic portion of the tumor and there is some gray material around it (Fig. 20.12). Zimmerman has described the gray material, the better differentiated portions of the tumor, as "fish flesh."

Often the pigment annulus that forms around the tumor vest is so dramatic that one would think the tumor had been photocoagulated. Telangiectatic vessels on the surface may be a response to irradiation or may be residual tumor vessels. Wolter has shown that the normal vascular framework of retinoblastoma has many microaneurysms and telangiectatic vessels in it. When many of these abnormal vessels are present, they are often interpreted as a sign of tumor growth when they are not that at all. Occasionally, a very large tumor, when irradiated, shrinks, breaks apart, and scatters gray material around the vitreous (Fig. 20.13). The clinical picture is frightening, and one is never sure whether that material is active or not.

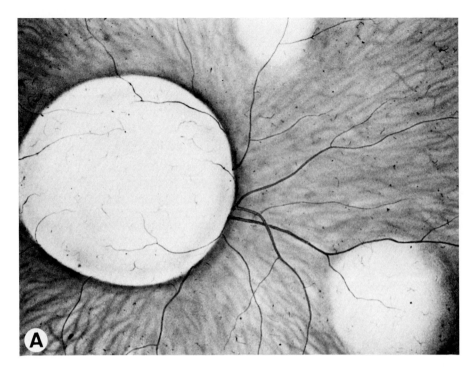

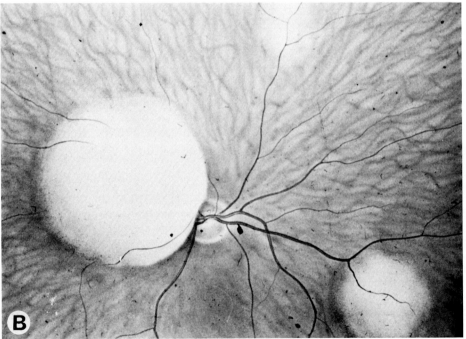

FIG. 20.11. Type 2 regression pattern. **A.** Before irradiation. **B.** After irradiation.

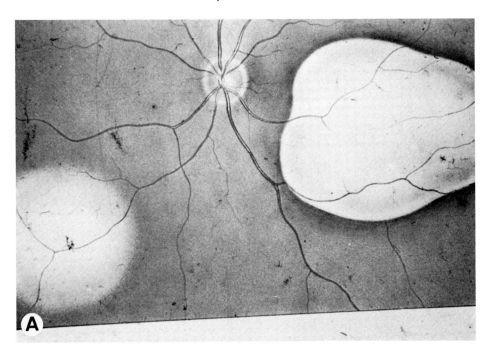

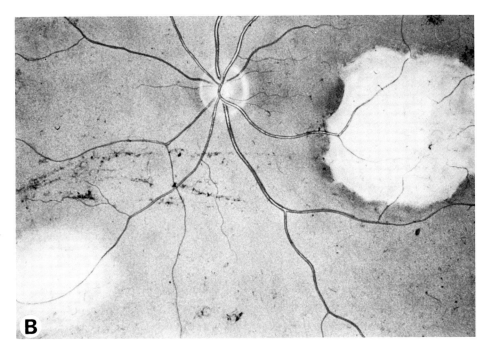

FIG. 20.12. Type 3 mixed regression pattern. **A.** Before irradiation. **B.** After irradiation. Note cottage cheese-like material and grayish "fish flesh."

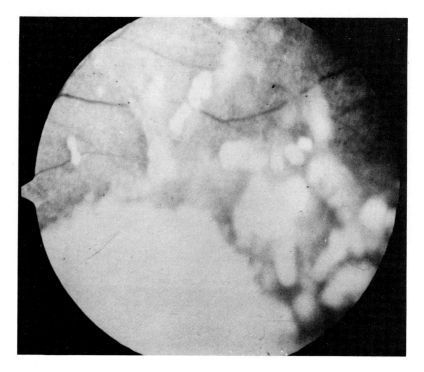

FIG. 20.13. Breakdown of a large tumor with material scattered in the vitreous after irradiation.

If there are any viable portions of the tumor, they may settle down on the lower part of the retina and establish implantation growths. This vitreous scattering must be followed very carefully; we often examine these children under anethesia once a month.

Complications

Vascular necrosis is the greatest problem in ocular irradiation (Fig. 20.14). The endothelium of the retinal vessels is damaged, and, unfortunately, the retinal vasculature is an end-arterial system. At dosage levels over 6000 rads, this problem is very serious. When hemorrhage into the vitreous is bad enough to cause secondary glaucoma, the eye hardly ever survives. Hemorrhages around the nervehead or in the retina and limited vitreous hemorrhage may absorb as the vessels repair themselves, and the eye may survive with useful vision. Dramatic salt-and-pepper stippling of the retina is especially marked when the retina is detached at the time of irradiation.

We increase the dose to 4500 rads in advanced cases because we really only have one chance to arrest this disease. There is probably at least a twofold difference in radioresponsiveness between one tumor and another. There is probably an equal variation between one individual and another in the response of normal tissues

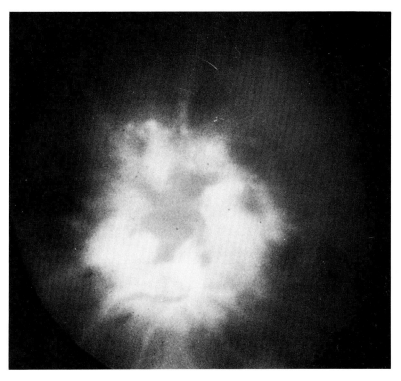

FIG. 20.14. Irradiation-induced vascular necrosis and hemorrhage around the optic nervehead.

to irradiation. That is, in certain sensitive individuals retinal vascular damage occurs at 3500 rads, although this degree of sensitivity is very rare. At 6000 rads, such damage occurs about 60 percent of the time, and at 8000 rads, about 90 percent of the time.

If a second course of external beam irradiation must be administered in an only eye with useful vision, the total dose is about 8000 rads. At this level there is a 90 percent chance of complications. Most eyes do not survive a total dose at that level, even if the two courses of irradiation have been separated by several years—long enough, one might think, to allow normal tissue repair.

A less common complication is cataract (Fig. 20.15), which is really no problem at all. In most cases, if the irradiation is properly administered, it does not occur; even if a cataract does develop, it does not appear for two or three years. In the rather large series of rhabdomyosarcomas of the orbit that we have treated with a lens dose of 5000 rads, the eyes do not get a cataract for two or three years. If the cataract does occur at a time when it is important to observe the fundus to see what the tumor is doing, the cataract has to be removed and there is a slight danger of tumor cells spreading after aspiration or phacoemulsification in an eye with active tumor.

Radiation dermatitis was a serious complication in the old series, but with

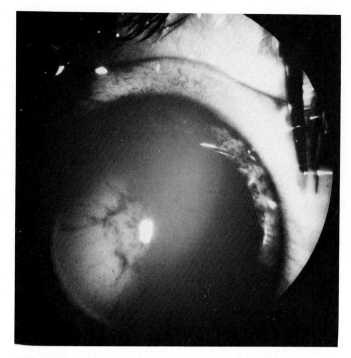

FIG. 20.15. Irradiation-induced stellate posterior subcapsular cataract.

supervoltage radiation neither dermatitis nor bone atrophy is a problem. The anterior segment is not irradiated with the technique we use, so glaucoma and anterior segment problems are very rare.

The problem of irradiation-induced tumors is one that is concerning us more and more. About eight or ten years ago, we were concerned by some late deaths in children with retinoblastoma. We usually feel that if children do well for two years after treatment of retinoblastoma they are cured, but some of these children were dying at 10 to 20 years of age. We reviewed these cases and found three possible causes of death. Some were dying of late metastasis of retinoblastoma. We think this event is very unusual, and indeed it is difficult to diagnose. As mentioned previously, retinoblastoma outside the eye does not look like retinoblastoma within the eye. Outside the eye it is a wild, anaplastic tissue with much more cytoplasm in the cells. It does not form rosettes. A pathologist may speculate on three or four possible origins of these tumor cells, and retinoblastoma will probably not be among the suggestions. The origin of many of these anaplastic tumors that arise later in life is not readily identifiable, so there is a possibility that some of them are truly late metastases.

Irradiation-induced tumor is another possible cause of late death in children with retinoblastoma. Other primary neoplasms not related to retinoblastoma itself or to the treatment of retinoblastoma developed in a number of patients. Six or eight osteogenic sarcomas occurred in the distal femur, a common location for osteosarcoma. We have seen several cases of Wilms' tumor, a thyroid tumor, rhabdomyosarcomas, and many other neoplasms. Some children with retinoblastoma have a deletion of the long arm of chromosome 13, and the others may well have a small chromosomal abnormality that we have not been able to detect by current methods of chromosome analysis. Nevertheless, some chromosomal anomaly predisposes these patients to retinoblastoma; it may also predispose them to osteogenic sarcoma later in life or to many other kinds of primary tumors. If this hypothesis is true, it represents one of the few times a genetic predisposition has been related to the development of neoplasms—not to a specific one, but to an underlying constitution that predisposes people to tumors. "Tumor diathesis" is a concept that has been popular for a long time. Certain families seem to be prone to cancers, and the above hypothesis may explain this phenomenon. We are very wary of administering radiation of any kind to children with bilateral retinoblastoma, and yet in most of these patients it is the only treatment that can control the tumor.

Chemotherapy

We have used chemotherapy in two different situations: as an adjunct to irradiation in the treatment of intraocular disease and as a method to reduce the mortality after unilateral enucleation.

Chemotherapy can be effective as an adjunct to irradiation in the treatment of advanced tumors. There are theoretical reasons to suppose that irradiation and chemotherapeutic agents work at different points in dividing chromosomes and that their effect would therefore be additive, or perhaps even synergistic. We used triethylenemelamine throughout the earlier series because it was a relatively safe and rapidly fixed alkylating agent. Dr. George Hyman labeled it with radioactive carbon and injected it into the internal carotid artery in an eye that was going to be removed. Differential counts of carbon 14 were taken in the tumor from the eye and in tissue from a bone marrow biopsy. The concentration of the fixed triethylenemelamine was higher in the tumor tissue than it was in the bone marrow; this finding was the rationale for using this particular drug intraarterially. When the drug has been given intravenously, the concentrations in both the eye tissue and the bone marrow have been the same. Although intraarterial administration has been effective, we have come to believe that the advantage it provides is probably not worth the neck dissection it necessitates. We now think that some of the newer, more easily administered agents may be just as effective.

The other use of chemotherapy is in reducing the mortality of the disease. We have not used it in this way in the past because the mortality rate of our patients has been only 18 percent. If we treat all children with chemotherapy, we will, ipso facto, poison 82 percent of them unnecessarily. We now have some clues, based on findings in the enucleated eye, as to which children will have a recurrence in the orbit. We treat these children with chemotherapy. We now have a new protocol in which children who have unilateral group 5 retinoblastoma and a normal fellow eye are treated by the classical enucleation procedure followed by chemotherapy; the chemotherapy consists of cyclophosphamide and vincristine used together in two-week courses for one year. We intend to compare the mortality in this series with an historical control to determine whether this type of chemotherapy does indeed reduce mortality from this disease. It will take four or five years to complete this study.

DIATHERMY

There is no question that diathermy can control small tumors, but it usually results in much more retinal damage than external beam irradiation (Fig. 20.16).

PHOTOCOAGULATION AND CRYOTHERAPY

Photocoagulation is a tremendously valuable adjunct in the treatment of retinoblastoma (Fig. 20.17). Indeed, in a child with retinoblastoma who has a germinal mutation, if the tumors are small they should be treated by photocoagulation or cryotherapy and not by external beam irradiation, if possible. In the majority of cases, however, these conditions are not met. One sees small retinoblastomas usually in only two circumstances: (1) a tiny tumor in the macula that causes an esotropia is noticed on routine fundus examination, or (2) a small tumor is found in a child with a family history of retinoblastoma (hereditary) who, from birth, routinely undergoes examination under anesthesia. When we do find these small tumors, we treat them first with photocoagulation or cryotherapy; we treat the larger tumors with cobalt plaques before proceeding to external beam irradiation to try to avoid the exposure to the mutagenic effects of irradiation. Photocoagulation can be performed all the way out to the ora serrata and up onto the pars plana with the use of the Searcey pick for fixation and indentation. There are almost no complications with photocoagulation when it is performed with the proper indications. Occasionally an exudative detachment or hemorrhage occurs. Unlike regression after irradiation, the whole tumor must disappear after photocoagulation or cryotherapy. If the tumor does not disappear entirely with one treatment, it must be retreated until it does.

The rationale for photocoagulation is based on the fact that retinoblastomas, at least during a considerable portion of their growth, depend entirely on the retinal circulation. If the circulation from the retina is interrupted with photocoagulation, the tumor shrinks away and disappears. If the tumor permeates Bruch's membrane and gets a good vascular component from the choroid, photocoagulation is not nearly as effective as otherwise. Heavy treatment with photocoagulation can obliterate the choroidal circulation entirely if it has a wide enough base, but perforating arteries from behind, especially the short ciliaries, is always a concern. If the tumor does not depend on the retinal circulation, photocoagulation will probably not be effective.

Cryotherapy and photocoagulation are roughly equivalent in the size of the tumor they can treat, ie, up to about 6 disk diameters without too much elevation. Cryotherapy destroys tissue by interrupting the microcirculation of the tumor itself and by intracellular ice crystal formation, with direct destruction of the tumor. It

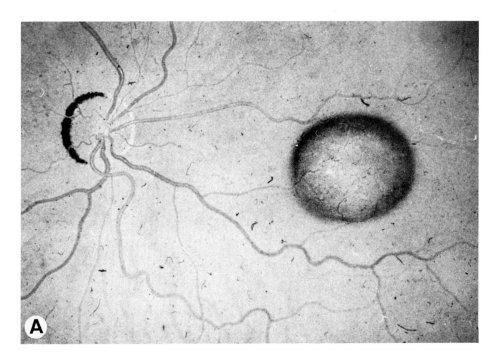

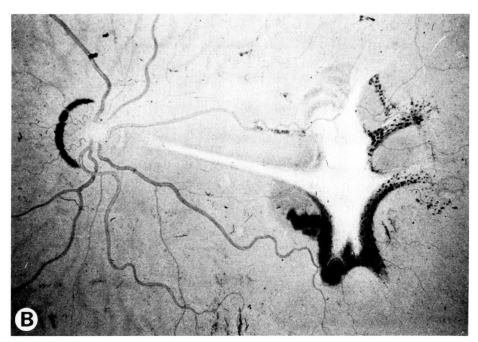

FIG. 20.16. Retinoblastoma treated by diathermy. **A.** Before treatment. **B.** After treatment resulting in marked macular fibrosis.

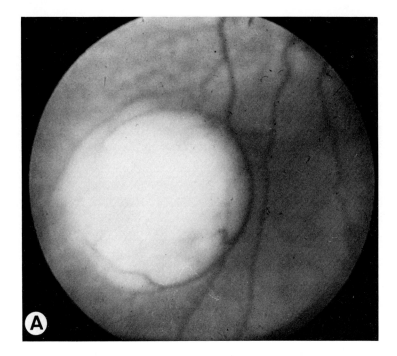

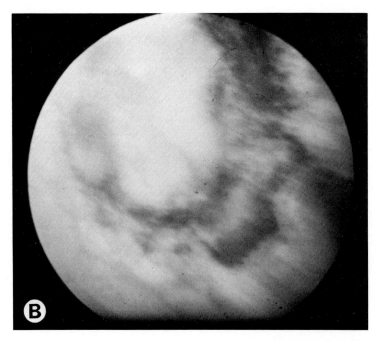

FIG. 20.17. Retinoblastoma treated by photcoagulation. **A.** Before treatment. **B.** After treatment.

has become popular to freeze three times, and there is some evidence that freezing, partial thawing, and refreezing does more damage to the cells than allowing them to heat up in between. There is no question that cryotherapy destroys small tumors. They can be treated transconjunctivally with good visualization through the indirect ophthalmoscope. Cryotherapy is somewhat easier than photocoagulation for an anterior lesion, but the methods are roughly interchangeable. One of the specific indications for cryotherapy is a tumor that has been treated with photocoagulation with obliteration of all retinal vessels but a persistent tumor vest.

COBALT 60 PLAQUES

Cobalt 60 plaques are very effective in the treatment of retinoblastoma. The basic indication in our series was a recurrence after external beam irradiation. If, in an eye with four or five tumors, one tumor recurs and it is too large to be treated by photocoagulation or cryotherapy, it may be effectively treated with a plaque. This treatment is especially suitable if there is choroidal extension, which presents several clinical signs: (1) rapid growth over a period of several weeks or a month or two; (2) very high pedunculation on a narrow base; and (3) a yellow color over the dome of the tumor. Moreover, a single tumor up to 10 or 12 mm in size should be treated with a plaque rather than external beam irradiation. The dose at the tumor apex is 4000 rads. In an average hemispheric tumor, the scleral dose is about 30,000 rads; the sclera generally takes this dose very well. If these tumors are pedunculated and highly elevated, by the time 4000 rads reaches the tumor apex, the base dose may be as high as 80,000 or 90,000 rads.

Lorenz E. Zimmerman

21 Ciliary Body Tumors in Children

In studying tumors of the ciliary epithelium, I have repeatedly been impressed by their remarkable polymorphism—a feature that I do not believe has been pointed out before. I believe it can be accounted for, at least in part, by the pluripotentiality of that part of the embryonic medullary epithelium that gives rise to the ciliary and iridic epithelium.

To obtain a better perspective, I have reviewed all such tumors that are on file in the Armed Forces Institute of Pathology Registry of Ophthalmic Pathology and have solicited additional cases from a number of other laboratories. It is the purpose of this presentation to summarize some of my observations, with emphasis on the remarkable histopathologic variations that may be encountered among these tumors. The follow-up studies are far from complete, so only limited information on the biologic behavior of these neoplasms will be included. Because of the selective nature of the case material used in this study, meaningful estimates of the relative frequency of the various tumors cannot be provided.

EMBRYOLOGIC, HISTOLOGIC, AND PATHOLOGIC CONSIDERATIONS

During early embryologic development in the human, between the fifth and eighth weeks, the medullary epithelium that forms the inner surface of the optic cup anteriorly is virtually an undifferentiated multinucleated membrane (Fig. 21.1), while the outer layer exhibits marked melanogenic activity.[1] The main evidence of differentiation in the inner layer at this early stage of development is the polarization that can be observed along both surfaces of the tissue. Along its outer surface, where the nonpigmented layer of medullary epithelium faces the pigment epithelium, development of an outer limiting membrane can be observed. Along its inner surface, the medullary epithelium appears to project protoplasmic processes that are in intimate contact with the vitreous. Stains for acid mucopolysaccharide reveal an abundance of hyaluronic acid along the inner vitreal surface of the medullary epithelium, but there is no evidence of the elaboration of mucopolysaccharide along its outer surface.

This report has been adapted and modified from the Norman McAlister Gregg Lecture, part I: The remarkable polymorphism of tumours of the ciliary epithelium. Trans Aust Coll Ophthalmol 2:114, 1970.

357

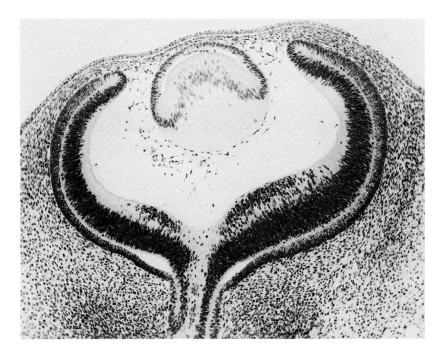

FIG. 21.1. Optic cup of human embryo at about the fifth week of gestation. The medullary epithelium anteriorly is a completely undifferentiated multilayered structure, except that the cells are polarized and an internal limiting membrane is readily visualized along the retinovitreal interface. ×77. (From Zimmerman: Trans Aust Coll Ophthalmol 2:114, 1970)

Later, as the iris and ciliary body begin to develop, the undifferentiated multi-nucleated medullary epithelium gradually gives rise to a layer of columnar or cuboidal cells that continue to exhibit evidence of the formation of both the extracellular fibrillar materials and the mucopolysaccharide of the vitreous along its inner surface. Subsequently, during the fetal stage of development, the primitive medullary epithelium disappears, having given rise to the various neuronal, photo-receptor, and glial elements of the sensory retina posteriorly, the nonpigmented cuboidal and columnar epithelium of the pars plicata and pars plana regions of the ciliary body, the two layers of pigmented epithelium of the iris, and the peculiar smooth muscles (dilator and sphincter) of the iris. In birds, the medullary epithelium also gives rise to the striated (skeletal) muscles of the iris. Whether the cortical cells of the vitreous that may be seen along the inner surface of the retina and ciliary body are also derived from the primitive medullary epithelium, or from the mesoderm associated with the hyaloid vessels, is uncertain. The ciliary epithelium may be observed to increase pathologically its production of cells, fibrils, and mucopolysaccharide. A prominent contribution to the formation of cyclitic membranes, for example, is this proliferation of ciliary epithelium accompanied by the deposition of collagenous fibrils and the accumulation of acid mucopolysaccharides. With microcyst and macrocyst formation, and in association with certain tumors, there is often evidence of the elaboration of these extracellular materials by the ciliary epithelium.[2]

CLASSIFICATION OF TUMORS
OF THE CILIARY EPITHELIUM

In the past we have not had a good classification of tumors of the ciliary epithelium. One can also criticize the names for individual tumors, just as Verhoeff[3] did in his discussion of Fralick and Wilder's description[4] of a tumor that they called "intraocular diktyoma and glioneuroma." Verhoeff was obviously distressed that the name he had suggested, "terato-neuroma," had been rejected by Fuchs, who preferred "diktyoma."[5] The latter term, referring to the network of interlacing sheets and cords of medullary epithelium observed in some of these tumors, is the one that has been most widely used over the years for the tumor that is today generally classified as a medulloepithelioma. The latter term, suggested by Grinker,[6] was based, at least in part, on a misconception. Grinker stated: "In the retina, medullary epithelium persists in almost undifferentiated form throughout adult life in the epithelium of the pars ciliaris retina, and it is from this tissue that medulloepitheliomas of the retina usually arise." Actually the mature ciliary epithelium is not poorly differentiated tissue, and the acquired tumors that arise from it do not closely resemble the medulloepitheliomas that arise from the embryonic medullary epithelium.

Nevertheless, certain authoritative writers such as Andersen[7] and Reese[8] have followed Grinker's suggestion, and include under the heading of medullepithelioma both embryonic and acquired tumors of the ciliary body. In Andersen's classification, the former are called "embryonal medulloepitheliomas." Both designations are objectionable. To better understand why they are objectionable, let me first refer to Willis' concept of medulloepitheliomas.[9] He would classify them among the embryonic tumors (eg, Wilms' tumor of the kidney, retinoblastoma, neuroblastoma, and embryonal rhabdomyosarcomas)—neoplasms that arise from embryonic or fetal tissues, or, in certain instances, from tissues that normally complete their differentiation after birth. Following this concept, the term "embryonal medulloepithelioma" becomes redundant (medulloepitheliomas are by definition embryonic neoplasms), and "adult medulloepithelioma" becomes contradictory. Reese discusses acquired tumors of the ciliary epithelium under two headings—"benign and malignant epitheliomas" and "adult-type medulloepitheliomas"—but he is not at all clear as to the criteria he uses to distinguish the two groups. It seems that the lesions he places in the category designated adult-type medulloepithelioma really belong with the benign and malignant epitheliomas.*

Duke-Elder and Perkins[10] tried to classify these tumors, but their classification is also objectionable on several grounds. They, too, place "adult epitheliomas" under the heading of medulloepitheliomas, and all these are grouped among the malignant neoplasms. They apparently do not recognize a benign form of medulloepithelioma. In addition, they place a tumor that they call "papillary cystadenoma" among the malignant neoplasms. If that tumor is malignant, then the name it has been given is inappropriate, because the name signifies a benign neoplasm. While criticizing the classifications proposed by others, I should also admit that the dis-

---

* In the third edition of his book, published in 1976 after this manuscript went to press, Reese had adopted the classification I proposed (Table 21.1).

cussion of these tumors that Hogan and I provided in our book on ophthalmic pathology[11] is very poor, and our classification of them is totally inadequate. These deficiencies will be corrected in our next edition.

To return again to Willis' comments on embryonic neoplasms, he points out that they may show heteroplastic formation of tissues that are not normally present in the affected organ.[9] For example, in Wilms' tumor of the kidney, in addition to embryonic renal structures, one may see the formation of rhabdomyoblasts and well-differentiated skeletal muscle by the tumor's mesenchyme. Among the ciliary body tumors that I believe to belong to the medulloepithelioma category, one may also see heteroplastic formation of such tissues as brain, cartilage, and skeletal muscle that are not normally present in the human eye. In the classification offered here, this group of medulloepitheliomas is designated by the term "teratoid," to put emphasis on their heteroplastic features. Some of these heteroplastic elements have been described previously. Andersen found cartilage in 20 percent of medulloepitheliomas,[7] and the presence of various tissues reminiscent of brain has been described many times. Only recently, however, has the formation of skeletal muscle been observed in the mesenchyme associated with these medulloepitheliomas.[12] Attempts have been made to take note of the heteroplastic elements in naming the tumors, though not in an entirely satisfactory manner. Fralick and Wilder,[4] for example, used the name "intraocular diktyoma and glioneuroma," which specifically emphasizes the glial and neuronal differentiation; but that name fails to indicate the cartilage that was present in the tumor.

From a conceptual point of view, it is logical (and probably correct) to assume that intraocular medulloepitheliomas are congenital neoplasms. At least the *analage* from which the tumors arise are undoubtedly present at birth, even though the clinical manifestations of the tumor that lead to its recognition may not develop until long after birth. In striking contrast, the group that other authors have called "adult medulloepitheliomas" I believe arise from fully differentiated ciliary epithelium that subsequently undergoes neoplastic change, not infrequently after having passed through a stage of nonneoplastic reactive hyperplasia (pseudoadenomatous hyperplasia). Thus, I suggest that these neuroepithelial tumors of the ciliary body be divided into two main groups, the congenital and the acquired, as presented in Table 21.1.

The fact that the vast majority of medulloepitheliomas arise from the ciliary region is a reflection of the fact that the primitive medullary epithelium remains incompletely differentiated in this region longer than elsewhere; however, rarely one may encounter typical benign and malignant medulloepitheliomas in the retina or even in the optic nervehead.[8]

The classification offered here applies to both the pigmented and the nonpigmented epithelial tumors. In many cases one cannot arbitrarily categorize a tumor as being pigmented or nonpigmented. While there are occasional tumors, particularly among the adenomas, that do appear to be purely pigmented or nonpigmented, the majority in both the congenital and the acquired groups show evidence of differentiation in both directions, with the formation of pigmented and nonpigmented epithelium. Nevertheless, the discussion of congenital tumors that follows will mainly be concerned with the predominantly nonpigmented tumors.

Table 21.1

Classification of Neuroepithelial
Tumors of the Ciliary Body

Congenital
    Glioneuroma
    Nonteratoid medulloepithelioma
      Benign
      Malignant
    Teratoid medulloepithelioma
      Benign
      Malignant
Acquired
    Pseudoadenomatous hyperplasia
    Adenoma
      Solid
      Papillary
      Pleomorphic
    Adenocarcinoma
      Solid
      Papillary
      Pleomorphic

CONGENITAL TUMORS

Glioneuroma

Glioneuroma is represented by only a few cases. One recorded by Kuhlenbeck and Haymaker[13] among a group of brain tumors contained neuronal as well as spongioblastic elements, and a remarkably similar case was reported by Spencer[14] in 1962. The former tumor was in a baby who was born with a slightly enlarged eye, in which the opaque cornea resembled sclera. At the age of two months, the blind eye was enucleated because an intraocular neoplasm was suspected. The tumor was really a benign choristomatous malformation of the entire anterior segment. On one side of the eye, the iris, ciliary body, and anterior choroid could not be identified. They were replaced by a large mass resembling brain tissue, which was adherent to the cornea and almost totally surrounded the cataractous lens. On the opposite side, a small, partially differentiated iris and ciliary body were present. In some planes of section one could trace direct continuity of the nonpigmented ciliary epithelium into the choristomatous mass behind the lens, while in other planes of section, the presence of tissue resembling brain tissue could be observed adjacent to the iridic pigment epithelium at the pupillary margin, where one would normally expect to see sphincter muscle. Some cleft-like spaces lined by ciliated neuroepithelial cells were present in the main mass attached to the cornea. In some, the lining cells resembled ependyma, while in others they were heavily pigmented. Ganglion cells and axis cylinders were present, but this tumor did not contain sheets and cords of embryonic medullary epithelium, the hallmark of the medulloepitheliomas.

Nonteratoid Medulloepithelioma

A nonteratoid medulloepithelioma is a tumor that is derived from the embryonic medullary epithelium and contains as its most significant component multilayered sheets and cords of poorly differentiated neuroepithelial cells (Figs. 21.2, 21.3). In some tumors, particularly the benign ones, these elements have a strikingly similar appearance to the normal embryonic retina and ciliary epithelium (Fig. 21.1), and they account for most of the tumor's mass. In others, particularly the malignant medulloepitheliomas and the teratoid medulloepitheliomas, structures resembling the embryonic medullary epithelium may form only an inconspicuous component of the tumor.

BENIGN NONTERATOID MEDULLOEPITHELIOMA. Benign nonteratoid medulloepitheliomas vary from small placoid tumors projecting into the posterior chamber from the inner surface of the ciliary epithelium in eyes that are otherwise relatively normal, to huge masses that have largely replaced much of the anterior segment of the eye. The latter frequently have produced such complications as glaucoma, cataract, and retinal detachment by the time the eye is enucleated. The larger tumors often appear to have developed in areas where the neuroepithelial layers are colobomatous, and the presence of a colobomatous defect makes possible spread of the tumor, even though it may be histologically benign, into the uvea.

These tumors also tend to have considerable myxoid stroma that extends onto

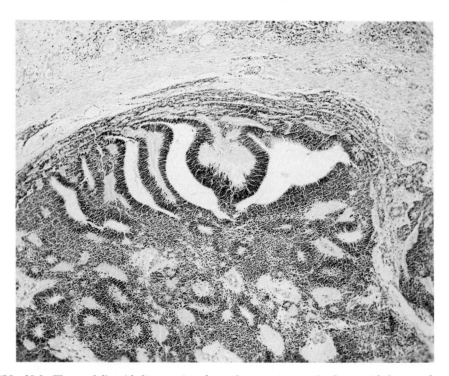

FIG. 21.2. The medulloepithelioma arises from the nonpigmented ciliary epithelium and produces intricate convolutions enclosing lumina of various shapes and sizes. The neoplasm is composed of structures resembling the medullary epithelium of the embryonic ciliary epithelium and retina. ×48. (From Zimmerman: Trans Am Ophthalmol Soc 69:210, 1971)

the posterior surface of the lens. In both its configuration and its microscopic appearance, this stromal tissue may resemble PHPV. The histologic relationship of the sheets and cords of medullary epithelium to this myxoid stroma is usually reminiscent of the relationship of the primitive retina and ciliary body to the vitreous being elaborated along the inner retinal surface. Just as the embryonic retina and ciliary epithelium are polarized at a very early stage in their differentiation, so are these analogous structures in the tumor (Figs. 21.2, 21.3). One surface of the neoplastic sheets and cords of medullary epithelium is analogous, developmentally and in its microscopic appearance, to the inner limiting membrane of the retina and ciliary epithelium. Protoplasmic extensions of the cells along this surface project into the relatively acellular, slightly fibrillar, myxoid tissue that seems to form the tumor's stroma. This tissue is rich in acid mucopolysaccharide that is sensitive to hyaluronidase.[2] The opposite surface of the neoplastic sheets of medullary epithelium forms a structure resembling the outer limiting membrane of the embryonic retina. No mucopolysaccharide is present along this surface.

Typically, the sheets are folded back upon themselves, forming enclosed or partially enclosed areas. Usually it is the surface analogous to the outer limiting membrane that forms the luminal surface of these tubular or slit-like spaces, and in such structures no acid mucopolysaccharide fills the lumen. The formations that have small lumina will usually appear empty, while larger ones may contain cellular debris or serous exudate. When the surface that is analogous to the inner limiting

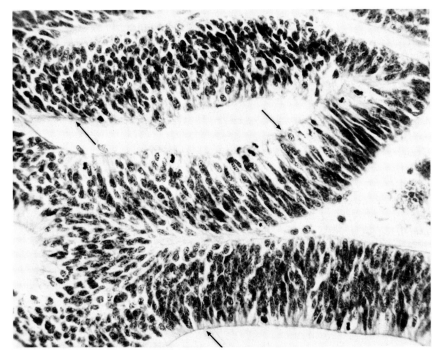

FIG. 21.3. Medulloepithelioma. The multicellular bands are polarized, forming a sharply defined structure analogous to the external limiting membrane of the retina along one surface (arrows). ×198. (From Zimmerman: Trans Am Ophthalmol Soc 69:210, 1971)

membrane forms the lining surface, the structure formed is not hollow, but rather is a solid mass of myxoid tissue surrounded by medullary epithelium. Such structures reminded Verhoeff of little embryonic eyes containing vitreous.[15] Since he considered the vitreous to always be vascular and of mesodermal derivation, he believed this tumor could best be described as "teratoneuroma." Subsequently it has been shown that the myxoid tissue contained within these "little eyes" formed by the tumor is not always vascular. Pieces of the primitive medullary epithelium may become separated from the main tumor and be carried by flow of aqueous into the posterior and anterior chambers, where they may remain free floating or become attached to the lens, iris, or cornea. Such structures clinically have been confused with parasitic cysts.[16, 17] Collins, in his discussion of the remarkable case recorded by Spicer and Greeves,[16] made some very pertinent comments:

> One of the most interesting points in this very interesting case, was the way in which it demonstrated how pathology helped to explain embryological processes. It used to be generally thought that the vitreous humour was of mesoblastic origin; but of late embryologists had regarded it as derived from neural epiblast: and this specimen bore out that view very conclusively.

If examination of the free-floating cysts in the anterior chamber in cases such as those reported by Spicer and Greeves and by Gifford reveals no mesenchymal elements and yet there is plenty of hyaluronic acid, this observation would provide compelling support in favor of the neuroepithelial origin of this mucoid material. In the great majority of cases, however, one does see some blood vessels as well as mesenchymal cells in the tissue that resembles primitive vitreous; hence it is impossible to exclude the possibility that some of the hyaluronic acid might be derived from the mesodermal tissue contained in the retrolental mass that resembles hyperplastic primary vitreous. The latter may be supplied by vessels arising from the ciliary body or choroid and entering the retrolental area via a colobomatous defect, but vascular connections may also be observed with the iris and tunica vasculosa lentis or, very rarely, with a patent hyaloid vessel.

MALIGNANT NONTERATOID MEDULLOEPITHELIOMA. Malignant nonteratoid medulloepitheliomas also contain areas in which the tumor produces sheets of poorly differentiated medullary epithelium and cords of tubular and papillary structures resembling, respectively, the embryonic retina and ciliary epithelium; but, in addition, there are areas in which the tumor exhibits more anaplasia than is found in the benign medulloepitheliomas. Even in those areas where the tumor forms sheets resembling embryonic retina, the constituent cells tend to be larger, the nuclei are more predominant and basophilic, and mitotic figures are more numerous. The most obvious difference, however, is that in the malignant medulloepitheliomas, one sees areas in which the neoplasm is composed of densely packed, small, dark cells with scanty cytoplasm. In such areas the tumors resemble retinoblastomas. In general, malignant medulloepitheliomas are more aggressive; one sees greater invasion of the iris, ciliary body, and anterior chamber, and destruction of the internal architecture of the globe. Extraocular extension and orbital invasion may be observed, and several cases are on record in which the tumor has proved lethal.[7, 18]

Even in such malignant tumors that have spread out of the eye, the neoplasm retains its typical tendency to form sheets and cords of polarized medullary epithelium, elaborating a hyaluronic acid-contained myxoid tissue resembling vitreous along one surface of these structures. I have seen such diagnostic areas in tumors that recurred in the orbit and invaded intracranially, and also in a tumor that metastasized to the cervical lymph nodes.

Teratoid Medulloepithelioma

Teratoid medulloepithelioma is the name I propose for a large group of medulloepitheliomas that exhibit differentiation into brain tissue or that contain other tissues, such as cartilage or striated muscle, not normally found in the human eye. These tumors must also, by definition, contain the sheets and cords of neuro-epithelial cells resembling embryonic medullary epithelium, embryonic retina, or embryonic ciliary epithelium.

BENIGN TERATOID MEDULLOEPITHELIOMA. Benign teratoid medulloepitheliomas vary greatly in their size and microscopic appearance. In some instances, most of the tumor appears to be a typical "pure" benign medulloepithelioma, and only a small island of cartilage contained in the mesenchymal stromal tissue places it in the "teratoid" group (Figs. 21.4, 21.5). In other cases, huge masses of chondroid tissue and large areas of myxoid mesenchymal stroma are observed, but the cords

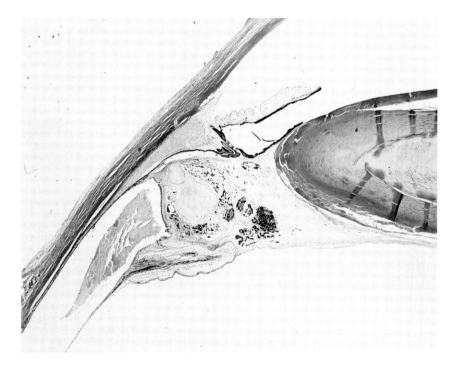

FIG. 21.4. Benign teratoid medulloepithelioma filling the posterior chamber on one side of the eye. Islands of hyaline cartilage are present, along with stellate and spindle-shaped mesenchymal cells. ×10. (From Zimmerman: Trans Aust Coll Ophthalmol 2:114, 1970)

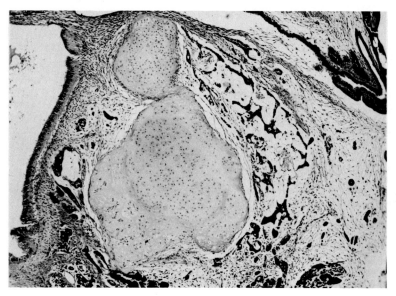

FIG. 21.5. Enlargement of area containing hyaline cartilage shown in Figure 21.4. ×33. (From Zimmerman: Trans Aust Coll Ophthalmol 2:114, 1970)

and sheets of medullary epithelium are only rather inconspicuously present. In still other tumors the main constituent of the mass resembles brain tissue, including such related histologic structures as ependyma and choroid plexus. Glial differentiation predominates, but ganglion cells and other neuronal elements are also observed.

MALIGNANT TERATOID MEDULLOEPITHELIOMA. Malignant teratoid medulloepitheliomas (Fig. 21.6) present an extremely variable microscopic appearance. At one end of the histopathologic spectrum are tumors that closely resemble the nonteratoid malignant medulloepitheliomas described earlier, except that they may contain an island of cartilage or show some tendency to form tissue resembling brain. At the other end of the spectrum are very pleomorphic and polymorphic tumors that are barely identifiable as being medulloepitheliomatous, for the formation of recognizable neuroepithelial structures may be minimal. In some of these tumors the presence of mesenchymal elements, including rhabdomyoblastic structures similar to those observed in embryonal rhabdomyosarcomas, may so dominate the microscopic picture that a relationship to the ciliary epithelium may be overlooked (Fig. 21.7). Several such tumors are described and illustrated in detail elsewhere.[12] As with other malignant medulloepitheliomas, these teratoid tumors may become extremely destructive and may prove lethal.

ACQUIRED TUMORS

All of the acquired tumors—the hyperplastic group, the adenoma, and the adenocarcinoma—are believed to be derivatives of the fully differentiated ciliary epithelium, not from the undifferentiated medullary epithelium that characterized the congenital tumors.

Pseudoadenomatous hyperplasia or Fuchs' adenoma is considered a senile

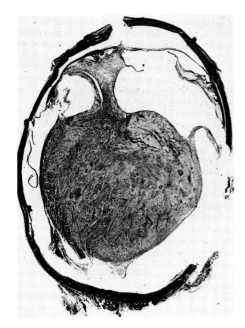

FIG. 21.6. Large polymorphic malignant teratoid medulloepithelioma. ×4. (From Zimmerman: Trans Aust Coll Ophthalmol 2:114, 1970)

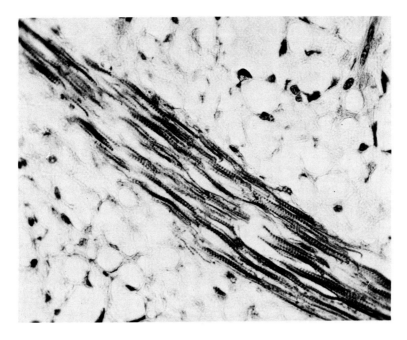

FIG 21.7. Evidence of rhabdomyoblastic differentiation is prominent throughout the mesenchymal portion of the tumor shown in Figure 21.6. Strap cells with cross striations are shown. Phosphotungstic and acid-hematoxylin, ×253. (From Zimmerman: Trans Aust Coll Ophthalmol 2:114, 1970)

hyperplastic lesion, never of any real clinical significance. It typically is a very small nodular proliferation in the pars plicata, where, as a rule, it escapes clinical detection. It is mainly of interest to the pathologist who uncovers it in the course of examination of an eye that has either been removed at autopsy or has been removed as a result of enucleation for some other disease.

Adenomas are benign proliferations of the ciliary epithelium that may be either solid or papillary. I have not yet recognized a pleomorphic adenoma, although this category is included in the classification anticipating that eventually we will see one because we have seen the malignant counterpart.

Adenocarcinomas, malignant tumors of the differentiated ciliary epithelium, may be solid, papillary, or pleomorphic. This diagnosis is made in cases where the tumor cells show significant mitotic activity and other evidence of anaplasia. Because acinar structures and mucin-containing goblet cells are often present, these tumors may be histologically confused with metastatic adenocarcinoma.

REFERENCES

1. Mann I: The Development of the Human Eye. New York, Grune & Stratton, 1950
2. Zimmerman LE, Fine BS: Production of hyaluronic acid by cysts and tumors of the ciliary epithelium. Arch Ophthalmol 72:365, 1964
3. Verhoeff FH, in discussion, Fralick FB, Wilder HC: Intraocular diktyoma and glioneuroma. Trans Am Ophthalmol Soc 47:317, 1949
4. Fralick FB, Wilder HC: Intraocular diktyoma and glioneuroma. Trans Am Ophthalmol Soc 47:317, 1949
5. Fuchs E: Wurcherungen und Geschwulste des Ziliarepithels. Albrecht von Graefes Arch Klin Exp Ophthalmol 68:534, 1908
6. Grinker RR: Gliomas of the retina, including the results of studies with silver impregnations. Arch Ophthalmol 5:920, 1931
7. Andersen SR: Medullo-epithelioma of the retina. Int Ophthalmol Clin 2:483, 1962
8. Reese AB: Tumors of the Eye, 2nd ed. New York, Hoeber, 1963
9. Willis RA: The Borderland of Embryology and Pathology, 2nd ed. Washington, DC, Butterworths, 1962
10. Duke-Elder S, Perkins ES: Diseases of the Uveal Tract. In Duke-Elder S (ed): System of Ophthalmology. London, Kimpton, 1966
11. Hogan MJ, Zimmerman LE: Ophthalmic Pathology, 2nd ed. Philadelphia, Saunders, 1962
12. Zimmerman LE, Font RL, Andersen SR: Rhabdomyosarcomatous differentiation in malignant medullo-epitheliomas of the ciliary body and retina. Read before the annual meeting of the Association for Research in Vision and Ophthalmology, Sarasota, Fla, 1970
13. Kuhlenbeck H, Haymaker W: Neuro-ectodermal tumours containing neoplastic neuronal elements: ganglioneuroma, spongioneuroblastoma and glioneuroma, with a clinicopathologic report of eleven cases, and a discussion of their origin and classification. Milit Surg 99:273, 1946
14. Spencer W: Presentation before the Ophthalmic Pathology Club, 1962
15. Verhoeff FH: A rare tumor arising from the pars ciliaris retina (teratoneuroma), of a nature hitherto unrecognized and its relation to the so-called clioma retina. Trans Am Ophthalmol Soc 10:351, 1904
16. Spicer WTH, Greeves RA: Multiple cysts in the anterior chamber derived from a congenital cystic growth of the ciliary epithelium. Proc R Soc Med 8:9, 1914
17. Gifford H: A cystic diktyoma. Surv Ophthalmol 11:557, 1966
18. De Buen S, Gonzalez-Angulo A: Diktyoma (embryonal medullo-epithelioma): review of the literature and report of a case. Am J Ophthalmol 49:606, 1960

Index